Women's Health in Autoimmune Diseases

Shefali Khanna Sharma
Editor

Women's Health in Autoimmune Diseases

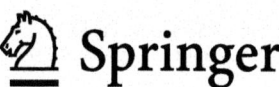
Springer

Editor
Shefali Khanna Sharma
Department of Internal Medicine
PGIMER
Chandigarh, India

ISBN 978-981-15-0113-5   ISBN 978-981-15-0114-2 (eBook)
https://doi.org/10.1007/978-981-15-0114-2

© Springer Nature Singapore Pte Ltd. 2020
This work is subject to copyright. All rights are reserved by the Publisher, whether the whole or part of the material is concerned, specifically the rights of translation, reprinting, reuse of illustrations, recitation, broadcasting, reproduction on microfilms or in any other physical way, and transmission or information storage and retrieval, electronic adaptation, computer software, or by similar or dissimilar methodology now known or hereafter developed.
The use of general descriptive names, registered names, trademarks, service marks, etc. in this publication does not imply, even in the absence of a specific statement, that such names are exempt from the relevant protective laws and regulations and therefore free for general use.
The publisher, the authors, and the editors are safe to assume that the advice and information in this book are believed to be true and accurate at the date of publication. Neither the publisher nor the authors or the editors give a warranty, expressed or implied, with respect to the material contained herein or for any errors or omissions that may have been made. The publisher remains neutral with regard to jurisdictional claims in published maps and institutional affiliations.

This Springer imprint is published by the registered company Springer Nature Singapore Pte Ltd.
The registered company address is: 152 Beach Road, #21-01/04 Gateway East, Singapore 189721, Singapore

My parents Raj Khanna and Sukhdev Khanna for their unconditional love and trust

My husband Sanjay Sharma for his support

My daughter Sania Sharma for her love and care

To my teachers, colleagues, and patients for enriching my life

Foreword

Autoimmune inflammatory rheumatic diseases (AIRD) include diseases like rheumatoid arthritis, lupus erythematosus, spondyloarthritis, psoriatic arthritis, scleroderma, sjogren's disease, antiphospholipid syndrome, and many others. Initial diagnosis is noted in children as early as 2 years of age and continues throughout adolescence into late adulthood affecting women through menopause. The burden of autoimmunity is several times higher in women with a female/male ratio of up to 9:1. The peak incidence often occurs during the reproductive years and may variably affect both fertility and pregnancy outcomes. Impacts on pregnancy can lead to early miscarriages, low birth weight infants, as well as adverse maternal outcomes with increased morbidity and mortality.

Furthermore, many of the conventional therapies for AIRDs may also affect fertility or are contraindicated during pregnancy. The advent of newer therapies, however, has led to improved disease management and increased the likelihood of safe, successful pregnancies. The care of women with autoimmune diseases will require a team approach that includes health care providers across a spectrum of specialties including primary care, rheumatology, obstetrics and gynecology, materno-fetal medicine, and pediatrics. Understanding the unique needs of female patients throughout the spectrum of their life experiences from menarche through menopause can lead to increased health and wellness with far-reaching impacts on the society as a whole.

This book, *Women's Health in Autoimmune Diseases*, provides insight into the pathophysiology, management of autoimmune inflammatory rheumatic diseases through the life journey of a woman, including pregnancy. It is an important landmark contribution to our understanding of the uniqueness of women living with autoimmune inflammatory rheumatic diseases and will serve as a roadmap for health care providers who are challenged with caring for this important sector of the population.

Association of Women in Rheumatology Grace C. Wright
New York, NY, USA

Preface

There is no dearth of books on rheumatology but none with a special focus on rheumatic diseases affecting women's health in autoimmune diseases and its bearing on pregnancy and pregnancy outcomes. This book aims to fill this important gap. Even while miscarriages, preterm deliveries, and neonatal mortality remain a concern, a successful pregnancy outcome is an achievable goal. Good pregnancy outcomes are possible with close prepregnancy counseling, risk stratification, early recognition of disease flares, and its complications, both medical and obstetric. Of the several issues that confront a physician, the timing of pregnancy is of utmost importance. The presence of active disease correlates directly with a higher risk of adverse pregnancy outcome. Thus, a pregnancy is best planned when the disease is quiescent. Further, the immune suppressants should be discontinued a few months before a planned pregnancy. Meticulous pregnancy care and the availability of a multidisciplinary team are cornerstones to optimize the maternal and fetal outcomes. We hope that this book will be beneficial for an internist in general, and a rheumatologist and obstetricians in particular, besides being helpful to other related health-care professionals. This endeavor would not have been possible without the invaluable contribution of esteemed authors. I earnestly hope that this book forms a useful addition to your shelves. Happy reading (!)

Chandigarh, India   Shefali Khanna Sharma

Contents

1. **Does Genetics Play a Role in Auto-immune Diseases?** 1
   Himanshi Chaudhary, Amit Rawat, and Surjit Singh

2. **Influence of Gender on Autoimmune Rheumatic Diseases** 17
   Arun Kumar Kedia and Vinod Ravindran

3. **Sex Bias in Systemic Lupus Erythematosus and Sjögren's Syndrome**. 29
   R. Hal Scofield and Valerie M. Harris

4. **Autoantibodies in Pregnancy** 45
   Gummadi Anjani and Amit Rawat

5. **Laboratory Testing for the Antiphospholipid Syndrome** 57
   Jasmina Ahluwalia and Saniya Sharma

6. **Fertility and Pregnancy in Autoimmune Diseases** 67
   Susheel Kumar

7. **Update on Use of Biologic and Targeted Synthetic Drugs in Pregnancy** 77
   Hanh Nguyen and Ian Giles

8. **Managing Menstrual Irregularities in AID** 93
   Rama Walia and Anshita Aggarwal

9. **Fertility Preservation in Women with Autoimmune Diseases Treated with Gonadotoxic Agents** 101
   Aashima Arora

10. **Preconception Care and Counseling in Autoimmune Disorders** 107
    Bharti Sharma and Shinjini Narang

11. **Effect of Pregnancy on Autoimmune Rheumatic Diseases** 113
    Hafis Muhammed and Amita Aggarwal

12. **Management of Lupus Flare During Pregnancy** 123
    Rajeswari Sankaralingam

13	**Lupus Nephritis and Pregnancy** .... Manish Rathi	143
14	**Pregnancy in Systemic Vasculitis**............................. Puneet Mashru and Chetan Mukhtyar	153
15	**Managing APLA During Pregnancy**........................... Arghya Chattopadhyay and Varun Dhir	163
16	**Managing Pregnancy in Systemic Sclerosis**...................... Shefali K. Sharma	175
17	**Management and Monitoring of Anti-Ro/La positive Mother**...... G. S. R. S. N. K. Naidu and M. B. Adarsh	181
18	**Management of Sjögren's Syndrome During Pregnancy**.......... Pulukool Sandhya	187
19	**Maternal Mortality and Morbidity in Autoimmune Diseases**....... Pooja Sikka and Rinnie Brar	197
20	**Anti-rheumatic Drugs in Pregnancy**........................... Ashok Kumar and Anunay Agarwal	203
21	**Nonsteroidal Anti-inflammatory Drug Use During Pregnancy and Lactation: Effects on Mother and Child** .... Ghan Shyam Pangtey and Niharika Agarwal	215
22	**Management of Neonate with Heart Block** .... Parag Barwad and Lipi Uppal	221
23	**Women Issues in Autoimmune Diseases: Compilation of Indian Data** .... Kaushik S. Bhojani	231
24	**Osteoporosis in Autoimmune Rheumatic Diseases** .... C. Godsave, R. Garner, and Ira Pande	241
25	**Menopause in Autoimmune Disease and Hormone Replacement Therapy**.. Ramandeep Bansal and Neelam Aggarwal	255
26	**Fibromyalgia**.. B. G. Dharmanand	269

About the Editor

Shefali K. Sharma is an Additional Professor in the Unit of Clinical Immunology and Rheumatology, Department of Internal Medicine, Postgraduate Institute of Medical Education and Research, Chandigarh, India. She is interested in rare rheumatological diseases like systemic sclerosis and CTD-ILD. She has a special interest in women's health in autoimmune diseases and has spearheaded the Indian Chapter of the Association of Women in Rheumatology.

She won the prestigious ARA-APLAR (Australian Rheumatology Association–Asia Pacific League of Associations for Rheumatology) International Fellowship, the Japanese College of Rheumatology (JCR) International Scholarship, and the Young Scientists International fellowship by Indian Council of Medical Research.

She is a Fellow of American College of Rheumatology and Indian College of Physicians and a Member of National Academy of Medical Sciences. She is an ardent researcher and has more than 80 research papers in various peer-reviewed international and national journals to her credit.

Does Genetics Play a Role in Auto-immune Diseases?

Himanshi Chaudhary, Amit Rawat, and Surjit Singh

Abstract

Eighty autoimmune diseases (AD) have been identified to date, and they affect 5–10% of the population. Familial clustering is evident in many autoimmune conditions. A higher concordance of disease association is seen among monozygotic twins as compared to dizygotic twins and other siblings. With advances in genetic diagnostic facilities, a variety of genetic studies have been developed which have established genetic associations with AD. This chapter aims at providing an overview of the genetic profile of AD and the main determinants which define the ultimate phenotypic manifestations of the genetic variants related to AD.

Keywords

Genetics · Autoimmune diseases · Autoimmunity

1.1 Introduction

Autoimmune diseases (AD) are a heterogeneous group of disorders characterized by a breach of self-immune tolerance. As a result, autoantibodies are generated and these result in damage to various organ systems. These autoantibodies are of two types: (1) organ-specific as in Type 1 DM, (2) autoantibodies targeting autoantigens in multiple organs and hence having multiorgan involvement (seen in SLE). Eighty autoimmune diseases have been identified till date and they affect 5–10% of the population. These diseases are of considerable public health significance [1]. The likely etiology is not clear and it has been postulated that a combination of genetic and environmental determinants decides the susceptibility of developing an autoimmune condition in an individual. Genetic factors have long been associated with the

H. Chaudhary · A. Rawat · S. Singh (✉)
Allergy Immunology Unit, Advanced Pediatric Centre, Post Graduate Institute of Medical Education and Research, Chandigarh, India

© Springer Nature Singapore Pte Ltd. 2020
S. K. Sharma (ed.), *Women's Health in Autoimmune Diseases*,
https://doi.org/10.1007/978-981-15-0114-2_1

pathogenesis of AD. These are believed to be responsible for the dysregulation of self-tolerance mechanisms. Familial clustering is evident in many autoimmune conditions. A higher concordance of disease association is seen among monozygotic twins as compared to dizygotic twins and other siblings. With advances in genetic diagnostic facilities, a variety of genetic studies have been developed which have established genetic associations with AD [2]. Over 130 GWAS have established AD-associated alleles [3–5]. The genes are involved in transcription of proteins for important cellular pathways (e.g., apoptosis of cellular fragments or immune complexes, regulation of innate and acquired immunity, generation of cytokines and chemokines). This chapter aims at providing an overview of the genetic profile of AD and the main determinants which define the ultimate phenotypic manifestations of the genetic variants related to AD.

1.2 Epidemiological Analysis of the Genetic Basis of AD

The worldwide prevalence of ADs is estimated to be 5–10% [6]. The American Autoimmune Related Disease Association (AARDA) has identified more than 100 ADs, thereby making it the third most common disease etiology in the USA [7]. The estimated prevalence of all ADs in the USA is 50 million and the likelihood of a woman developing an AD is two to ten times more than men [7]. As per estimates, women account for 58% of all diagnosed AD in the USA [8]. There has been an increase of 19% in the occurrence of ADs worldwide [9]. ADs have been seen to cluster in families [10], and their co-occurrence in the same individuals has been shown to be higher than what can be expected by chance [11]. The familial clustering is well known in association with Rheumatoid arthritis (RA), systemic sclerosis (SSc), autoimmune thyroid disease (AITD), and systemic lupus erythematosus (SLE) [12]. AITD is the most common disease encountered among first-degree relatives. Familial occurrence of celiac disease (CD), (MS), primary biliary cirrhosis (PBC), multiple sclerosis, and antiphospholipid syndrome (APS) has also been noted although concordance among family members is less. There are also reports of co-aggregation of multiple AD among family members (i.e., polyautoimmunity) which means that different ADs are seen in different members of the same family. Type 1 diabetes mellitus (T1D), SSc, and SLE share susceptibility gene polymorphisms and can be seen to affect different members of the same family. Sjogren syndrome (SS) may occur with other ADs such as RA, SSc, AITD, and SLE suggesting common genetic pathways. ADs do not follow the classical Mendelian pattern of inheritance. These genetic factors are influenced by environmental influences which lead to a multifactorial model whereby genetically predisposed individuals come in contact with some environmental trigger which ultimately leads to the development of AD.

1.2.1 Approach to Genetic Analysis of Diseases

The human genome comprises of a set of 46 chromosomes with 22 pairs of autosomes and one pair of sex chromosomes. It contains both protein-coding and noncoding DNA. There are an estimated 3.3 billion base pairs in the haploid genome [13]. Protein coding sequence comprises a fraction of the entire genome (approximately 1.5%) with an estimated 19,000–20,000 human protein-coding genes [14]. Genetic variations are defined as differences in allelic sequences within the population which are inheritable. Genetic variations between individuals are limited to 0.1–0.4% of the genome and can be present in two major forms:

1. *Microsatellites*: These are a sequence of highly repetitive DNA motifs that have a higher mutation rate than the rest of the DNA. Their main application is in determining relatability between individuals and populations [15]. They are not present in the coding region.
2. *Single nucleotide polymorphisms (SNPs)* are point mutations in nucleotides at specific locations in the genome which occur at a much higher frequency than the rest of the DNA. These are the modern unit of genetic variation. These can occur without changing the amino acid sequence in the genome and are then referred to as sense mutations. Non-sense SNPs lead to alteration in the protein products of the gene by changing the sequence of amino acids. These are the most abundant forms of genetic variations in the human genome [16].

Pathogenic variations have been identified in the causative relation of autoimmune disease through three basic approaches:

(a) Candidate gene association studies
(b) Linkage analysis in affected families, and
(c) Genome-wide association studies (GWAS)

Candidate gene studies are the most commonly performed genetic studies (Fig. 1.1). These are relatively inexpensive and quick to perform and identify polymorphisms in genes already known to be related to the disease phenotype. The genes selected have a known physiological relevance to the disease. The verification of the association is done by observing its occurrence in stratified case–control studies. These have high statistical power for making a diagnosis. There are certain limitations to this method. These can only identify genes which are already known in association with the disease. Second is the problem with population stratification. There could be systematic differences in allele frequency in populations likely due to different ancestries and an association could be detected due to the structural similarities of the population and not because of the polymorphism per se [17].

Linkage analysis is a genetic method that maps a pathogenic variant on chromosomal segments which is likely to harbor genes for the trait (Fig. 1.2). Linkage studies have been successful in the identification of various diseases with Mendelian inheritance like Huntington's disease (HD) and cystic fibrosis (CF) [18]. Linkage

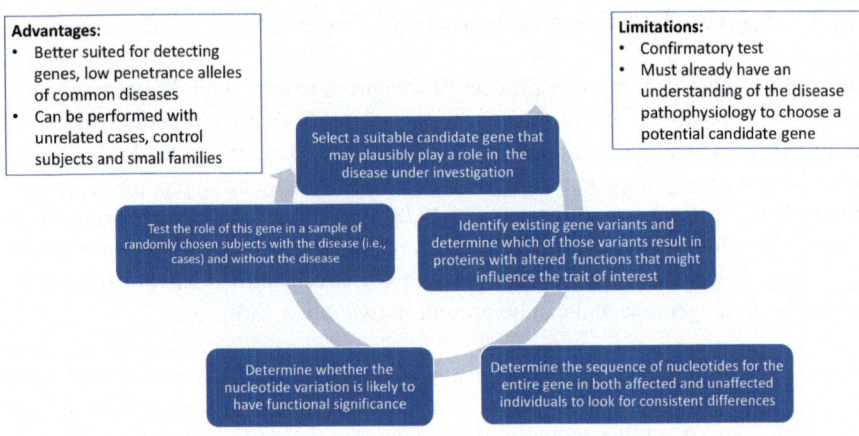

Fig. 1.1 Candidate gene association studies

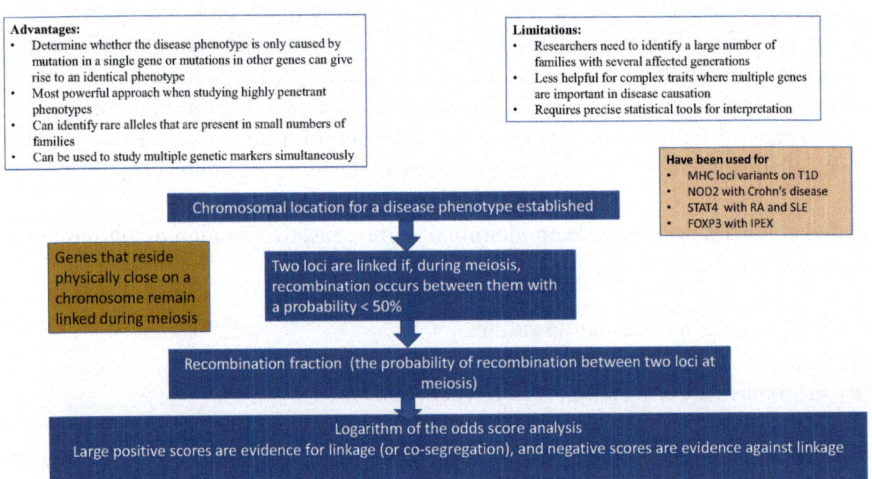

Fig. 1.2 Genome-wide linkage studies

analysis combined with positional cloning has identified causal mutations of a large number of AD. Tomer et al. have shown linkage association of some major histocompatibility complex (MHC) loci variants to AITD [19]. The associations of *STAT4* (signal transducer and activator of transcription 4) with RA and SLE, *FOXP3* with immune dysregulation, polyendocrinopathy, enteropathy, X-linked (IPEX) syndrome and *NOD2* (nucleotide binding and oligomerization domain 2) with Crohn's disease are already known [20–22]. However, the familial aggregation of the autoimmune conditions is not very common and hence linkage analytic studies have not been very fruitful in determining genetic risks within families.

Genetic diagnostics have been revolutionized by *GWAS* which is a relatively new way for scientists to identify common genetic variations associated with human diseases (Fig. 1.3). These identify SNPs within the genome which occur at a higher

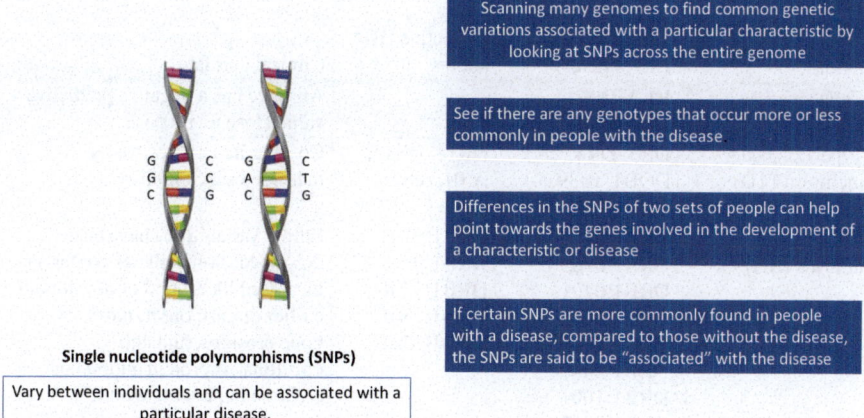

Fig. 1.3 Genome-wide association studies

frequency in the diseased individual than healthy people. Hundreds of thousands of SNPs can be evaluated at the same time and are a comparatively cost-effective way of genetic testing [23]. GWASs are based on the principle of linkage disequilibrium (LD), which determines a nonrandom association of alleles at different loci in relation to a disease in a given population. Linkage disequilibrium refers to the independent and nonrandom association of different disease-causing alleles in a population [24]. These studies are usually followed up with further studies to ascertain the causative variant.

1.3 Mechanisms Underlying Autoimmune Disorders

ADs have been shown to be associated with different types of cellular dysfunctions that hamper the smooth functioning of the immune system. Human leukocyte antigen (HLA) genes have long been studied with ADs, e.g., HLA-B27 in spondyloarthritis, HLA-B51 in Behcet disease, HLADQ2/DQ8 in celiac disease, and HLA-DRB1 in RA. There are also reports of association of non-HLA genes, including cytotoxic T lymphocyte-associated antigen-4 (CTLA4) gene, protein tyrosine phosphate non-receptor type 22 (PTPN22), and other autoimmune susceptibility loci with AD.

1.3.1 Role of Human Leukocyte Antigens (HLAs) in Autoimmune Diseases

The most studied association of genetic factors for ADs are genes located in the MHC and, in particular, loci from human leukocyte antigen (HLA) class I and class II. Genetic associations between HLA and AD have been reported since the early 1970s (Table 1.1) [25].

Table 1.1 HLA genes associated with AD

Disease	Predisposing HLA alleles	Protective HLA alleles	Clinical corelate
Celiac disease	HLA-DQ2, HLA-DQ8		Absence has a negative predictive value close to 100%
Type 1 diabetes mellitus (T1D)	DR3, DR4, DQB1, B*39, B*18, A*24	DR14, DR15, A*01, A*11, A*31	Co-inherited alleles confer increased susceptibility
Rheumatoid arthritis (RA)	DRB1*0101 DRB1*0102 DRB1*0401 DRB1*0404 DRB1*0405 DRB1*0408 DRB1*1001 DRB1*1402	DRB1*0103 DRB1*07 DRB1*1201 DRB1*1301 DRB1*1501	Ethnic variabilities have been described; Some alleles confer an increased likelihood of developing earlier disease onset, more severe bone erosions, and anti-citrullinated protein antibodies (ACPA) in patients with RA
Multiple sclerosis (MS)	HLA-DRB1, HLA-DQB1, DR15, C*05, C*15	DR14	Some alleles associated with a younger age at onset, worse Expanded Disability Status Scale (EDSS) score, and a more disabling disease
Systemic lupus erythematosus (SLE)	HLA-DR3, DR8, DR15		Associated with more severe disease course and development of renal complications
Ankylosing spondylitis (AS)	HLA-B*2701, *2702, *2704, *2705		Positive association between HLA-B27 and male sex, family history, uveitis, peripheral joint involvement, and hip involvement
Sjogren syndrome (SS)	DQA1*05:01, DQB1*02:01, DRB1*03:01, DQA2		Strongest signal of genetic association with primary SS
Dermatomyositis (DM)	HLA-DP1*17, DQA1*0104, HLA-DRB1*07		Association with severity of pulmonary and esophageal complications
Myasthenia Gravis	HLA-DRB1*03, HLA-DRB1*01		HLA-DRB1*03 associated with early onset MG, HLA-DRB1*01 with late onset disease, HLA-DRB1*10 allele associated with thymoma-associated MG
Addison's disease	DRB1*03:01 and DRB1*04:04		Strongest association observed for the *DRB1* locus
Graves' disease	DR3, DRB1*08, C*07, B*08	C*16, C*03, B*44, DR7, HLA-DRB1*07:01	Ethnic variabilities described in disease susceptibility
Antiphospholipid antibody syndrome	HLA-DR4, DR7, DQB1*0302, and DRw53		Ethnic variabilities described in disease susceptibility
Sarcoidosis	*DRB1* and *DQB1*		Ethnic variabilities described in disease susceptibility

The HLA complex spans approximately 4 Mb on chromosome 6. It contains around 250 genes, out of which 40% have a role in the functioning of the immune system [26]. An extensive list of AD has been associated with different variants of the HLA genes, particularly, class II genes. HLA A1-B8 region is a haplotype that covers several MHC class 1 alleles. Common haplotypes are seen across the population as a result of descent from a common ancestor. There are many gene alleles in the haplotype, and they have been studied across different populations in association with AD. In Europe, A1-B8 is found as a part of the HLA A1-B8-DR3-DQ2 haplotype. In Africa and India, A1-B8 is associated with other genes and other variants of A*01 and B*08. A1-B8 haplotype has been associated with a number of ADs like CD, Autoimmune hepatitis, Cushing syndrome, myasthenia gravis, and primary biliary cirrhosis. HLA genes have been known to be affected by epigenetic regulation through environmental factors. The exact pathology of how HLA affects the development of AD remains unclear. In certain conditions like RA and T1D, ethnic variations in susceptibility to these diseases have also been established in Caucasians [27].

1.3.1.1 Celiac Disease (CD)
CD has a strong genetic basis. The concordance rates in monozygotic twins are 90% as compared to 10% in first-degree relatives. The strongest described association is with HLA. HLA-DQ2 (encoded by HLA-DQA1*05:01-DQB1*02:01) or HLA-DQ8 (encoded by DQA1*03:01-DQB1*03:02) has been shown to be expressed in 30%–35% of the populations where CD is prevalent [28]. Gluten, the pathogenic antigen in CD, binds to the pockets of a CD-risk DQ heterodimer (encoded by the DQ2.2, DQ2.5, and DQ8 haplotypes) after being processed in the gut. This stimulates the production of gliadin-specific CD4 T cells in the intestinal epithelium which triggers immunity and produces intestinal inflammation. This association has also been confirmed by MHC fine mapping, which indicated strong independent associations of HLA genes with CD risk [29]. Their absence has been regarded as a negative predictive value for CD that is close to 100% [30].

1.3.1.2 Type 1 Diabetes Mellitus (T1D)
HLA association with T1D is the most complex. The number of alleles found in association with T1D in the DR and DQ loci is high. Some of the alleles when co-inherited confer increased susceptibility to T1D while some modify the relative risk of developing the disease. In European descendants, the highest risk is conferred by HLA-DQB1*03:02, DR3-DQA1*05-DQB1*02, and DR4-DQA1*03-DQB1*03:02 haplotypes [31, 32]. Heterozygosity of these loci confers the strongest genotypic risk for T1D [33].

1.3.1.3 Rheumatoid Arthritis (RA)
The association between HLA and RA has been extensively analyzed. A strong association between RA and DRB1*04:01, *04:04, *01:01, and *10:01 has been reported and confirmed in numerous studies [34, 35]. Ethnic variabilities have also been described in this association. These include HLA-DRB1*04:01, *04:04, and *04:08 in Caucasians [35–37]; HLADRB1*04:05 in Spaniards and Japanese; HLA-DRB1*01:01 and *01:02 in Israelis; HLA-DRB1*14:02 in some Native Americans

such as Pima and Yakima Indians; HLA-DRB1*10:01 in Greeks; and HLA-DRB1*01:01, *04:01, *04:04, and *04:05 in Latin Americans [38]. Some of these alleles confer an increase in the likelihood of developing earlier disease onset [39], more severe bone erosions and anti-citrullinated protein antibodies (ACPA) in patients with RA [40].

1.3.1.4 Multiple Sclerosis (MS)

It is an autoimmune neurological disorder characterized by the presence of autoreactive T cells that react against various proteins of the nervous system. HLA-DRB1*15:01 and HLA-DQB1*06:02 alleles are mainly described in association with risk for MS among Caucasians and Latin Americans [41]. HLA-DRB1*15 has been associated with a younger age at onset, worse Expanded Disability Status Scale (EDSS) score, and a more disabling disease in patients with MS. HLA-DRB1*13:03, 08:01, 03:01, 15:03, 04:05 alleles confer a detrimental and HLA-DRB1*14:01, 07:11, 02:01, 01:08 a protective role in MS [42].

1.3.1.5 Systemic Lupus Erythematosus (SLE)

Multiple HLA alleles have been discovered through GWAS in SLE in both European and Asian populations. HLA-DR4, DR11, DR14 alleles have been shown to have to be protective against SLE and HLA-DR3, DR9, DR15 is associated with high disease susceptibility. HLA-DR4 and DR11 alleles have been shown to be protective for lupus nephritis, and DR3 and DR15 may have a high risk of developing renal complications in SLE [43].

1.3.1.6 Other Autoimmune Conditions

HLA-B27 has been observed in 96% of patients suffering from AS [44]. HLA-B alleles (HLA-B*51:01, B*47:01, and B*13:02) have also been described as risk alleles for AS [45].

A recent meta-analysis has identified associations between HLA Class II and SS [46]. An analysis of more than a thousand cases of SS from 23 studies across different populations was done. Risk associations were found in HLA DQA1*05:01, DQB1*02:01, and DRB1*03:01 alleles for the disease [41]. In Dermatomyositis (DM), GWAS have identified significant susceptibility with variants located in the MHC class II region, with HLA-DP1*17 being the most significant [47]. Strong independent associations to the class I locus have been reported for IBD, psoriasis, AS, and Graves' disease [48, 49]. Haplotypes DR3-DQA1*05-DQB1*02 and DR4-DQA1*03-DQB1*03:02 in Europeans and DR9-DQA1*03-DQB1*03:03 and DR4-DQA1*03-DQB1*04:01 in the Japanese population have been known to predispose to other AD (e.g., autoimmune polyglandular syndrome type II [50], CD [51], and antineutrophil cytoplasmic antibody-associated vasculitis (AAV)) [52].

Understanding of these genetic associations offers the potential to identify disease susceptibility in individuals at risk of ADs. This would be a major step toward developing new treatments and preventing manifestations of disease in genetically predisposed individuals.

Table 1.2 Non-HLA genes associated with AD

SLE	FCGR2A, IFIH1. STAT4, ATG16L1, TMEM39A, TNIP1, PRDM1, ATG5, TNFAIP3, IRF5, TNPO3, TRAF1-C5, KIAA1542, IRF7, SLC15A4, ITGAM, ITGAX, IRF8, IKZF3, TYK2, HIC2, UBE2L3 TLR7, TLR8, IRAK1, TREX1, TNFAIP3, SIAE
RA	TNFRSF14, MMEL1, REL, ANKRD55, IL6ST, TNFAIP3, TRAF1-C5, HIC2, UBE2L3
CD	TNFRSF14, MMEL1, REL, IRF4, TNFAIP3, HIC2, UBE2L3, TLR7, TLR8
T1D	IFIH1, STAT4, KIAA0350, TYK2, C1QTNF6
PSO	STAT4, TNIP1, TNFAIP3
IBD	FCGR2A, STAT4, ATG16L1, IRGM, IRF5, TNPO3, TNFSF15, NOD2, TNFRSF6B
Sarcoidosis	ACE, CCR-2, CXCR-5, CR-1,

SLE systemic lupus erythematosus, *RA* rheumatoid arthritis, *CD* celiac disease, *T1D* type 1 diabetes mellitus, *PSO* psoriasis, *IBD* inflammatory bowel disease

1.3.2 Non-HLA Genes

The breach of self-tolerance among T and B lymphocyte clones is the hallmark of autoimmunity. Several genes have been identified which have an impact on the adaptive immune system. These susceptibility alleles may affect the production, activation, and regulation of immune cell lineages and predispose to the development of AD (Table 1.2).

1.3.2.1 Genes Impacting T-Cell Activation and Signaling
Any abnormality in the differentiation of naïve T cells into functional subsets can be a trigger for the development of AD. The abnormal signaling secondary to genetic polymorphisms impacts T-cell differentiation and hence predispose to autoimmune conditions.

(a) PTPN22 (protein tyrosine phosphatase, non-receptor type 22) encodes a protein tyrosine phosphatase that dephosphorylates key downstream signaling molecules in T-cell differentiation. Associations of PTPN22 have been described with susceptibility to T1DM, RA, AITD, SLE, and JIA [53].
(b) Protein tyrosine phosphatase, non-receptor type 2 (PTPN2), which is also an intracellular tyrosine phosphatase, has also been associated with CD and T1D [54].
(c) CTLA4, a key negative regulatory molecule impacts antigen-driven activation of T cells. CTLA4 polymorphisms are reported in association with T1D, IBD, RA, CD, MS, and SLE [55].
(d) SH2B3 (SH2B adaptor protein 3) gene is involved in the negative regulation of T-cell receptor signaling. It has been described in association with T1D, CD, and SLE.
(e) TAGAP (T-cell activation GTPase-activating protein) is associated with CD, T1D, and RA.

(f) CD226 is a type I transmembrane receptor of the immunoglobulin superfamily expressed on the surface of lymphocytes and involved in T-cell activation and differentiation. A missense variation is associated with T1D, MS, AITD, RA, AAV, and SL.
(g) The TNFSF4 [tumor necrosis factor (ligand) superfamily member 4] binds to the surface of APC by its receptor (TNFRSF4). Genetic variants in the promoter of TNFSF4 have been seen in cases of monogenic SLE. TNFSF4 and TNFRSF9 are involved in T-cell activation and are implicated in CD.

1.3.2.2 Susceptibility Genes Impacting B-Cell Activation
(a) BANK1 (B-cell scaffold protein with ankyrin repeats 1) gene is involved in the transmission of B-cell receptor signaling and affects B-cell receptor-induced calcium mobilization required for activation of B cells. Allelic variants in BANK1 are associated with SLE.
(b) BLK (B lymphoid tyrosine kinase) encodes a tyrosine kinase that has a role in B-cell signal transduction. The variants rs2248932 and/or rs13277113 in BLK have been studied in association with SLE, RA, AS, and SSc.
(c) CD40 (CD40 molecule) plays a crucial role in the activation and differentiation of B lymphocytes. CD40 has been described in association with susceptibility to RA, MS, and IBD.

1.3.2.3 Genes Affecting Helper T Cells
CD3 helper T cells (Th1 and Th2 subsets) have a definite role in the generation of autoimmunity. Th1 cells have a pathogenic association with T1D, MS, and RA.

(a) IL18RAP, STAT1-STAT4, STAT3, and IL12A impact the differentiation of Th1 and Th2 cells, and have polymorphisms associated with AD.
(b) IL12B encodes the p40 subunit of the heterodimeric cytokines IL-12 and IL-23. IL12B variants are associated with T1D, MS, psoriasis, and IBD.
(c) CD58 and CD6 instruct the production of co-stimulatory molecules that are involved in the pathway of signaling of T cells and their differentiation. These molecules have a pathogenic role in MS and RA.
(d) Th17 has been known to have a role in the pathogenesis of various ADs. IL-17 levels have been shown to be elevated in patients with active SLE, MS, and RA.
(e) Treg (Regulatory T cells) are involved in the maintenance of immunological tolerance. IL-2 is required for the differentiation of Tregs. IL2RA variants are associated with RA, T1D, MS, and IBD, and IL2RB is associated with RA and T1D. IL7RA variations have been shown to be associated with IBD and MS.

1.3.2.4 TNF Receptor Superfamily Genes Associated with ADs
(a) The upregulation of TNFSF15 on macrophages and CD4+/CD8+ lymphocytes of the intestinal lamina propria has been shown in relation with IBD.
(b) TNFRSF14, another member of TNF-receptor superfamily, is associated with RA and CD.

(c) TNFRSF6B, encoding a decoy receptor that prevents Fas-induced apoptosis, is associated with IBD, RA, SLE, PSO, and CD.

1.3.2.5 Genes Involved in Innate Immunity

The dysregulation of the innate immune system plays an important part in the development of autoimmune phenomena. Abnormalities in signaling through toll-like receptor (TLR) pathways appear to be fundamental. The autoimmune susceptibility loci in innate immunity pathways include TNIP1 (TNFAIP3 interacting protein 1): associated with psoriasis, IRF8 (interferon regulatory factor 8): (associated with MS and SLE), TYK2 (tyrosine kinase 2) (associated with MS and T1D), and TNFAIP3. MIF (macrophage migration inhibitory factor) is a cytokine that is expressed by many immune cells, and polymorphisms in MIF have been shown in association with multiple AD. Genetic polymorphisms throughout the Toll-like receptor (TLR) and NOD-like receptor (NLR) pathways are associated with susceptibility to AD-like SLE and IBD. Variants in CLEC16A (C-type lectin domain family 16-member A) gene are associated with T1D and MS. Members of the interferon regulatory factor (IRF) family of transcription factors play a crucial role in the activation of transcription through the TLR pathway and have been linked to various AD-like SLE, RA, SS, IBD, and MS.

1.4 The Intersection of Autoimmunity and Primary Immunodeficiency

Autoimmunity is frequently observed in settings of primary immunodeficiency (PID). This is due to impaired regulatory functions within the immune system resulting in failure to maintain self-tolerance. Autoimmunity has been well described in association with Wiskott-Aldrich syndrome (WAS), monogenic forms of common variable immunodeficiency (CVID) like IKBKG, CTLA4, NFKB1, GATA2, CD40LG, and TAZ, and chronic granulomatous disease (CGD) [56]. GWAS conducted on autoimmune conditions have identified genes that overlap with some PIDs. In the largest GWAS on RA in European and Asian patients, 377 candidate genes were identified to be associated with RA. Among these genes, certain genes overlap with PID genes (e.g., caspase 8 [CASP8], caspase 10 [CASP10], autoimmune regulator [AIRE], and IL-2 receptor a [IL2RA] genes were identified [57]). Similarly, monogenic inheritance is well known in cases of SLE. Early disease onset in the background of a significant family history of SLE is likely to involve monogenic defects. These genetic aberrations disrupt the equilibrium of the immune system and generate autoimmunity [58]. Three groups of PID have been described in association with SLE:

1. Defects of complement pathway (C1Q, C3, C4), which prevent proper disposal of apoptotic tissue in the cells along with defective clearance of microbes.
2. Selective and partial defects in immunoglobulin synthesis.
3. Chronic granulomatous disease especially in carriers of X-linked trait.

These increase the susceptibility of the affected individual toward a host of infections with a wide severity spectrum. Jesus et al. have reported a 28% incidence of some form of PID in a consecutive cohort of 300 adult SLE patients [59].

It has been recommended that patients with autoimmunity targeting multiple organ systems should be investigated for underlying PID. Also, in patients with PIDs, an early assessment for risk of autoimmunity/inflammation should be carried out [60].

1.5 Conclusion

The various genetic studies conducted in AD have strengthened our understanding of autoimmunity in many dimensions. A host of susceptibility genes have been described in relation with AD which can predict an individual's susceptibility toward the development of the disease, the age of onset, the severity of illness, likely complication, and response to therapy. These molecular clues can even help ascertain the risk of autoimmunity among other family members so that preventive measures can be enforced early in life. A better understanding of susceptibility alleles will pave way for the development of target-based therapeutics in the future whereby treatment customized toward modifications of the individual genetic abnormality is instituted to the patients.

References

1. Jacobson DL, Gange SJ, Rose NR, Graham NM (1997) Epidemiology and estimated population burden of selected autoimmune diseases in the United States. Clin Immunol Immunopathol 84(3):223–243
2. Dai Y, Zhang L, Hu C, Zhang Y (2010) Genome-wide analysis of histone H3 lysine 4 trimethylation by ChIP-chip in peripheral blood mononuclear cells of systemic lupus erythematosus patients. Clin Exp Rheumatol 28(2):158–168
3. Barreiro LB, Quintana-Murci L (2010) From evolutionary genetics to human immunology: how selection shapes host defence genes. Nat Rev Genet 11(1):17–30
4. Zhernakova A, Elbers CC, Ferwerda B, Romanos J, Trynka G, Dubois PC et al (2010) Evolutionary and functional analysis of celiac risk loci reveals SH2B3 as a protective factor against bacterial infection. Am J Hum Genet 86(6):970–977
5. Ramos PS, Shaftman SR, Ward RC, Langefeld CD (2014) Genes associated with SLE are targets of recent positive selection. Autoimmune Dis 2014:203435. [cited 6 Mar 2019]. Available from: https://www.ncbi.nlm.nih.gov/pmc/articles/PMC3920976/
6. Autoimmune Statistics. The Autoimmune Registry. [cited 10 Mar 2019]. Available from: http://www.autoimmuneregistry.org/autoimmune-statistics
7. Autoimmune Disease Statistics•AARDA (2016) AARDA. [cited 10 Mar 2019]. Available from: https://www.aarda.org/news-information/statistics/
8. Women & Autoimmunity•AARDA (2016) AARDA. [cited 10 Mar 2019]. Available from: https://www.aarda.org/who-we-help/patients/women-and-autoimmunity/
9. (PDF) The world incidence and prevalence of autoimmune diseases is increasing. ResearchGate. [cited 10 Mar 2019]. Available from: https://www.researchgate.net/publication/294419057_The_World_Incidence_and_Prevalence_of_Autoimmune_Diseases_is_Increasing

10. Torfs CP, King MC, Huey B, Malmgren J, Grumet FC (1986) Genetic interrelationship between insulin-dependent diabetes mellitus, the autoimmune thyroid diseases, and rheumatoid arthritis. Am J Hum Genet 38(2):170–187
11. Eaton WW, Rose NR, Kalaydjian A, Pedersen MG, Mortensen PB (2007) Epidemiology of autoimmune diseases in Denmark. J Autoimmun 29(1):1–9
12. Somers EC, Thomas SL, Smeeth L, Hall AJ (2006) Autoimmune diseases co-occurring within individuals and within families: a systematic review. Epidemiol Camb Mass 17(2):202–217
13. Lander ES, Linton LM, Birren B, Nusbaum C, Zody MC, Baldwin J et al (2001) Initial sequencing and analysis of the human genome. Nature 409(6822):860–921
14. Ezkurdia I, Juan D, Rodriguez JM et al (2014) Multiple evidence strands suggest that there may be as few as 19,000 human protein-coding genes. Hum Mol Genet. 23(22):5866–5878. https://doi.org/10.1093/hmg/ddu309
15. Bagshaw ATM (2017) Functional mechanisms of microsatellite DNA in eukaryotic genomes. Genome Biol Evol 9(9):2428–2443
16. Charlon T, Martínez-Bueno M, Bossini-Castillo L, Carmona FD, Cara AD, Wojcik J et al (2016) Single nucleotide polymorphism clustering in systemic autoimmune diseases. PLoS One 11(8):e0160270
17. Patnala R, Clements J, Batra J (2013) Candidate gene association studies: a comprehensive guide to useful in silico tools. BMC Genet 14:39
18. FutureLearn. The applications of genetic linkage and association analysis. FutureLearn. [cited 18 Mar 2019]. Available from: https://www.futurelearn.com/courses/translational-research/0/steps/14199
19. Tomer Y, Ban Y, Concepcion E, Barbesino G, Villanueva R, Greenberg DA et al (2003) Common and unique susceptibility loci in graves and hashimoto diseases: results of whole-genome screening in a data set of 102 multiplex families. Am J Hum Genet 73(4):736–747
20. Hugot JP, Chamaillard M, Zouali H, Lesage S, Cézard JP, Belaiche J et al (2001) Association of NOD2 leucine-rich repeat variants with susceptibility to Crohn's disease. Nature 411(6837):599–603
21. Ogura Y, Bonen DK, Inohara N, Nicolae DL, Chen FF, Ramos R et al (2001) A frameshift mutation in NOD2 associated with susceptibility to Crohn's disease. Nature 411(6837):603–606
22. Remmers EF, Plenge RM, Lee AT, Graham RR, Hom G, Behrens TW et al (2007) STAT4 and the risk of rheumatoid arthritis and systemic lupus erythematosus. N Engl J Med 357(10):977–986
23. Wang MH, Cordell HJ, Van Steen K (2019) Statistical methods for genome-wide association studies. Semin Cancer Biol. 55:53–60. https://doi.org/10.1016/j.semcancer.2018.04.008
24. Visscher PM, Wray NR, Zhang Q, Sklar P, McCarthy MI, Brown MA et al (2017) 10 Years of GWAS discovery: biology, function, and translation. Am J Hum Genet 101(1):5–22
25. McDevitt HO, Bodmer WF (1974) HL-A, immune-response genes, and disease. Lancet 303(7869):1269–1275
26. The MHC Sequencing Consortium (1999) Complete sequence and gene map of a human major histocompatibility complex. Nature 401(6756):921–923
27. Castiblanco J, Arcos-Burgos M, Anaya J-M (2013) Introduction to genetics of autoimmune diseases. El Rosario University Press, Bogota. [cited 10 May 2019]. Available from: https://www.ncbi.nlm.nih.gov/books/NBK459433/
28. Wolters VM, Wijmenga C (2008) Genetic background of celiac disease and its clinical implications. Am J Gastroenterol 103(1):190–195
29. Gutierrez-Achury J, Zhernakova A, Pulit SL, Trynka G, Hunt KA, Romanos J et al (2015) Fine mapping in the MHC region accounts for 18% additional genetic risk for celiac disease. Nat Genet 47(6):577–578
30. Pallav K, Kabbani T, Tariq S, Vanga R, Kelly CP, Leffler DA (2014) Clinical utility of celiac disease-associated HLA testing. Dig Dis Sci 59(9):2199–2206
31. Thomson G, Valdes AM, Noble JA, Kockum I, Grote MN, Najman J et al (2007) Relative predispositional effects of HLA class II DRB1-DQB1 haplotypes and genotypes on type 1 diabetes: a meta-analysis. Tissue Antigens 70(2):110–127

32. Koeleman BPC, Lie BA, Undlien DE, Dudbridge F, Thorsby E, de Vries RRP et al (2004) Genotype effects and epistasis in type 1 diabetes and HLA-DQ trans dimer associations with disease. Genes Immun 5(5):381–388
33. Corper AL, Stratmann T, Apostolopoulos V, Scott CA, Garcia KC, Kang AS et al (2000) A structural framework for deciphering the link between I-Ag7 and autoimmune diabetes. Science 288(5465):505–511
34. Gregersen PK, Silver J, Winchester RJ (1987) The shared epitope hypothesis. An approach to understanding the molecular genetics of susceptibility to rheumatoid arthritis. Arthritis Rheum 30(11):1205–1213
35. Mackie SL, Taylor JC, Martin SG, YEAR Consortium, UKRAG Consortium, Wordsworth P et al (2012) A spectrum of susceptibility to rheumatoid arthritis within HLA-DRB1: stratification by autoantibody status in a large UK population. Genes Immun 13(2):120–128
36. Zanelli E, Breedveld FC, de Vries RR (2000) HLA class II association with rheumatoid arthritis: facts and interpretations. Hum Immunol 61(12):1254–1261
37. Auger I, Toussirot E, Roudier J (1997) Molecular mechanisms involved in the association of HLA-DR4 and rheumatoid arthritis. Immunol Res 16(1):121–126
38. Newton JL, Harney SMJ, Wordsworth BP, Brown MA (2004) A review of the MHC genetics of rheumatoid arthritis. Genes Immun 5(3):151–157
39. Weyand CM, Goronzy JJ (2000) Association of MHC and rheumatoid arthritis:HLA polymorphisms in phenotypic variants of rheumatoid arthritis. Arthritis Res 2(3):212–216
40. Kampstra ASB, Toes REM (2017) HLA class II and rheumatoid arthritis: the bumpy road of revelation. Immunogenetics 69(8):597–603
41. Cruz-Tapias P, Pérez-Fernández OM, Rojas-Villarraga A, Rodríguez-Rodríguez A, Arango M-T, Anaya J-M (2012) Shared HLA class II in six autoimmune diseases in Latin America: a meta-analysis. Autoimmun Dis 2012:569728. [cited 20 Mar 2019]. Available from: https://www.hindawi.com/journals/ad/2012/569728/
42. Stamatelos P, Anagnostouli MC (2017) HLA-genotype in multiple sclerosis: the role in disease onset, clinical course, cognitive status and response to treatment: a clear step towards personalized therapeutics
43. Niu Z, Zhang P, Tong Y (2015) Value of HLA-DR genotype in systemic lupus erythematosus and lupus nephritis: a meta-analysis. Int J Rheum Dis 18:17–28. https://doi.org/10.1111/1756-185X.12528
44. Buxton SE, Benjamin RJ, Clayberger C, Parham P, Krensky AM (1992) Anchoring pockets in human histocompatibility complex leukocyte antigen (HLA) class I molecules: analysis of the conserved B ("45") pocket of HLA-B27. J Exp Med 175(3):809–820
45. Cortes A, Pulit SL, Leo PJ et al (2015) Major histocompatibility complex associations of ankylosing spondylitis are complex and involve further epistasis with ERAP1. Nat Commun 6, 7146 . Published 2015 May 21. https://doi.org/10.1038/ncomms8146
46. Nakken B, Jonsson R, Brokstad KA, Omholt K, Nerland AH, Haga HJ et al (2001) Associations of MHC class II alleles in Norwegian primary Sjögren's syndrome patients: implications for development of autoantibodies to the Ro52 autoantigen. Scand J Immunol 54(4):428–433
47. Li L, Chen S, Wen X, Wang Q, Lv G, Li J et al (2017) Positive association between ANKRD55 polymorphism 7731626 and dermatomyositis/polymyositis with interstitial lung disease in Chinese Han population. Biomed Res Int 2017:2905987. [cited 11 Mar 2019]. Available from: https://www.ncbi.nlm.nih.gov/pmc/articles/PMC5392395/
48. Umapathy S, Pawar A, Mitra R, Khuperkar D, Devaraj JP, Ghosh K et al (2011) HLA-A and HLA-B alleles associated in psoriasis patients from Mumbai, Western India. Indian J Dermatol 56(5):497–500
49. Díaz-Peña R, López-Vázquez A, López-Larrea C (2012) Old and new HLA associations with ankylosing spondylitis. Tissue Antigens 80(3):205–213
50. Weinstock C, Matheis N, Barkia S, Haager M-C, Janson A, Marković A et al (2011) Autoimmune polyglandular syndrome type 2 shows the same HLA class II pattern as type 1 diabetes. Tissue Antigens 77(4):317–324

51. Sollid LM, Markussen G, Ek J, Gjerde H, Vartdal F, Thorsby E (1989) Evidence for a primary association of celiac disease to a particular HLA-DQ alpha/beta heterodimer. J Exp Med 169(1):345–350
52. Tsuchiya N (2013) Genetics of ANCA-associated vasculitis in Japan: a role for HLA-DRB1*09:01 haplotype. Clin Exp Nephrol. 17(5):628–630. https://doi.org/10.1007/s10157-012-0691-6
53. Pradhan V, Borse V, Ghosh K (2010) PTPN22 gene polymorphisms in autoimmune diseases with special reference to systemic lupus erythematosus disease susceptibility. J Postgrad Med 56(3):239–242
54. Buckner J. Linking genetic variation in the PTPN2 gene to autoimmune disease susceptibility. Benaroya Research Institute at Virginia Mason, Seattle, WA. [cited 20 Mar 2019]. Available from: http://grantome.com/grant/NIH/R03-DA027013-01
55. Walker LSK (2015) CTLA-4 and autoimmunity: new twists in the tale. Trends Immunol 36(12):760–762
56. Rae W, Ward D, Mattocks CJ, Gao Y, Pengelly RJ, Patel SV et al (2017) Autoimmunity/inflammation in a monogenic primary immunodeficiency cohort. Clin Transl Immunol 6(9):e155
57. Okada Y, Kim K, Han B, Pillai NE, Ong RT-H, Saw W-Y et al (2014) Risk for ACPA-positive rheumatoid arthritis is driven by shared HLA amino acid polymorphisms in Asian and European populations. Hum Mol Genet 23(25):6916–6926
58. Primary immunodeficiency association with systemic lupus erythematosus: review of literature and lessons learned by the Rheumatology Division of a tertiary university hospital at São Paulo, Brazil | Elsevier Enhanced Reader. [cited 23 May 2019]. Available from: https://reader.elsevier.com/reader/sd/pii/S2255502115000644?token=BB8776B4DBE7920B2CF2DDD653DBBBC3B3CEDB72E7FE26C45C80F31B8DD2A34C4A17792CB9367E7BFFC829357FEDD0AB
59. Jesus AA, Liphaus BL, Silva CA, Bando SY, Andrade LEC, Coutinho A et al (2011) Complement and antibody primary immunodeficiency in juvenile systemic lupus erythematosus patients. Lupus 20(12):1275–1284
60. Grimbacher B, Warnatz K, Yong PFK, Korganow A-S, Peter H-H (2016) The crossroads of autoimmunity and immunodeficiency: Lessons from polygenic traits and monogenic defects. J Allergy Clin Immunol 137(1):3–17
61. Bennett CL, Christie J, Ramsdell F, Brunkow ME, Ferguson PJ, Whitesell L et al (2001) The immune dysregulation, polyendocrinopathy, enteropathy, X-linked syndrome (IPEX) is caused by mutations of FOXP3. Nat Genet 27(1):20–21
62. Solovieff N, Cotsapas C, Lee PH, Purcell SM, Smoller JW (2013) Pleiotropy in complex traits: challenges and strategies. Nat Rev Genet 14(7):483–495
63. Ahmad T, Marshall SE, Jewell D (2006) Genetics of inflammatory bowel disease: the role of the HLA complex. World J Gastroenterol 12(23):3628–3635
64. Allannic H, Fauchet R, Lorcy Y, Heim J, Gueguen M, Leguerrier AM et al (1980) HLA and Graves' disease: an association with HLA-DRw3. J Clin Endocrinol Metab 51(4):863–867
65. Goudey B, Abraham G, Kikianty E, Wang Q, Rawlinson D, Shi F et al (2017) Interactions within the MHC contribute to the genetic architecture of celiac disease. PLoS One 12(3):e0172826
66. Wei JC et al (2015) Interaction between HLA-B60 and HLA-B27 as a better predictor of ankylosing spondylitis in a Taiwanese population. PLoS One 10:e0137189. [cited 20 Mar 2019]. Available from: https://www.ncbi.nlm.nih.gov/pubmed/26469786

Influence of Gender on Autoimmune Rheumatic Diseases

Arun Kumar Kedia and Vinod Ravindran

Abstract

Females, while enjoying the advantage of being protected from infections due to their immunoreactivity, are at a higher risk of autoimmune diseases due to the same mechanism. This sexual dimorphism of the immune response in the background of a skewed prevalence of autoimmune diseases in females and the knowledge of the immunomodulatory function of sex steroids indicate a major role of sex hormones as important mediators of the observed clinical gender differences. Recent studies also point toward the reciprocal influence of the sex hormones and microbiome composition in the human body, contributing to the differences in the immune response between females and males. Based on available data, it appears that sex is an important variable to address in future research which may eventually lead to more sex-specific therapy for patients with these diseases. In this narrative review, we appraise how gender has an impact on various autoimmune rheumatic diseases with regard to incidence, disease course, severity, response to treatment, and pathogenesis.

Keywords

Sex · Rheumatoid arthritis · Lupus · Sex hormones · Pregnancy

---

A. K. Kedia
Lifeworth Hospital, Raipur, Chhattisgarh, India

V. Ravindran (✉)
Centre for Rheumatology, Calicut, Kerala, India

2.1 Introduction

Autoimmune diseases of all organ sites and system affect approximately 8% of the population, around 78% of which are females [1, 2]. This gender difference is wide, ranging from 2:1 to 9:1 (Table 2.1), with women predominating in most of the major autoimmune rheumatic diseases (AIRDs) [1, 2]. The major AIRDs are generally observed in the late teens to the early forties, coinciding with the greatest hormonal level changes in females. With advancing age, this ratio between females to males decreases and for certain diseases like rheumatoid arthritis (RA), males outnumber females after the age of 75 years. This gender difference is almost universal and is maintained across various geographical locations and ethnicity.

Both experimental and clinical observations suggest that autoimmunity is influenced by gender. Females have a higher immune reactivity than males as evidenced by the higher antigen presenting capacity and mitogenic response of lymphocytes and monocytes, a higher immunoglobulin level, enhanced antibody production, and a higher homograft rejection rate in females. Males, on the other hand, are more prone to infections. Thus the enhanced immunoreactivity in females is a boon in that it provides a better protection against infections but at the cost of enhanced autoreactivity which contributes to autoimmunity. This sexual dimorphism of the immune response in the background of a skewed prevalence of autoimmune diseases in females and the knowledge of the modulatory effects of sex steroids in immune function in vitro points toward the need to discuss the role of sex hormones mainly estrogen, progesterone, and testosterone as primary mediators of the sex differences [3]. Recent studies also suggest that the hormonal status of the host can shape microbiome composition and reciprocally the microbiome may exert various influences over host sex hormone levels, contributing to the differences in the immune response between females and males. There is a wealth of clinical and experimental data on the gender differences in autoimmune diseases, and it appears that sex is an important variable to address in future research which may eventually lead to more gender-specific therapy for patients with these diseases. In this narrative review, we appraise how gender has an impact on various autoimmune rheumatic diseases with regard to incidence, disease course, severity, response to treatment, and pathogenesis.

Table 2.1 Gender-based prevalence in autoimmune diseases

Autoimmune disease	Female/male ratio
Ankylosing spondylitis	1:3
Antiphospholipid antibody syndrome	5:1
Rheumatoid arthritis	3:1
Sjogrens syndrome	9:1
Systemic sclerosis	5:1
Systemic lupus erythematosus	9:1
Psoriasis	1:1

2.2 Rheumatoid Arthritis

Rheumatoid arthritis affects females thrice as often as males and has a peak incidence at the age of 45–55 years which also coincides with the perimenopausal years which suggests a possible association between estrogen deficiency and the disease onset. In the Nurses Health Study cohort, there was no clear association between the age of menarche, parity, regularity of menses or oral contraceptive pill use and RA risk [4]. A few studies have also shown that the relative risk for developing RA is twofold among nulliparous compared to parous women and that currently pregnant women may have a reduced risk of developing RA during pregnancy. Subsequently an increased risk of developing RA after a woman's first pregnancy has also been reported. However, pregnancy has an ameliorating effect on the disease activity while the disease tends to flare up in the immediate postpartum period suggesting the role of breastfeeding in inducing the disease. Postmenopausal hormone use did not show any difference in RA incidence between those who did or did not receive hormones. Breastfeeding for more than 24 months was found to be associated with protective effect against RA risk [4]. RA probably does not affect fertility, although a decrease in fecundity prior to disease onset has been described [5]. There is no evidence that RA increases risk of spontaneous abortions, preterm labor, or preeclampsia [6].

After the age of 45, the incidence of RA in men increases rapidly and approaches to that of age-matched women. Below 45, men are protected against RA probably due to their higher levels of androgens. However in men, tobacco use has been associated with a higher relative risk of RA, in particular seropositive cases.

With regard to the severity of the disease, several studies have shown that both sexes have similar disease severity at the time of diagnosis, but men are more likely to achieve remission early in the course of RA. This also implies that men have a better response to the therapy. The DANBIO registry which compared sex-based differences in response to anti-TNF therapy demonstrated that the treatment response occurred more quickly in men [7]. However, there have been contradictory results in other studies stating that both sexes had almost similar DAS28 scores although women reported subjectively worse symptoms [8]. Thus, so far sex-specific treatment algorithms cannot be made unless the outcomes are shown to differ by sex and by medication.

Influence of hormonal factors in the pathogenesis in RA is relevant in view of female preponderance in its prevalence. But the peak age corresponding to postmenopausal period also suggests factors other than estrogens and progesterone. In general, higher disease activity in females with a significantly elevated estrogen levels in synovial fluid in RA patients indicate E2 as a detrimental factor in disease activity [9]. Not only the increased estrogen level but also the differential expression of estrogen receptors on immune cells might be implicated in the pathogenesis. Conversely, androgen levels show an inverse relation with disease onset and severity accounting for the decreased incidence in young men and decreased severe course of the disease as compared to age-matched women [10]. Men with RA have lower levels of testosterone, DHEA, and estrone, while estradiol is increased and correlates with inflammatory indices [11]. Progesterone, like estrogen, also stimulates a switch from a Th1 to a Th2 predominant immune response. Progesterone-induced suppression of Th1 response and induction of regulatory T cells could account for the observed decrease in RA activity during pregnancy [12].

Very little information on genetic influence in sex disparities in RA exist. The rarity of RA in individuals with Klinefelter's syndrome suggests that the extra X chromosome does not confer an added risk. Only one study found an association with single nucleotide polymorphisms of the X-encoded genes TIMP1 and ILR9 [13]. Transmission of the X chromosome from mother *vs* father was found unlikely to account for sex differences in disease prevalence [14]. To date, no studies have focused on epigenetic modification of the inactivated X chromosome as related to RA susceptibility.

2.3 Systemic Lupus Erythematosus (SLE)

Lupus is probably the most extensively studied autoimmune disease with respect to gender differences. The female to male ratio cited commonly as 9:1 characterizes incident cases during the childbearing years. The ratio is much lower both prior to puberty and post menopause. Male prevalence varies from 4% to 30% in different series, with higher prevalence in studies considering familial aggregates of the disease. These skewed findings suggest a strong possibility of hormonal influence on the disease. Exogenous or endogenous estrogen may have a triggering effect on the disease development. Age <10 at menarche, oral contraceptive (OC) pills, and post-menopausal HRT have been associated with a higher relative risk of SLE [15]. Estrogen containing OC pills pose greater risk with a strong dose–response relationship between estrogen dose and development of lupus. The highest risk of developing SLE was observed during the first 2 years of OC pills exposure. Breastfeeding has not been found to be associated with increased risk of SLE.

Pregnancy and SLE flares are well known. On the contrary, it may be diagnosed during pregnancy for the first time. Women with active SLE at the time of conception are at increased risk for adverse maternal and fetal outcomes [16, 17]. Breast feeding has not been found to be associated with flares. Studies in humans have found that breastfeeding was associated with a decreased risk of SLE (OR = 0.6), and the risk was further reduced with an increasing number of babies fed and an increasing total time of breastfeeding [18].

There is a distinct impact of gender on disease manifestations, and this difference has been noted to be almost the same in different geographic regions across the globe. Even though male SLE is relatively uncommon, men develop the typical manifestations with a different prognosis. Skin manifestations, serositis, neurological complications, thrombocytopenia, and renal involvement have been found to be more common in men, and males are likely to have more severe renal and cardiorespiratory involvement. Arthritis was more commonly observed in females. Thus males tend to have more severe disease than the females. Sex-based differences in mortality are difficult to study, and different studies conclude differently.

Female sex hormones are crucial regulators of lupus activity. Estrogens, both endogenous and exogenous, may act in conjunction with other factors to override immune tolerance to self-antigens. In the B cell dominant cascade, both the hormones are immune stimulators that affect maturation of autoreactive B cells as well as autoantibody secretion while progesterone is an immuno-suppressor. Estrogen leads to the survival and activation of autoreactive B cells with a marginal zone phenotype whereas prolactin induces self-reactive B cells with a follicular zone phenotype. Thus these two hormones allow autoreactive B cells to escape the normal mechanisms of tolerance and mature to fully functional antibody secreting B cells that can cause clinically apparent lupus [19]. Experimental studies in murine models of lupus have also shown that estrogens have stimulating while androgens have ameliorating effects [20]. The recent SELENA study indicated that estrogen replacement therapy in postmenopausal SLE patients induced a slightly increased number of mild flares. Similarly, ovarian stimulation by hormonal manipulations may also cause an induction of a lupus flare [21].

Prolactin also plays an important role. Almost 30% patients with SLE have mild to moderate hyperprolactinemia. This hormone induces the production of anti-dsDNA antibody by peripheral blood monocytes as well as interferon-gamma. It also causes breaking of tolerance by impairing negative selection of autoreactive B cells and by allowing for their maturation into fully functional B cells with follicular phenotype [22]. Prolactin also regulates the maturation of precursor T cells to CD34+ T cells, decreases apoptosis of B cells and increases immunoglobulin production [23].

There is a complex but definite implications of androgens in the pathogenesis of Lupus. Female SLE patients have accelerated oxidation of testosterone which may have immunomodulatory effect since testosterone suppresses anti-dsDNA production. Male SLE patients have elevated serum 16-hydroxyestrone and estrone concentrations leading to estrogen/androgen imbalance, while some men also have functional hypoandrogenism with low levels of testosterone and elevated luteinizing hormone (LH). Female patients have lower plasma androgen levels than their healthy counterparts.

Not only female hormones but also specific genetic factors involving chromosome X have been implicated in the development of Lupus. The X chromosome includes genes that are crucial in determining sex hormone levels and in maintaining tolerance. The presence of a second X chromosome in females may be important for SLE pathogenesis. Skewed X inactivation can lead to the survival of autoreactive T cells which may be a factor in the pathogenesis [24]. Incomplete X inactivation leading to expression of gene products from both the maternal and paternal X chromosomes and thus doubling of X-encoded proteins has also been explored in the pathogenesis. The relevant genes of interest in SLE encoded on X chromosome are gene for CD40 ligand, IRAK1, Foxp3, TLR7, and MECP2. All of these have been associated with increased risk for developing SLE, and any of these could be over-expressed in women due to incomplete X inactivation [25]. Two studies have suggested a dose effect of the X chromosome as evidenced by a more than tenfold increased prevalence of genotype 47XXY (Klinefelter's syndrome) compared to 46XY in men with SLE [26, 27]. Klinefelter's syndrome men were found to have fewer severe manifestations than normal karyotype men with SLE. Also the females have a lower threshold to develop SLE, yet men have more severe disease when they develop SLE. This difference can be explained probably by the protective effect of the second X chromosome in terms of disease severity or an increased estrogen to androgen ratio. The increased susceptibility could be explained by an X chromosome gene–dose effect.

Epigenetic modification of the genes on the inactive X chromosome in females has also been proposed as a possible mechanism for increased female prevalence. Women, but not men, with active SLE had demethylation of the gene for and increased expression of CD40 ligand, which raises the possibility that demethylation of the inactive X chromosome may be related to disease activity. Men have been found to have a higher number of SLE risk alleles and more T cell DNA demethylation during SLE flares compared to women [28]. Moreover, translocation from the telomeric end of the X chromosome onto the Y chromosome results in a Yaa (Y linked autoimmune accelerator) mutant mice in experiments which develop features of Lupus, indicating the role of TLR7 and TLR8 gene on X chromosome in the pathogenesis of Lupus [29].

2.4 Systemic Sclerosis

This autoimmune disease is characterized by three key pathogenic features: (1) vasculopathy with endothelial dysfunction, (2) immune system activation and dysregulation, and (3) collagen overproduction with fibrosis.

The overall female to male ratio in systemic sclerosis (SSc) is 3:1 or greater and the incidence is highest in the childbearing age. In females, it occurs at a younger age and is more likely to be of the limited cutaneous type with anticentromere antibody and improved survival. In contrast, male patients present at an older age are more likely to be cigarette smokers, have diffuse cutaneous involvement, antitopoisomerase I and anti-U3RNP antibody, pulmonary fibrosis, and reduced survival. Overlap syndromes are equally frequent but while the females have a higher frequency of overlap with SLE, the males have overlap with myositis [30].

A Swedish study showed that nulliparity was associated with an increased risk of SSc, while an increasing number of births were associated with decreased risk [31]. An Italian study also showed that parous women have a reduced risk of SSc and that the risk reduced with increasing number of children. Women who had a history of abortive pregnancies were also at a decreased risk [32]. Differences have also been found in the age of onset, disease severity, course, and cause of death in women who develop SSc prior to pregnancy compared with those who develop the disease after pregnancy [33]. Role of breastfeeding and the risk of SSc have very limited data.

The key hormone to the pathogenesis of SSc is estradiol. Estradiol (E2) promotes the development of a fibrotic phenotype in human skin. Serum E2 levels were found elevated in postmenopausal female patients with early diffuse cutaneous SSc compared to healthy postmenopausal female controls, suggesting an important role of estrogens in the pathogenesis of skin thickening and organ fibrosis [34]. Elevated estradiol may also underlie worse prognosis in males. Increased estradiol level was associated with an increased risk of all-cause mortality in men [35]. High prolactin and low DHEA levels have been observed in patients with SSc; however the mechanisms by which they affect the immune system in SSc remain unclear [36].

In addition, the female preponderance in SSc is thought to be due to genetic or epigenetic differences and X chromosome gene reactivation or skewed chromosome inactivation. Skewed X chromosome inactivation was observed in 64% of patients with SSc as compared with 8% in the controls [37]. Also the rate of monosomy X in white blood cell subpopulation was significantly higher in patients with SSc when compared with healthy females. These data provide evidence for chromosome instability in women with SSc and that haplo-insufficiency for X-linked genes may be a critical factor for female preponderance. Other genetic factors could also be implicated in gender differences. Coexistence of SSc with Klinefelter syndrome like that in SLE has been reported though rare. Similarly a case report of a phenotypic male SSc patient with hypogonadism having an XX sex chromosome has been reported where it was shown that the patient had a 46XX, Xp22.3 (SRY+) gene translocation [38].

2.5 Sjogrens Syndrome

Primary Sjogrens syndrome (SS) is characterized by chronic inflammation and progressive destruction of exocrine salivary and lacrimal glands leading to symptoms of dryness and extraglandular manifestations (EGM) like ILD, cutaneous vasculitis, and lymphadenopathy. The majority of patients are women with an estimated female to male ratio of 9–14 to 1. The difference in incidence further extends to differences in clinical presentation as well. In general, men present with a more severe disease phenotype. EGM follow typical sex difference predominance with thyroiditis, Raynaud's phenomenon, depression, and myalgia occurring more frequently in women, while lymphoma and lung diseases more frequently in men. Gender differences in serological markers and autoantibody are not consistent and perhaps more research is needed in this area whether sex differences in autoantibody levels exist [39].

Both clinical and experimental studies have shown sex hormones to be a major influence in the immunopathogenesis of SS. A complex interplay between estrogen, testosterone, androgens, and prolactin accounts for the increased incidence in women especially in the postmenopausal period. Estrogens' central role in driving a Th2-type skewed immune response that activates B cells and elevates autoantibody and immune complex levels could be the major contributing factor in women after triggers like infection. In the context of genetic, epigenetic, and environmental influences, the rapid decline in estrogen (E2) levels prior to menopause leads to reduced glandular cell health. Death of glandular cells via apoptosis provides self-antigens for presentation to the immune system to promote autoimmune disease. At the same time the protective effects of higher estrogen levels on inflammation disappear allowing increased activation of the innate immune pathways. In contrast, low levels of estrogen continue to increase the level and different types of autoantibodies with age. Pregnancy and other AID further increase the risk of developing SS. Not only does estrogen increase the prolactin levels but also they work together to increase autoantibody levels. This could also explain for the appearance of SS during childbearing years. Thus prolactin may work with high estrogen levels to increase the risk for SS in premenopausal women. The role of sex hormones may not be so straightforward. Both estrogen and androgens are needed for normal exocrine gland function, and reduced levels of DHEA have been noted in salivary glands of patients with SS.

Another hypothesis proposed for the increased incidence in women is through microchimerism which is defined as the presence of nonhost stem cells or their progeny in an individual at a low level and can occur as early as 6 weeks into pregnancy. Initial evidence of its involvement in SS comes from a number of reports of patients developing SS-type disease following blood transfusion, stem cell transplantation, or during GVH disease. However interesting this theory may appear, its role in the pathogenesis of SS still needs more research so as to determine whether it really could skew the prevalence toward women.

2.6 Ankylosing Spondylitis

Ankylosing spondylitis, previously thought to be a male predominant disease, has now been shown to have a male to female ratio of 3:1 as against 9:1 in the older data. This gender variation is much more evident in AS compared to undifferentiated SpA or non-radiographic SpA. Age of onset is nearly the same in both sexes; however the diagnosis is delayed in females by 1–2 years. Females on average have lesser ankylosis of the spine on radiography and therefore lesser damage compared to males. Thus it is assumed that females with AS have a milder form of the disease than males. Despite this, women have more functional limitations for a given radiographic damage. Moreover, women are more likely to present cervical spine involvement, whereas men tend to complain more frequently about lumbar pain [40].

Pregnancy does not improve the symptoms of AS. Two prospective studies have shown active disease during the first and early second trimester with a flare around 20 weeks of pregnancy [41, 42]. Anterior Uveitis can flare up during this period. Disease activity may decrease during the third trimester. Only 20% of patients improve from pain, particularly those who have a history of peripheral symptoms. In patients with multiple pregnancies, no uniform pattern regarding remission or flare is seen. Complete remission never occurs in any patients with pure axial disease. Postpartum flare (4–12 weeks after delivery) is seen in 50–80% patients, and episodes of acute peripheral arthritis or anterior uveitis rise up to three times after delivery [43]. Pregnancy outcomes remain similar to healthy women with regard to miscarriage, stillbirth, prematurity, and IUGR. However, Cesarean section is performed more in patients with AS.

The genetic risk factors appear to be the same and prevalence of HLA-B27 positivity is similar in both sexes. No linkage of the X chromosome with susceptibility to AS has been found so far. In a study by Tsui et al., a direct genetic difference in the ankylosis homologue (ANKH) gene between men and women was reported which could account for the differences in radiological progression observed in the two sexes [44]. Distinct sexual dimorphism in the immunological profile of patients has also been reported. Male AS patients display an elevated Th17 axis. However, it still remains unclear whether this is a basic sex-related pathogenic mechanism or a reflection of higher level of inflammation in males. But aforementioned observations point to the importance of addressing sex in future AS research especially in the ongoing clinical trials with anti-IL17 agents.

2.7 Psoriatic Arthritis

Few studies have investigated the role of gender in psoriatic arthritis (PsA) and the results are variable. While some studies report a male predominance, others suggest a more equal distribution between sexes. Clinical manifestations differ, with males more frequently having axial or oligo-articular involvement and females more poly-articular disease. With regard to severity, men are reported to have a more aggressive radiographic progression. Women are found to be more disabled perhaps due to a different pain perception as well as fatigue which is also higher in the female sex. Sex differences are seen even in the outcomes of PsA treatment options with men requiring more aggressive treatment and more frequent prescription of biologicals. Women show a better treatment response and a better prognosis with lower rates of radiographic progression [45].

Genetics represents a major risk factor for psoriasis and PsA, with the former being associated mainly with HLA-Cw06 and the second with HLA B27, and this knowledge may provide further help in choosing the therapy as patients carrying the HLA-Cw06 allele seem to respond better to Ustekinumab. Women may benefit more with this drug as they are reported to carry the HLA-Cw06 allele more frequently; in contrast HLA B27 is more frequent in men [46].

2.8 Conclusion

Female predominance in autoimmune rheumatic diseases is well recognized. In the pursuit to explain the differences for this female preponderance, most of the research has focused on the role of hormones, both exogenous (e.g., OC pills) and fluctuations in endogenous hormone levels related to menarche, menstruation, pregnancy, and breastfeeding. Other reasons include genetic and epigenetic differences, both direct (influence of genes on sex chromosomes) and indirect (e.g., microchimerism) as well as gender differences in environmental exposure due to lifestyle factors. A greater understanding of both these influences will emerge with the intensive research efforts in these areas permitted by newer technologies. It is also of prime importance to thoroughly elucidate sex differences in the basic immune response, both innate and adaptive. More research about the immune system functioning and a deeper understanding of the immunological mechanisms behind these diseases may form the basis for personalized medicine in future. It is also important to determine the mechanisms by which the primary sex hormones (estrogen, progesterone, and testosterone) affect immune function and to extend mechanistic studies to other sexually dimorphic hormones like prolactin, growth hormone, and insulin-like growth factor. It would also be insightful to understand the effects of naturally fluctuating hormone concentrations on the immune and autoimmune response. The contribution of genetics to sex differences in autoimmune diseases needs further research, so also the interaction between genetic and environmental factors needs deeper studies. Research also needs to be expanded in the field of gut microbiata. The differences in gut microbiata composition between males and females are a cause, or a consequence of gender-specific differences in immune system is not yet completely known and gender might be considered in the development of strategies in future to target gut microbiata in different disorders. The current though limited evidence for gender-based response to various therapies in autoimmune rheumatic diseases provide impetus for future research. This may pave the way for more accurate individualized treatment and also in employing sex hormones as adjuvants in treatment.

Compliance with Ethical Standards

Funding None.

Conflict of Interest Arun Kumar Kedia declares that he has no conflict of interest. Vinod Ravindran declares that he has no conflict of interest.

Ethical Approval This article does not contain any studies with human participants performed by any of the authors.

References

1. Whitcare CC (2001) Sex differences in autoimmune diseases. Nat Immunol 2:777–780
2. Moroni L, Bianchi I, Lleo A (2012) Geoepidemiology, gender and autoimmune diseases. Autoimmun Rev 11:A386–A392
3. Cincinelli G, Generali E, Dudam R, Ravindran V, Selmi C (2018) Why women or why not men? Sex and autoimmune diseases. Indian J Rheumatol 13:44–50
4. Karlson EW et al (2004) Do breast feeding and other reproductive factors influence future risk of rheumatoid arthritis? Results from the Nurses Health Study. Arthritis Rheum 50:3458–3467

5. Nelson JL et al (1993) Fecundity before disease onset in women with rheumatoid arthritis. Arthritis Rheum 36:7–14
6. Nelson JL, Ostensen M (1997) Pregnancy and rheumatoid arthritis. Rheum Dis Clin N Am 23:195–212
7. Jawaheer D, Olsen J, Hetland ML (2012) Sex differences in response to anti-tumor necrosis factor therapy in early and established rheumatoid arthritis, results from the DANBIO registry. J Rheumatol 39:46–53
8. Sokka T et al (2009) Women men and rheumatoid arthritis: analyses of disease activity, disease characteristics and treatments in the QUEST-RA study. Arthritis Res Ther 11:R7
9. Castagnetta LA, Carruba G, Granata OM et al (2003) Increased estrogen formation and estrogen to androgen ration in the synovial fluid of patients with rheumatoid arthritis. J Rheumatol 30:2597–2605
10. Cutolo M (2009) Androgens in rheumatoid arthritis: when are they effectors? Arthritis Res Ther 11:126
11. Tengstrand B, Carlstorm K, Tsai F et al (2003) Abnormal levels of serum DHEA, estrone and estradiol in men with rheumatoid arthritis: high correlation between serum estradiol and current degree of inflammation. J Rheumatol 30:2338–2343
12. Hughes GC (2012) Progesterone and autoimmune diseases. Autoimmun Rev 11:A502–A514
13. Burkhardt J et al (2009) Association of the X chromosomal genes TIMP1 and ILR 9 with rheumatoid arthritis. J Rheumatol 36:2149–2157
14. Somers EC et al (2013) Paternal history of lupus and rheumatoid arthritis and risk in offspring in a nationwide cohort study: does sex matter? Ann Rheum Dis 72:525–529
15. Costenbader KH, Feskanich D, Stampfer MJ, Karlson EW (2007) Reproductive and menopausal factors and risk of systemic lupus erythematosus in women. Arthritis Rheum 56:1251–1262
16. Clowse ME et al (2005) The impact of increased lupus activity on obstetric outcomes. Arthritis Rheum 52:514–521
17. Mohan MC, Ravindran V (2016) Lupus pregnancies: an Indian perspective. Indian J Rheumatol 11:S2135–S2138
18. Cooper GS, Dooley MA, Treadwell EL, St Clair EW, Gilkeson GS (2002) Hormonal and reproductive risk factors for the development of systemic lupus erythematosus—results of a population based case-control study. Arthritis Rheum 46:1830–1839
19. Grimaldi CM, Hill L, Xu X, Peeva E, Diamond B (2005) Hormonal modulation of B cell development and repertoire selection. Mol Immunol 42:811–820
20. Roubinian J, Talal N, Greenspan J, Goodman J, Siiteri P (1978) Effect of castration and sex hormone treatment on survival, anti nucleic acid antibodies, and glomeruolonephritis in NZB/NZW F1 mice. J Exp Med 147:1568–1583
21. Ben-Chetrit A, Ben-Chetrit E (1994) Systemic lupus erythematosus induced by ovulation induction treatment. Arthritis Rheum 37:1614–1617
22. Peeva E, Michael D, Cleary J et al (2003) Prolactin modulates the naïve B cell repertoire. J Clin Invest 111:275–283
23. Cohen-Solal JF et al (2008) Hormonal regulation of B cell function and systemic lupus erythematosus. Lupus 17:528–532
24. Chtinis S et al (2000) The role of X chromosome inactivation in female predisposition to autoimmunity. Arthritis Res 2:399–406
25. Costenbader KH, Bermas B, Tedesch SK (2013) Sexual disparities in the incidence and course of SLE and RA. Clin Immunol 149:211–218
26. Dillon S et al (2011) Klinefelter syndrome among men with SLE. Acta Paediatr 100:819–823
27. Scofield RH et al (2008) Klinefelters syndrome (46 XXY) in male SLE patients: support for the notion of a gene-dose effect from the X chromosome. Arthritis Rheum 58:2511–2517
28. Sawalha AH et al (2012) Sex specific differences in the relationship between genetic susceptibility, T cell DNA demethylation and Lupus flare activity. J Autoimmun 38:216–222
29. Santiago-Raber ML, Kikuchi S, Borel P et al (2008) Evidence for genes in addition to TLR7 in the Yaa translocation linked with acceleration of SLE. J Immunol 181:1556–1562

30. Christine P, Thomas AM, Maryl L, Bedda LR, Carol AFB (2016) Gender differences in systemic sclerosis: relationship to clinical features, serologic status and outcomes. J Scleroderma Relat Disord 1:177–240
31. Lambe M, Bjornadal L, Neregard P, Nyren O, Cooper GS (2004) Childbearing and the risk of scleroderma: a population based study in Sweden. Am J Epidemiol 159:162–166
32. Pisa FE, Bovenzi M, Romeo L, Tonello A, Biasi D, Bambara LM, Betta A, Barbone F (2002) Reproductive factors and the risk of scleroderma: an Italian case control study. Arthritis Rheum 46:451–456
33. Arlett CM, Rasheed M, Russo KE, Sawaya HH, Jimenez SA (2002) Influence of prior pregnancies on disease course and cause of death in systemic sclerosis. Ann Rheum Dis 61:346–350
34. Aida-Yasuoka K, Peoples C, Yasuoka H et al (2013) Estradiol promotes the development of a fibrotic phenotype and is increased in the serum of patients with systemic sclerosis. Arthritis Res Ther 15:R10
35. Vermeulen A, Kaufmann JM et al (2002) Estradiol in elderly men. Aging Male 5:98–102
36. Straub RH, Zeuner M, Lock G, Scholmerich J, Lang B (1997) High prolactin and low DHEA sulphate serum levels in patients with severe systemic sclerosis. Br J Rheumatol 36:426–432
37. Invernizzi P, Miozzi M, Selmi C, Persani L, Battezzati PM, Zuin M et al (2005) X-chromosome monosomy: a common mechanism for autoimmune diseases. J Immunol 175:575–578
38. Velasco G, Savarese V, Sandorfi N, Jimenez SA, Jabbour S (2011) 46XX SRY positive male syndrome presenting with primary hypogonadism in the setting of scleroderma. Endocr Pract 17:95–98
39. Ramírez Sepúlveda JI, Kvarnström M, Brauner S, Baldini C, Wahren-Herlenius M (2017) Difference in clinical presentation between women and men in incident primary Sjögren's syndrome. Biol Sex Differ 8:16
40. Landi M, Maldonado-Ficco H, Perez-Alamino R et al (2016) Gender differences among patients with primary ankylosing spondylitis and spondylitis associated with psoriasis and inflammatory bowel disease in an iberoamerican spondyloarthritis cohort. Medicine (Baltimore) 95:e5652
41. Ostensen M, Fuhrer L, Mathieu R, Seitz M, Villiger PM (2004) A prospective study of pregnant patients with rheumatoid arthritis and ankylosing spondylitis using validated clinical instruments. Ann Rheum Dis 63:1212–1217
42. Wallenius M, Skomsvoll JF, Irgens LM, Salvesen KA et al (2011) Pregnancy and delivery in women with chronic inflammatory arthritides with a specific focus on the first birth. Arthritis Rheum 63:1534–1542
43. Katz PP (2006) Childbearing decisions and family size among women with rheumatoid arthritis. Arthritis Rheum 55:217–223
44. Tsui HW et al (2005) ANKH variants associated with ankylosing spondylitis: gender differences. Arthritis Res Ther 7:513–525
45. Elena G, Carlo A et al (2016) Sex differences in the treatment of psoriatic arthritis: a systematic literature review IMAJ. Vol 18:203–208
46. Chiu HY, Wang TS, Chan CC et al (2014) Human leukocyte antigen Cw06 as a predictor for clinical response to ustekinumab, an interleukin-12/23 blocker in Chinese patients with psoriasis: a retrospective analysis. Br J Dermatol 171:1181–1188

Sex Bias in Systemic Lupus Erythematosus and Sjögren's Syndrome

R. Hal Scofield and Valerie M. Harris

Abstract

Systemic lupus erythematosus (SLE) is an autoimmune disease with protean manifestations in both clinical and immunological domains. Sjögren's syndrome is another rheumatic, inflammatory autoimmune disease that is related to SLE at the level of clinical and serological manifestations as well as underlying pathophysiological mechanisms. For both diseases there are clearly genetic and environmental contributions to the risk of disease, but the etiology is largely undefined. Both SLE and Sjögren's syndrome predominately affect women compared to men at a ratio of at least 10:1. The mechanism by which female-bias is mediated has not been fully elucidated. Sex steroids, estrogens and androgens, do not differ between SLE patients and controls with another chronic disease. Elevated levels of prolactin are found in the sera of some women with either SLE or Sjögren's syndrome, but a cause and effect relationship is not established. The transcription factor vestigial-like family member 3 (VGLL3) may regulate sex-biased gene expression in a way that promotes autoimmunity. The X chromosome aneuploidies 47,XXY and 47,XXX are found in excess among men and women, respectively, with SLE or Sjögren's syndrome. X chromosome genes that escape X inactivation, such as TLR7 and CXorf21, may mediate the

X chromosome dose effect found in these diseases through effects of TLR7 signaling. Other X chromosome abnormalities including acquired X monosomy and skewed inactivation have not been found in SLE. The theory that genes escaping from X inactivation leads to increased intracellular protein concentration and subsequently to autoimmunity is untested. Thus, relatively new research has identified pathways other than sex hormones for female sex bias in these diseases. There may in fact be more than one mechanism by which autoimmune disease affects mostly women.

Keywords
Innate immunity · Toll-like receptors · X chromosome · Lysosome pH

3.1 Systemic Lupus Erythematosus

Credit for the description of systemic lupus erythematosus (SLE) is commonly given to Libman and Sacks who found similar heart valve lesions in patients with the characteristic rash of lupus erythematosus [1]. However, lupus erythematosus was first described as a systemic illness by Moriz Kaposi in 1875 when he described patients with the lupus erythematosus rash who also had kidney disease and arthritis [2]. In the twenty-first century, SLE is considered a, if not the, prototype autoimmune disease. And, while many disease features might lead to classification as autoimmune, key components are a lymphocytic infiltration of involved organs and antibodies binding self in the serum of patients.

SLE can affect most any organ but common features include arthritis, rash, hematological deficiencies, and glomerulonephritis. A large percentage of patients have circulating autoantibodies that bind ribonucleoprotein complexes [3]. The epidemiology of SLE has been studied throughout the world [4]. In general, those of European origin are less commonly affected than those of African or Asian origin. Recent population-based epidemiology in the United States confirms that Black Americans are about four times more likely to have SLE than White Americans [5, 6].

Monogenic forms of SLE caused by mutations in C1q, C2, C4, or DNAase I serve to show that, in large measure, SLE (and its murine models) can be considered an immune reaction to abnormal apoptosis [7]. Nonetheless, specific etiology of SLE remains elusive. Studies of large patient cohorts demonstrate that infection with Epstein-Barr virus is necessary but not sufficient for the disease to occur [8–11]. A recent comprehensive study of the EBV transcription factor EBNA2 proposes a mechanism by which EBV infection might predispose to SLE [12]. The disease is, at least in part, genetic as demonstrated by family and twin studies [13]. And, while some 100 genomic intervals have been found to have genetic association, the pathophysiological mechanism by which most of these genetic polymorphisms increase the risk of SLE is unknown [14].

However, there are immune pathways that are implicated in SLE pathogenesis. One such pathway involves the lysosomal toll-like receptors (TLRs) and the production of interferon [15]. The TLR7 and TLR8 signaling pathways are an integral part of the innate immune system, and therefore are first-line immune defense against viruses. Single-stranded nucleic acids are bound by these receptors. Subsequently, downstream signaling leads to interferon and other cytokine production. As mentioned above, the SLE antigens are most commonly ribonucleoprotein complexes, such as the spliceosome from which the SLE antigens Sm and nRNP are derived. Thus, binding of self-RNA (perhaps derived from apoptotic debris not cleared in a nonimmunogenic manner) could give rise to autoantibodies [16, 17]. This model of SLE pathogenesis is strongly supported by animal models in which abrogation of the TLR7 pathway ameliorates disease [18]. Interestingly though, both autoantibodies and increased action of interferon are present prior to the onset of clinical disease [19], and the trigger or triggers that produce clinical disease are not known.

3.2 Sjögren's Syndrome

First described by the Swedish ophthalmologist Henrik Sjögren in his doctoral dissertation of 1937 [20], the disease is related both clinically and serologically to SLE. The most common clinical feature of Sjögren's syndrome is sicca—severe dry mouth and dry eyes [21]. Typically, but not always, these patients have a lymphocytic infiltration of the salivary gland but not complete destruction of these exocrine glands [22]. Other (extra-glandular) manifestations include arthritis, cutaneous vasculitis, interstitial kidney disease, interstitial lung disease, and hematological deficiencies. Especially when ascertained by highly sensitive methods, a large percentage of Sjögren's syndrome patients have autoantibodies binding the Ro (or SSB) and/or La (or SSB) ribonucleoproteins [23]. SLE patients also commonly, but not as frequently as Sjögren's patients, have these same autoantibodies circulating in the blood [3].

Similar to SLE, the etiology of Sjögren's syndrome is not completely known, but the available data indicate that much like the clinical and serological manifestations, underlying pathophysiological mechanisms are shared between Sjögren's syndrome and SLE. There are serological and other data suggesting a connection to EBV infection [24, 25], but the recent data concerning EBNA2 binding of SLE genetic risk alleles did not study Sjögren's syndrome. The genetics of the disease is less well studied than those of SLE, but many risk alleles are common to the two diseases [26]. Interferon is involved in the pathogenesis of Sjögren's syndrome as evidenced by increased expression of interferon-regulated genes in peripheral blood cells [27], a finding also present among SLE patients [28–30].

3.3 Sex Bias of SLE and Sjögren's Syndrome

In cohorts of SLE patients assembled across the globe, the ratio of women to men is about 10:1 [4]. As noted above, there are now population-based epidemiological data for SLE which give good estimates for the prevalence and incidence of the disease among women [6]. However because of smaller numbers, these estimates

Table 3.1 Hypotheses for the sex bias of SLE and Sjögren's, diseases that disproportionally affect women

Sex steroid hormones
Prolactin
Sex-biased transcription factor LL
X chromosome number
X chromosome mosaicism
X dose compensation with abnormal cytosolic protein concentration
Acquired X monosomy

are not nearly as robust for men. The sex bias of SLE is greatest in childbearing years; however, even in prepubertal children, girls are over-represented by up to 5 to 1 [31]. In addition, while the average onset is in the fourth decade of life, SLE continues to appear in both sexes at ages when women are postmenopausal. And, at these ages, women still outnumber men. Thus, the female bias of SLE does differ across the stages of sexual development but remains present before sexual maturity as well as after loss of ovarian sex hormone secretion in women. There are fewer epidemiological data for Sjögren's syndrome, but virtually all cohorts of patients have a female:male ratio of at least 10:1 with many series approaching 15:1. Pediatric onset of Sjögren's syndrome is rare [32], and the age of onset in adults is substantially older than the age of SLE onset [33]. Thus, much of the onset of disease is postmenopausal in women. Without question, similar to many autoimmune diseases, there is a strong predilection for women to be affected by both SLE and Sjögren's syndrome, with the sex bias of the latter, despite the later in life onset, being as skewed as any of the autoimmune diseases.

There are a number of proposed, theorized, and studied explanations for the sex bias of these diseases (Table 3.1), which we will now discussed individually.

3.4 Factors Studied as an Explanation of SLE and Sjögren's Sex Bias

3.4.1 Sex Steroids

The sex steroid hormones, namely androgens and estrogens, have clear and well-described effects on the immune system, which have been reviewed in detail [34, 35]. Nevertheless, a brief review of these effects is in order prior to describing studies of sex steroid hormones in SLE and Sjögren's syndrome. For instance there is a reduction of TLR7 signaling in plasmacytoid dendritic cells from postmenopausal women, which is restored with estrogen therapy [36]. In fact, estrogen receptors are widely distributed on immune cells, including T cells. However, estrogen receptor α protein levels are lower in women with SLE compared to healthy controls, while serum estradiol levels were not different. Changed gene expression was noted in cultured peripheral blood T cells when treated with an estrogen receptor α antagonist [37]. Animal data implicate estrogen receptor α in pathogenesis that involves both B cells and T cells, but these data are mixed with estrogen receptor α not ameliorating murine lupus in some models [38–41]. *In vitro* autoantibody production by SLE patient peripheral blood cells is enhanced by estrogen treatment [42] as is expression of the Ro antigen by epidermal cells [43].

Levels of sex hormones among subjects with SLE are definitely abnormal. However, as noted by Mok at the beginning of the twenty-first century [44], most of the existing data do not allow a conclusion as to cause and effect. Almost all investigations are cross-sectional, cohort studies; thus, the subjects have had the disease for variable periods of time. Naturally, effects of the disease and its treatment [45] produce altered sex steroid hormones. There have only been a few studies on inception cohorts. In one study of men at the onset of SLE, androgen and estrogen levels were not different from healthy controls [46]. In the only study in which SLE men were compared to a diseased control group (namely men with congestive heart failure), while both patient groups had low testosterone levels, there were no difference between the groups [47]. Thus, these findings suggest that similar to other chronic diseases, SLE affects sex steroid hormones.

Unfortunately, there are fewer data concerning sex steroid hormones among Sjögren's syndrome subjects or in animal models of the disease [48, 49]. One study showed that disease activity was associated with higher serum testosterone concentrations, but there was no association with estrogen concentrations [50]. Another small study of 17 patients and 19 controls showed no difference in estrogen or progesterone levels [51]. Oophorectomy of Sjögren's-prone mice accelerated lacrimal gland's lymphocytic infiltration, and estrogen replacement therapy prevented this change [52]. There are exocrine gland-derived sex steroid hormones, notably dihydrotestosterone, which is lower in men and postmenopausal women. Konttinen and colleagues speculate that lower intra-glandular dihydrotestosterone may have effects on the gland rather than the immune system [53, 54].

Prolactin has also been examined in SLE, but Sjögren's syndrome is studied much less extensively. A recent meta-analysis showed that higher serum prolactin levels are associated with higher disease activity in SLE [55]. Furthermore, prolactin levels are associated with levels of particular cytokines in the serum of SLE patients [56]. Mildly elevated prolactin is found in some SLE patients. This finding has been replicated many times [57, 58] as well as in animal model of SLE [59, 60]. In addition, two studies have found statistically significantly elevated prolactin levels in women with Sjögren's syndrome with about 20% of these women having a value above 20 ng/ml [61, 62]. There was no correlation to disease activity or manifestations except those diagnosed below age 45 were more likely to have an elevated prolactin in one study of 110 patients [61]. Treatment with bromocriptine, a dopamine agonist that decreases prolactin secretion, has proven effective in SLE [63–68].

Thus, elevated prolactin is found among SLE patients, especially those with active disease. Similar to the data concerning sex steroid hormones, these association data do not allow a conclusion with regard to cause and effect. In fact, given the data that inflammatory cytokines increase secretion of prolactin from pituitary lactotroph cells, that prolactin is highest in active disease, and that serum prolactin in SLE is associated with serum cytokine levels, we conclude that elevated prolactin is likely caused by the disease. Given its many functions in the immune system (reviewed in [57]), our conclusion does not preclude prolactin acting as an enhancer of SLE, however.

3.4.2 A Sex-Biased Transcription Factor

Liang and colleagues studied sex-bias gene expression and co-expression patterns in human skin and found interesting results that may impact sex bias of autoimmune disease [69]. This study found increased expression of the transcription factor vestigial-like family member 3 (VGLL3) in female skin. Female cells had increased nuclear localization of VGLL3 protein than male cells. A number of genes important in inflammation were regulated by this transcription factor, and, thus, co-expressed. These included *TNFSF13B*, which encodes BAFF and *ITGAM*, both of which contain SLE risk allele single nucleotide polymorphisms (SNPs) [69]. Sex hormones did not regulate expression of any of these genes. A subsequent study by this same group found that overexpression of VGLL3 in the skin led to a lupus-like rash and systemic autoimmunity associated with B cell expansion, autoantibodies, and immune complex disease [70]. The relationship of these provocative findings to the sex bias of SLE and Sjögren's syndrome remains to be defined.

3.4.3 X Chromosome Aneuploidies

Sex chromosome abnormalities are relatively common in the population based on several karyotype studies of consecutive live births. About 1 in 500 live male births have 47,XXY (Klinefelter's syndrome), while about 1 in 1000 live female births carry a 47,XXX karyotype [71–73]. The original description of Klinefelter's syndrome was in 1942 from the Harvard Medical School [74], and while there are certainly clinical manifestations among 47,XXY men including immunological abnormalities [75], most in fact are undiagnosed [73]. Meanwhile, most women with 47,XXX are undiagnosed and largely asymptomatic. In particular, there are no sex hormone abnormalities in these women [76, 77]. Turner first described the syndrome that bears his name at the University of Oklahoma Health Science Center in 1938 [78]. Almost all women with Turner's syndrome are diagnosed owing to short stature and/or absence of menses. Complex mosaics such as 45,X/46,XX/47,XXX without a Turner's syndrome phenotype may be as rare as 1 in 25,000 live female births [71–73].

There have been numerous case reports of 47,XXY found in SLE patients [79–84], and a smaller number in Sjögren's syndrome [84–87]. Likewise, few are reports of 47,XXX in both of these diseases [85, 88, 89]. And, there is a report of a 46,XX boy with SLE [90]. But, while these case reports are of interest, such data does not constitute evidence of association or causation.

We collected about 3300 SLE patients for family and genetics studies and found an SLE man with 47,XXY early in this effort. This led us to systematically study Klinefelter's syndrome among the men with SLE in this cohort, which is the largest group of SLE men ever assembled [91]. Among a little over 300 SLE men, we found that about 1 in 30 had 47,XXY, almost all of them undiagnosed [92]. We calculated that men with Klinefelter's syndrome have the same prevalence of SLE as women in their same ethnic group using Bayes' theorem. We also had one men in this cohort who was 46,XX [93, 94]. When we examine the mechanism of the abnormal X and Y chromosome meiosis crossover leading to the transference of the *sry* gene (whose protein product is the testes determining factor) to one of the X chromosomes, we found the specifics to differ from the previously reported patient [90]. Thus, we conclude that no pseudoautosomal X gene could be responsible for the association [93]. We also studied a large cohort of men with Sjögren's syndrome [95] for 47,XXY and found highly similar results. In particular, 4 of these 136 men had Klinefelter's syndrome. Thus, Klinefelter's syndrome is found in excess among men with either Sjögren's syndrome or SLE. The latter finding has now been replicated by another group also studying SLE genetics [96]. Unlike abnormal sex steroid hormones and elevated prolactin, the diseases cannot cause supernumerary X chromosomes. Thus, these data suggest a causative role, as do the 47,XXX data discussed below.

Once the association of Klinefelter's syndrome with SLE and Sjögren's syndrome was established, we turned to women. In both SLE and Sjögren's syndrome, we found two- to threefold excess 47,XXX [88]. We found only a single patient with Turner's syndrome and SLE [97]. No women in the Sjögren's syndrome cohort had Turner's syndrome. Because Turner's syndrome is more rare (1 in 2500 live female births) than either trisomy X or 47,XXY, our data do not demonstrate a statistical decrease of Turner's syndrome among SLE and Sjögren's syndrome women, but there is no increase. Thus, the risk of SLE and Sjögren's varies not on the basis of biological sex but instead on the basis of the X chromosome complement. A doubling of the number from 1 to 2 increases risk by tenfold, while a 50% increase (from 2 to 3) increases risk by two- to threefold (Fig. 3.1).

We also examined women for rarer X chromosome abnormalities. Among SLE patients, we found three patients with the rare mosaic 45,X/46,XX/47,XXX [98]. Each of these subjects had about 94% 46,XX cells and 3% each of the abnormal cell types. This very rare X chromosome aneuploidy is likely the result of a mitotic non-disjunction of the X chromosome at a very early stage of embryonic

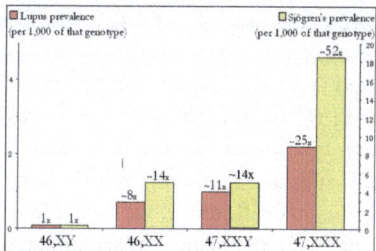

Fig. 3.1 Risk of SLE and Sjögren's syndrome related to the number of X chromosomes. While the data do not convincingly demonstrate it, we hypothesize that Turner's syndrome women (45,XO) segregate with 46,XY men in terms of risk of these two diseases

development. Among the Sjögren's syndrome women, we found a single subject with 45,X/46,XX/47,XXX in whom the triplication of the X chromosome was only partial, involving distal Xp. Another Sjögren's syndrome subject also had a partial triplication of distal Xp but no mosaicism [98]. While this finding was only in these two individuals, these data imply that the gene or genes mediating the X chromosome dose effect may lie on distal Xp.

Of interest, study of murine models of SLE in 40,XX male, 40,XY male, 40,XX female, and 40,XY female mice supports the idea that risk of SLE varies according to the number of X chromosomes and not according to biologic or phenotypic sex, or sex hormones [99, 100]. In point of fact, in these studies of two different female-biased lupus models, risk and severity of disease tracked with number of X chromosomes in these animals in which sex is determined by an *sry* gene that is translocated from the Y chromosome to an autosome [101–103]. Thus, in murine and human SLE (and human Sjögren's syndrome), risk varies with the number of X chromosomes.

3.4.4 TLR7 and CXorf21

While Forsdyke proposes a global function of proteins encoded by X chromosome genes in immune tolerance (discussed below), we are considering function of specific genes on the X chromosome that escape X inactivation. Such genes have higher expression in female cells than male cells. In particular, our studies are concentrated on two genes that not only escape X inactivation but also are located on distal Xp and contain SLE-associated risk alleles—namely *TLR7* and *CXorf21*. As discussed above, the TLR7 signaling pathway, which is initiated by TLR7 recognition of single-stranded RNA and ends with interferon and other cytokine production, is critical to SLE pathogenesis [15, 17]. A component of this pathway is SLC15a4, which regulates lysosomal antigen processing, TLR7 cytokine secretion, antibody production, and lysosomal pH [18, 104]. Knockout of the SLC15a4 gene ameliorates murine SLE [18, 105]. Furthermore, SLC15a4 is a binding partner of CXorf21 on the surface of the endolysosome [106].

We found that the CXorf21 protein is expressed in monocytes, B cells, and dendritic cells with expression roughly doubled in female cells compared to male cells. In studies of CXorf21 function of CXorf21, we found difference between male and female primary human monocytes. Knockdown of CXorf21 expression with CRISPR-Cas9 resulted in an abrogation of interferon, TNFα, and IL6 production after treatment with a TLR7 ligand. This effect was present in female cells only, however [107]. In addition, lysosomal pH was increased; therefore less conducive to lysosomal antigen processing and signaling, with CXorf21 knockdown. In more detailed work concerning this pH difference, we found lower endolysosomal pH in female monocytes, B cells, and dendritic cells compared to male cells but no difference between male and female NK and T cells, which do no express CXorf21 [108]. The CXorf21 sequence contains a putative short chain dehydrogenase reductase domain. If this is functional, then CXorf21 may supply hydrogen ion to

SLC15a4 for transport into the endolysome, and/or supply NADP to the NOX2 complex (see Fig. 3.2). Differences in either between the sexes would lead to differences in TLR7 signaling.

Thus, endolysosomal signaling is regulated in a sex-dependent manner by CXorf21, which is expressed more highly in female cells because the gene encoding this protein escapes X inactivation. These data are consistent with female-bias expression of TLR7 and CXorf21 based on X chromosome number mediating some part of the sex bias of SLE and Sjögren's syndrome as well as fundamental difference between immunity in men and women, especially related to interferon.

3.4.5 Other X Chromosome Factors

When two X chromosomes are present, one is randomly inactivated in each cell at the blastocyst stage of embryonic development. Because there are a small number of cells at this point of development, random inactivation can favor one X chromosome over the other such that there is a skewing with one of the X chromosomes inactivated in >90% of cells. Such skewing is in fact common in the general population [109]. Nonetheless, excess skewing of X inactivation has been found in several

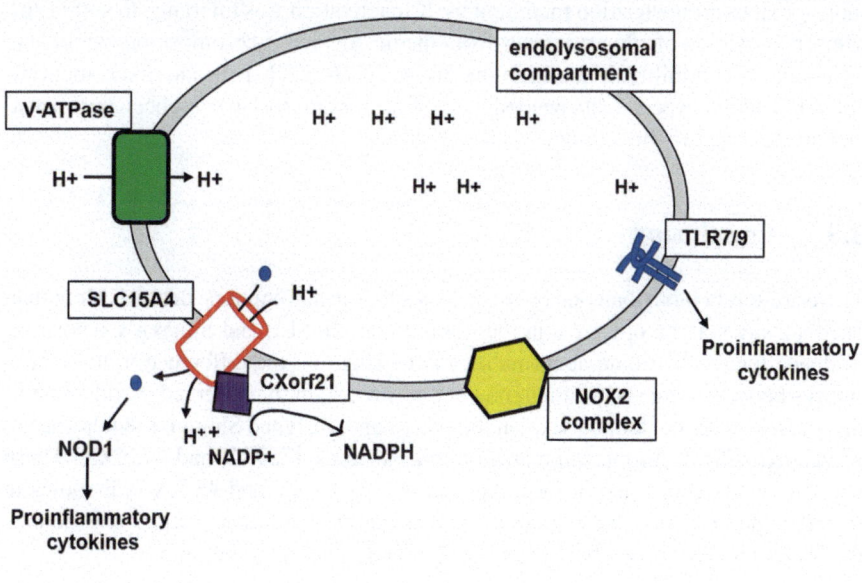

Fig. 3.2 Diagram of the putative function of CXorf21, which contains an SLE risk allele, in relationship to the function of SLC15a4, NOX2, TLR7, all of which contain SLE-risk alleles. SLC15a4 and CXorf21 are known binding partners. We propose that differential CXorf21 expression between those with different numbers of X chromosomes leads to functional differences in TLR7 signaling, which is known to be critical to SLE and Sjögren's syndrome pathoetiology

autoimmune diseases including scleroderma [110, 111], autoimmune thyroid disease [112–115], and female-biased juvenile idiopathic arthritis [116]. However, excess extreme skewing of X inactivation has not been found in SLE [117, 118], and is not studied among subjects with Sjögren's syndrome. So, while there is no evidence of skewed X inactivation of peripheral blood cells from those with SLE or Sjögren's syndrome, skewed X inactivation in the thymus is still possible and might influence T cell tolerance [118].

Turner's syndrome patients (female 45,XO) are at higher risk of type 1 diabetes, celiac disease, and autoimmune thyroid disease. This risk is associated with particular karyotypes including an X isochrome [119–121]. Acquired X monosomy in peripheral blood mononuclear cells of women has been studied in autoimmune disease. Increased acquired X monosomy is found in primary biliary cirrhosis, scleroderma, and autoimmune thyroid disease [122, 123], but not in SLE [88, 124]. Once again, Sjögren's syndrome has not been studied except in our study of X chromosome aneuploides, which found excess 47,XXX (see above) but did not identify subjects with 45,XO [88].

Forsdyke has proposed another theory that rests on a consideration of total protein concentration, which would differ between male and female mammals if not for dose compensation for the difference between possession of one or two X chromosomes [125]. Thus, Forsdyke hypothesizes that the underlying reason for X chromosome dose compensation mediated by X inactivation was tolerance to self [126]. Thus, reactivation of silenced genes from the inactivated X chromosome would lead to female susceptibility to autoimmune disease [126, 127]. Thus far, this is theoretical only and the experiments needed to test this hypothesis have not been performed and are not clear to the authors.

3.5 Conclusion

There are surely more than one pathway to sex bias in autoimmune disease. More than one pathway may be operative in the same illness. In SLE and Sjögren's syndrome, evidence for sex hormone abnormalities is lacking, but the difference in these substances between men and women may yet play a role in the observed predilection of these diseases for the female sex. On the other hand, SLE and Sjögren's syndrome are associated with X chromosome aneuploidies such as 47,XXY and 47,XXX. These uncommon situations may inform the situation of 46,XY and 46,XX individuals in regard to the sex bias of these illnesses. Genes that escape X inactivation may mediate the X chromosome dose effect found in SLE and Sjögren's syndrome.

References

1. Libman E, Sacks B (1924) A hitherto undescribed form of valvular and mural endocarditis. Arch Intern Med 33(6):701–737
2. Kaposi M (1875) Lupus eythematosus. In: Hebra F (ed) On diseases of the skin including the exanthemata IV. The New Syndenham Society, London, pp 14–35

3. Kurien BT, Scofield RH (2006) Autoantibody determination in the diagnosis of systemic lupus erythematosus. Scand J Immunol 64(3):227–235
4. Borchers AT, Naguwa SM, Shoenfeld Y, Gershwin ME (2010) The geoepidemiology of systemic lupus erythematosus. Autoimmun Rev 9(5):A277–A287
5. Dall'Era M, Cisternas MG, Snipes K, Herrinton LJ, Gordon C, Helmick CG (2017) The incidence and prevalence of systemic lupus erythematosus in San Francisco County, California: the California Lupus Surveillance Project. Arthritis Rheumatol (Hoboken, NJ) 69(10):1996–2005
6. Lim SS, Drenkard C (2015) Epidemiology of lupus: an update. Curr Opin Rheumatol 27(5):427–432
7. Costa-Reis P, Sullivan KE (2017) Monogenic lupus: it's all new! Curr Opin Immunol 49:87–95
8. McClain MT, Heinlen LD, Dennis GJ, Roebuck J, Harley JB, James JA (2005) Early events in lupus humoral autoimmunity suggest initiation through molecular mimicry. Nat Med 11(1):85–89
9. James JA, Robertson JM (2012) Lupus and Epstein-Barr. Curr Opin Rheumatol 24(4):383–388
10. James JA, Neas BR, Moser KL, Hall T, Bruner GR, Sestak AL et al (2001) Systemic lupus erythematosus in adults is associated with previous Epstein-Barr virus exposure. Arthritis Rheum 44(5):1122–1126
11. James JA, Kaufman KM, Farris AD, Taylor-Albert E, Lehman TJ, Harley JB (1997) An increased prevalence of Epstein-Barr virus infection in young patients suggests a possible etiology for systemic lupus erythematosus. J Clin Invest 100(12):3019–3026
12. Harley JB, Chen X, Pujato M, Miller D, Maddox A, Forney C et al (2018) Transcription factors operate across disease loci, with EBNA2 implicated in autoimmunity. Nat Genet 50(5):699–707
13. Block SR (2006) A brief history of twins. Lupus 15(2):61–64
14. Saeed M (2017) Lupus pathobiology based on genomics. Immunogenetics 69(1):1–12
15. Crowl JT, Gray EE, Pestal K, Volkman HE, Stetson DB (2017) Intracellular nucleic acid detection in autoimmunity. Annu Rev Immunol 35:313–336
16. Magna M, Pisetsky DS (2015) The role of cell death in the pathogenesis of SLE: is pyroptosis the missing link? Scand J Immunol 82(3):218–224
17. Tsokos GC, Lo MS, Costa Reis P, Sullivan KE (2016) New insights into the immunopathogenesis of systemic lupus erythematosus. Nat Rev Rheumatol 12(12):716–730
18. Kobayashi T, Shimabukuro-Demoto S, Yoshida-Sugitani R, Furuyama-Tanaka K, Karyu H, Sugiura Y et al (2014) The histidine transporter SLC15A4 coordinates mTOR-dependent inflammatory responses and pathogenic antibody production. Immunity 41(3):375–388
19. Arbuckle MR, McClain MT, Rubertone MV, Scofield RH, Dennis GJ, James JA et al (2003) Development of autoantibodies before the clinical onset of systemic lupus erythematosus. N Engl J Med 349(16):1526–1533
20. Wollheim FA (1986) Henrik Sjogren and Sjogren's syndrome. Scand J Rheumatol Suppl 61:11–16
21. Baer AN, Walitt B (2018) Update on Sjogren syndrome and other causes of sicca in older adults. Rheum Dis Clin N Am 44(3):419–436
22. Campos J, Hillen MR, Barone F (2016) Salivary gland pathology in Sjögren's syndrome. Rheum Dis Clin N Am 42(3):473–483
23. Fayyaz A, Kurien BT, Scofield RH (2016) Autoantibodies in Sjogren's syndrome. Rheum Dis Clin N Am 42(3):419–434
24. Mariette X (1995) Sjogren's syndrome and virus. Ann Med Int (Paris) 146(4):243–246
25. Igoe A, Scofield RH (2013) Autoimmunity and infection in Sjogren's syndrome. Curr Opin Rheumatol 25(4):480–487
26. Scofield RH (2009) Genetics of systemic lupus erythematosus and Sjogren's syndrome. Curr Opin Rheumatol 21(5):448–453
27. Emamian ES, Leon JM, Lessard CJ, Grandits M, Baechler EC, Gaffney PM et al (2009) Peripheral blood gene expression profiling in Sjogren's syndrome. Genes Immun 10(4):285–296

28. Banchereau J, Pascual V (2006) Type I interferon in systemic lupus erythematosus and other autoimmune diseases. Immunity 25(3):383–392
29. Baechler EC, Batliwalla FM, Karypis G, Gaffney PM, Ortmann WA, Espe KJ et al (2003) Interferon-inducible gene expression signature in peripheral blood cells of patients with severe lupus. Proc Natl Acad Sci U S A 100(5):2610–2615
30. Bennett L, Palucka AK, Arce E, Cantrell V, Borvak J, Banchereau J et al (2003) Interferon and granulopoiesis signatures in systemic lupus erythematosus blood. J Exp Med 197(6):711–723
31. Brunner HI, Gladman DD, Ibanez D, Urowitz MD, Silverman ED (2008) Difference in disease features between childhood-onset and adult-onset systemic lupus erythematosus. Arthritis Rheum 58(2):556–562
32. Tarvin SE, O'Neil KM (2018) Systemic lupus erythematosus, Sjogren syndrome, and mixed connective tissue disease in children and adolescents. Pediatr Clin N Am 65(4):711–737
33. Qin B, Wang J, Yang Z, Yang M, Ma N, Huang F et al (2015) Epidemiology of primary Sjogren's syndrome: a systematic review and meta-analysis. Ann Rheum Dis 74(11):1983–1989
34. Sakiani S, Olsen NJ, Kovacs WJ (2013) Gonadal steroids and humoral immunity. Nat Rev Endocrinol 9(1):56–62
35. Rubinow KB (2018) An intracrine view of sex steroids, immunity, and metabolic regulation. Mol Metab 15:92–103
36. Seillet C, Laffont S, Tremollieres F, Rouquie N, Ribot C, Arnal JF et al (2012) The TLR-mediated response of plasmacytoid dendritic cells is positively regulated by estradiol in vivo through cell-intrinsic estrogen receptor alpha signaling. Blood 119(2):454–464
37. Rider V, Abdou NI, Kimler BF, Lu N, Brown S, Fridley BL (2018) Gender bias in human systemic lupus erythematosus: a problem of steroid receptor action? Front Immunol 9:611
38. Fan H, Zhao G, Ren D, Liu F, Dong G, Hou Y (2017) Gender differences of B cell signature related to estrogen-induced IFI44L/BAFF in systemic lupus erythematosus. Immunol Lett 181:71–78
39. Tabor DE, Gould KA (2017) Estrogen receptor alpha promotes lupus in (NZBxNZW)F1 mice in a B cell intrinsic manner. Clin Immunol 174:41–52
40. Cunningham MA, Richard ML, Wirth JR, Scott JL, Eudaly J, Ruiz P et al (2019) Novel mechanism for estrogen receptor alpha modulation of murine lupus. J Autoimmun 97:59–69
41. Scott JL, Wirth JR, Eudaly J, Ruiz P, Cunningham MA (2017) Complete knockout of estrogen receptor alpha is not directly protective in murine lupus. Clin Immunol 183:132–141
42. Kanda N, Tsuchida T, Tamaki K (1999) Estrogen enhancement of anti-double-stranded DNA antibody and immunoglobulin G production in peripheral blood mononuclear cells from patients with systemic lupus erythematosus. Arthritis Rheum 42(2):328–337
43. Sakabe K, Yoshida T, Furuya H, Kayama F, Chan EK (1998) Estrogenic xenobiotics increase expression of SS-A/Ro autoantigens in cultured human epidermal cells. Acta Derm Venereol 78(6):420–423
44. Mok CC, Lau CS (2000) Profile of sex hormones in male patients with systemic lupus erythematosus. Lupus 9(4):252–257
45. Arnaud L, Nordin A, Lundholm H, Svenungsson E, Hellbacher E, Wikner J et al (2017) Effect of corticosteroids and cyclophosphamide on sex hormone profiles in male patients with systemic lupus erythematosus or systemic sclerosis. Arthritis Rheumatol 69(6):1272–1279
46. Chang DM, Chang CC, Kuo SY, Chu SJ, Chang ML (1999) Hormonal profiles and immunological studies of male lupus in Taiwan. Clin Rheumatol 18(2):158–162
47. Mackworth-Young CG, Parke AL, Morley KD, Fotherby K, Hughes GR (1983) Sex hormones in male patients with systemic lupus erythematosus: a comparison with other disease groups. Eur J Rheumatol Inflamm 6(3):228–232
48. Suzuki T, Schaumberg DA, Sullivan BD, Liu M, Richards SM, Sullivan RM et al (2002) Do estrogen and progesterone play a role in the dry eye of Sjogren's syndrome? Ann N Y Acad Sci 966:223–225
49. Mavragani CP, Fragoulis GE, Moutsopoulos HM (2012) Endocrine alterations in primary Sjogren's syndrome: an overview. J Autoimmun 39(4):354–358

50. Brennan MT, Sankar V, Leakan RA, Grisius MM, Collins MT, Fox PC et al (2003) Sex steroid hormones in primary Sjogren's syndrome. J Rheumatol 30(6):1267–1271
51. Taiym S, Haghighat N, Al-Hashimi I (2004) A comparison of the hormone levels in patients with Sjogren's syndrome and healthy controls. Oral Surg Oral Med Oral Pathol Oral Radiol Endod 97(5):579–583
52. Mostafa S, Seamon V, Azzarolo AM (2012) Influence of sex hormones and genetic predisposition in Sjogren's syndrome: a new clue to the immunopathogenesis of dry eye disease. Exp Eye Res 96(1):88–97
53. Konttinen YT, Stegajev V, Al-Samadi A, Porola P, Hietanen J, Ainola M (2015) Sjogren's syndrome and extragonadal sex steroid formation: a clue to a better disease control? J Steroid Biochem Mol Biol 145:237–244
54. Konttinen YT, Fuellen G, Bing Y, Porola P, Stegaev V, Trokovic N et al (2012) Sex steroids in Sjogren's syndrome. J Autoimmun 39(1–2):49–56
55. Song GG, Lee YH (2017) Circulating prolactin level in systemic lupus erythematosus and its correlation with disease activity: a meta-analysis. Lupus 26(12):1260–1268
56. Wan Asyraf WA, Mohd Shahrir MS, Asrul W, Norasyikin AW, Hanita O, Kong WY et al (2018) The association between serum prolactin levels and interleukin-6 and systemic lupus erythematosus activity. Reumatismo 70(4):241–250
57. Jara LJ, Medina G, Saavedra MA, Vera-Lastra O, Torres-Aguilar H, Navarro C et al (2017) Prolactin has a pathogenic role in systemic lupus erythematosus. Immunol Res 65(2):512–523
58. Walker SE, Allen SH, McMurray RW (1993) Prolactin and autoimmune disease. Trends Endocrinol Metab 4(5):147–151
59. McMurray R, Keisler D, Izui S, Walker SE (1994) Hyperprolactinemia in male NZB/NZW (B/W) F1 mice: accelerated autoimmune disease with normal circulating testosterone. Clin Immunol Immunopathol 71(3):338–343
60. Walker SE, Keisler D, Komatireddy GR, McMurray RW (1998) The effects of prolactin in animal models of SLE. Scand J Rheumatol Suppl 107:31–32
61. Haga HJ, Rygh T (1999) The prevalence of hyperprolactinemia in patients with primary Sjogren's syndrome. J Rheumatol 26(6):1291–1295
62. El Miedany YM, Ahmed I, Moustafa H, El Baddini M (2004) Hyperprolactinemia in Sjogren's syndrome: a patient subset or a disease manifestation? Joint Bone Spine 71(3):203–208
63. McMurray RW, Weidensaul D, Allen SH, Walker SE (1995) Efficacy of bromocriptine in an open label therapeutic trial for systemic lupus erythematosus. J Rheumatol 22(11):2084–2091
64. Qian Q, Liuqin L, Hao L, Shiwen Y, Zhongping Z, Dongying C et al (2015) The effects of bromocriptine on preventing postpartum flare in systemic lupus erythematosus patients from South China. J Immunol Res 2015:316965
65. Walker SE (2001) Bromocriptine treatment of systemic lupus erythematosus. Lupus 10(10):762–768
66. Jara LJ, Cruz-Cruz P, Saavedra MA, Medina G, Garcia-Flores A, Angeles U et al (2007) Bromocriptine during pregnancy in systemic lupus erythematosus: a pilot clinical trial. Ann N Y Acad Sci 1110:297–304
67. Peeva E, Grimaldi C, Spatz L, Diamond B (2000) Bromocriptine restores tolerance in estrogen-treated mice. J Clin Invest 106(11):1373–1379
68. McMurray RW (2001) Bromocriptine in rheumatic and autoimmune diseases. Semin Arthritis Rheum 31(1):21–32
69. Liang Y, Tsoi LC, Xing X, Beamer MA, Swindell WR, Sarkar MK et al (2017) A gene network regulated by the transcription factor VGLL3 as a promoter of sex-biased autoimmune diseases. Nat Immunol 18(2):152–160
70. Billi AC, Gharaee-Kermani M, Fullmer J, Tsoi LC, Hill BD, Gruszka D et al (2019) The female-biased factor VGLL3 drives cutaneous and systemic autoimmunity. JCI Insight 4(8):127291
71. Goad WB, Robinson A, Puck TT (1976) Incidence of aneuploidy in a human population. Am J Hum Genet 28(1):62–68

72. Nielsen J, Wohlert M (1991) Chromosome abnormalities found among 34,910 newborn children: results from a 13-year incidence study in Arhus, Denmark. Hum Genet 87(1):81–83
73. Abramsky L, Chapple J (1997) 47,XXY (Klinefelter syndrome) and 47,XYY: estimated rates of and indication for postnatal diagnosis with implications for prenatal counselling. Prenat Diagn 17(4):363–368
74. Klinefelter HF, Reifenstein EC, Albright F (1942) Syndrome characterized by gynecomastisa, aspermatogenesis without a-leydigism, and increased excietion of follicle-stimulating hormone. J Clin Endocrinol 2(11):615–627
75. Kocar IH, Yesilova Z, Ozata M, Turan M, Sengul A, Ozdemir I (2000) The effect of testosterone replacement treatment on immunological features of patients with Klinefelter's syndrome. Clin Exp Immunol 121(3):448–452
76. Otter M, Schrander-Stumpel C, Curfs LMG (2010) Triple X syndrome: a review of the literature. Eur J Hum Genet 18(3):265–271
77. Tartaglia NR, Howell S, Sutherland A, Wilson R, Wilson L (2010) A review of trisomy X (47,XXX). Orphanet J Rare Dis 5:8
78. Turner HH (1938) A syndrome of infantilism, congenital webbed neck, and cubitus valgus. Endocrinology 23(5):566–574
79. Lue Y, Jentsch JD, Wang C, Rao PN, Hikim AP, Salameh W et al (2005) XXY mice exhibit gonadal and behavioral phenotypes similar to Klinefelter syndrome. Endocrinology 146(9):4148–4154
80. Michalski JP, Snyder SM, McLeod RL, Talal N (1978) Monozygotic twins with Klinefelter's syndrome discordant for systemic lupus erythematosus and symptomatic myasthenia gravis. Arthritis Rheum 21(3):306–309
81. Lahita RG, Bradlow HL (1987) Klinefelter's syndrome: hormone metabolism in hypogonadal males with systemic lupus erythematosus. J Rheumatol Suppl 14(Suppl 13):154–157
82. Jimenez-Balderas FJ, Tapia-Serrano R, Fonseca ME, Arellano J, Beltran A, Yanez P et al (2001) High frequency of association of rheumatic/autoimmune diseases and untreated male hypogonadism with severe testicular dysfunction. Arthritis Res 3(6):362–367
83. Ortiz-Neu C, LeRoy EC (1969) The coincidence of Klinefelter's syndrome and systemic lupus erythematosus. Arthritis Rheum 12(3):241–246
84. Seminog OO, Seminog AB, Yeates D, Goldacre MJ (2015) Associations between Klinefelter's syndrome and autoimmune diseases: English national record linkage studies. Autoimmunity 48(2):125–128
85. Fujimoto M, Ikeda K, Nakamura T, Iwamoto T, Furuta S, Nakajima H (2015) Development of mixed connective tissue disease and Sjogren's syndrome in a patient with trisomy X. Lupus 24(11):1217–1220
86. Ishihara K, Yoshimura M, Nakao H, Kanakura Y, Kanayama Y, Matsuzawa Y (1994) T cell abnormalities in mixed connective tissue disease complicated with Klinefelter's syndrome. Intern Med 33(11):714–717
87. Tsung SH, Heckman MG (1974) Klinefelter syndrome, immunological disorders, and malignant neoplasm: report of a case. Arch Pathol Lab Med 98(5):351–354
88. Liu K, Kurien BT, Zimmerman SL, Kaufman KM, Taft DH, Kottyan LC et al (2016) X chromosome dose and sex bias in autoimmune diseases: increased prevalence of 47,XXX in systemic lupus erythematosus and Sjogren's syndrome. Arthritis Rheumatol (Hoboken, NJ) 68(5):1290–1300
89. Slae M, Heshin-Bekenstein M, Simckes A, Heimer G, Engelhard D, Eisenstein EM (2014) Female polysomy-X and systemic lupus erythematosus. Semin Arthritis Rheum 43(4):508–512
90. Chagnon P, Schneider R, Hebert J, Fortin PR, Provost S, Belisle C et al (2006) Identification and characterization of an Xp22.33;Yp11.2 translocation causing a triplication of several genes of the pseudoautosomal region 1 in an XX male patient with severe systemic lupus erythematosus. Arthritis Rheum 54(4):1270–1278
91. Rasmussen A, Sevier S, Kelly JA, Glenn SB, Aberle T, Cooney CM et al (2011) The lupus family registry and repository. Rheumatology (Oxford) 50(1):47–59

92. Scofield RH, Bruner GR, Namjou B, Kimberly RP, Ramsey-Goldman R, Petri M et al (2008) Klinefelter's syndrome (47,XXY) in male systemic lupus erythematosus patients: support for the notion of a gene-dose effect from the X chromosome. Arthritis Rheum 58(8):2511–2517
93. Dillon SP, Kurien BT, Li S, Bruner GR, Kaufman KM, Harley JB et al (2012) Sex chromosome aneuploidies among men with systemic lupus erythematosus. J Autoimmun 38(2–3):J129–J134
94. Dillon S, Aggarwal R, Harding JW, Li LJ, Weissman MH, Li S et al (2011) Klinefelter's syndrome (47,XXY) among men with systemic lupus erythematosus. Acta Paediatr 100(6):819–823
95. Lessard CJ, Li H, Adrianto I, Ice JA, Rasmussen A, Grundahl KM et al (2013) Variants at multiple loci implicated in both innate and adaptive immune responses are associated with Sjogren's syndrome. Nat Genet 45(11):1284–1292
96. Morris DL, Sheng Y, Zhang Y, Wang YF, Zhu Z, Tombleson P et al (2016) Genome-wide association meta-analysis in Chinese and European individuals identifies ten new loci associated with systemic lupus erythematosus. Nat Genet 48(8):940–946
97. Cooney CM, Bruner GR, Aberle T, Namjou-Khales B, Myers LK, Feo L et al (2009) 46,X,del(X)(q13) Turner's syndrome women with systemic lupus erythematosus in a pedigree multiplex for SLE. Genes Immun 10(5):478–481
98. Sharma R, Harris VM, Cavett J, Kurien BT, Liu K, Koelsch KA et al (2017) Rare X chromosome abnormalities in systemic lupus erythematosus and Sjogren's syndrome. Arthritis Rheumatol (Hoboken, NJ) 69(11):2187–2192
99. Sasidhar MV, Itoh N, Gold SM, Lawson GW, Voskuhl RR (2012) The XX sex chromosome complement in mice is associated with increased spontaneous lupus compared with XY. Ann Rheum Dis 71(8):1418–1422
100. Smith-Bouvier DL, Divekar AA, Sasidhar M, Du S, Tiwari-Woodruff SK, King JK et al (2008) A role for sex chromosome complement in the female bias in autoimmune disease. J Exp Med 205(5):1099–1108
101. Arnold AP (2009) Mouse models for evaluating sex chromosome effects that cause sex differences in non-gonadal tissues. J Neuroendocrinol 21(4):377–386
102. Burgoyne PS, Arnold AP (2016) A primer on the use of mouse models for identifying direct sex chromosome effects that cause sex differences in non-gonadal tissues. Biol Sex Differ 7:68
103. Itoh Y, Mackie R, Kampf K, Domadia S, Brown JD, O'Neill R et al (2015) Four core genotypes mouse model: localization of the Sry transgene and bioassay for testicular hormone levels. BMC Res Notes 8:69
104. Lee J, Tattoli I, Wojtal KA, Vavricka SR, Philpott DJ, Girardin SE (2009) pH-dependent internalization of muramyl peptides from early endosomes enables Nod1 and Nod2 signaling. J Biol Chem 284(35):23818–23829
105. Baccala R, Gonzalez-Quintial R, Blasius AL, Rimann I, Ozato K, Kono DH et al (2013) Essential requirement for IRF8 and SLC15A4 implicates plasmacytoid dendritic cells in the pathogenesis of lupus. Proc Natl Acad Sci U S A 110(8):2940–2945
106. Henikoff S, Henikoff JG (1991) Automated assembly of protein blocks for database searching. Nucleic Acids Res 19(23):6565–6572
107. Harris VM, Harley IWT, Kurien BT, Koelsch KA, Scofield RH (2019) The lupus risk gene CXorf21regulates lysosomal pH in a sex dependent manner. Front Immunol 10:578, https://doi.org/10.3389/fimmu.2019.00578
108. Harris VM, Harley ITW, Kurien BT, Koelsch KA, Scofield RH (2019) Lysosomal pH is regulated in a sex dependent manner in immune cells expressing CXorf21. Front Immunol 10:578
109. Shvetsova E, Sofronova A, Monajemi R, Gagalova K, HHM D, White SJ et al (2019) Skewed X-inactivation is common in the general female population. Eur J Hum Genet 27(3):455–465
110. Ozbalkan Z, Bagislar S, Kiraz S, Akyerli CB, Ozer HT, Yavuz S et al (2005) Skewed X chromosome inactivation in blood cells of women with scleroderma. Arthritis Rheum 52(5):1564–1570

111. Broen JC, Wolvers-Tettero IL, Geurts-van Bon L, Vonk MC, Coenen MJ, Lafyatis R et al (2010) Skewed X chromosomal inactivation impacts T regulatory cell function in systemic sclerosis. Ann Rheum Dis 69(12):2213–2216
112. Santiwatana S, Mahachoklertwattana P (2018) Skewed X chromosome inactivation in girls and female adolescents with autoimmune thyroid disease. Clin Endocrinol (Oxf) 89(6):863–869
113. Simmonds MJ, Kavvoura FK, Brand OJ, Newby PR, Jackson LE, Hargreaves CE et al (2014) Skewed X chromosome inactivation and female preponderance in autoimmune thyroid disease: an association study and meta-analysis. J Clin Endocrinol Metab 99(1):E127–E131
114. Brix TH, Knudsen GP, Kristiansen M, Kyvik KO, Orstavik KH, Hegedus L (2005) High frequency of skewed X-chromosome inactivation in females with autoimmune thyroid disease: a possible explanation for the female predisposition to thyroid autoimmunity. J Clin Endocrinol Metab 90(11):5949–5953
115. Ozcelik T, Uz E, Akyerli CB, Bagislar S, Mustafa CA, Gursoy A et al (2006) Evidence from autoimmune thyroiditis of skewed X-chromosome inactivation in female predisposition to autoimmunity. Eur J Hum Genet 14(6):791–797
116. Uz E, Mustafa C, Topaloglu R, Bilginer Y, Dursun A, Kasapcopur O et al (2009) Increased frequency of extremely skewed X chromosome inactivation in juvenile idiopathic arthritis. Arthritis Rheum 60(11):3410–3412
117. Huang Q, Parfitt A, Grennan DM, Manolios N (1997) X-chromosome inactivation in monozygotic twins with systemic lupus erythematosus. Autoimmunity 26(2):85–93
118. Chitnis S, Monteiro J, Glass D, Apatoff B, Salmon J, Concannon P et al (2000) The role of X-chromosome inactivation in female predisposition to autoimmunity. Arthritis Res 2(5):399–406
119. Hamza RT, Raof NA, Abdallah KO (2013) Prevalence of multiple forms of autoimmunity in Egyptian patients with Turner syndrome: relation to karyotype. J Pediatr Endocrinol Metab 26(5–6):545–550
120. Elsheikh M, Wass JA, Conway GS (2001) Autoimmune thyroid syndrome in women with Turner's syndrome—the association with karyotype. Clin Endocrinol (Oxf) 55(2):223–226
121. Jorgensen KT, Rostgaard K, Bache I, Biggar RJ, Nielsen NM, Tommerup N et al (2010) Autoimmune diseases in women with Turner's syndrome. Arthritis Rheum 62(3):658–666
122. Invernizzi P, Miozzo M, Selmi C, Persani L, Battezzati PM, Zuin M et al (2005) X chromosome monosomy: a common mechanism for autoimmune diseases. J Immunol 175(1):575–578
123. Invernizzi P (2007) The X chromosome in female-predominant autoimmune diseases. Ann N Y Acad Sci 1110:57–64
124. Invernizzi P, Miozzo M, Oertelt-Prigione S, Meroni PL, Persani L, Selmi C et al (2007) X monosomy in female systemic lupus erythematosus. Ann N Y Acad Sci 1110:84–91
125. Forsdyke DR (1994) Relationship of X chromosome dosage compensation to intracellular self/not-self discrimination: a resolution of Muller's paradox? J Theor Biol 167(1):7–12
126. Forsdyke DR (2009) X chromosome reactivation perturbs intracellular self/not-self discrimination. Immunol Cell Biol 87(7):525–528
127. Forsdyke DR (2012) Ohno's hypothesis and Muller's paradox: sex chromosome dosage compensation may serve collective gene functions. BioEssays 34(11):930–933

Autoantibodies in Pregnancy

Gummadi Anjani and Amit Rawat

Abstract

Autoantibodies are immunoglobulins with specificity against self-antigens due to the presence of autoreactive T and B lymphocytes. Pregnancy is complicated by many diseases and vice versa. Various antibodies in mother during pregnancy are involved in maternal-fetal interactions, and the levels of various circulating antibodies in pregnancy may play a crucial role in the outcome of pregnancy, intrauterine fetal death or stillbirth, intrauterine growth restriction, pre-term birth, and so on. This chapter gives a brief review of the most commonly detected antibodies in pregnancy.

Keywords

Autoantibodies · Pregnancy outcome · Antinuclear antibody · Maternal antibody

4.1 Introduction

Autoantibodies are immunoglobulins with specificity against self-antigens due to the presence of autoreactive T and B lymphocytes. The presence of auto-reactive lymphocyte clones is an antithesis to the tenet of immune tolerance. Testing for autoantibodies is the most common diagnostic tool used for suspected autoimmune diseases. However, the mere presence of autoantibodies does not always denote autoimmune disease or predict its development in the future. Self-reactive natural autoantibodies are also seen in healthy individuals. Natural autoantibodies are IgM isotype antibodies with restricted repertoire, produced independent of antigen exposure and T cell help. They are low-affinity, poly-specific antibodies produced by

---

G. Anjani · A. Rawat (✉)
Department of Pediatrics, Post Graduate Institute of Medical Education and Research, Chandigarh, India

© Springer Nature Singapore Pte Ltd. 2020
S. K. Sharma (ed.), *Women's Health in Autoimmune Diseases*,
https://doi.org/10.1007/978-981-15-0114-2_4

B1B lymphocytes. They prevent high-affinity, detrimental IgG class autoantibodies from binding to self-antigens by blocking their antigenic determinants. They serve diverse immunological functions such as providing innate immune protection and scavenging effete cells and apoptotic cell debris, thus ensuring the removal of putative autoantigens.

Pregnancy may be complicated by many diseases and vice versa. Antibodies in the mother during pregnancy are involved in maternal–fetal interactions. The presence and levels of various circulating antibodies in pregnancy may play a crucial role in the outcome of pregnancy [1] as these can cross the placental barrier and cause damage to the fetus. So, assessment of these antibodies becomes essential in an appropriate clinical setting. Examples include fetal thyroid goiter in response to maternal Graves' disease, fetal heart block due to maternal anti-Ro and anti-La antibodies, fetal arthrogryposis multiplex congenita in association with maternal myasthenia gravis, and fetal brain hemorrhage due to maternal autoimmune thrombocytopenia [2].

Certain autoantibodies which are found in autoimmune diseases can impair fertility, lead to pregnancy loss, intrauterine fetal death, or stillbirth, intrauterine growth restriction, preterm birth, and so on. Many autoantibodies have been associated with impaired fertility, and it is still not completely clear which antibody panel should be assessed in the management of pregnancy complications. In the absence of specific antibodies that are pathognomonic of pregnancy failure, it seems that a group of antibodies is more significant than any one antibody, and it may be more appropriate to assess a panel of antibodies rather than one antibody. Although many autoantibodies have been associated with reproductive failure, it is still not clear which antibodies should be assessed in the evaluation and management of infertility and RPL.

4.2 Antinuclear Antibody (ANA)

Autoimmune processes have been implicated in the pathogenesis of recurrent pregnancy loss (RPL). ANA is one of the contributory antibodies, and multiple studies have supported this notion. ANA positive cases showed significantly higher number of RPL and lower number of successful pregnancies [3]. Contrarily, studies have also shown that serologic parameters of autoimmunity are not elevated in women with RPL and are not associated with clinical characteristics of affected women [4]. Disappearance of ANA in early pregnancy could have a favorable prognostic value in the successive pregnancy [5]. Hence, ANA test is a potential prognostic tool for this condition which merits further research.

Antinuclear antibodies were detected in 31.8% of patients with a history of miscarriages but only in 5.7% of healthy patients with no fetal losses or autoimmunity by Cubillos et al. [6].

An increased prevalence of ANA was found in patients with autoimmune disease in Shoenfeld et al.'s [7] study. However, their prevalence was not increased in patients with infertility or recurrent pregnancy.

4.3 Anti-Ro/La Antibodies

Congenital heart block (CHB) is an autoantibody-mediated disorder presumably caused by placental transmission of maternal autoantibodies to Ro/SSA and La/SSB ribonucleoproteins. In a study with 163 pregnant women positive for anti-Ro/SSA 52 kDa and/or anti-Ro/SSA 60 kDa and/or anti-La/SSB antibodies using ELISA, 24 children born to these mothers developed CHB, and 139 had a favorable outcome [8]. These findings suggest that fetal echocardiography should be performed in all pregnant women with anti-Ro or anti-La autoantibodies.

4.4 Anticentromere Antibody

Anticentromere antibody is commonly detected in patients with limited forms of systemic sclerosis particularly CREST (Calcinosis cutis, Raynaud's phenomenon, esophageal dysmotility, sclerodactyly, and telangiectasia) syndrome. However, in recent years anticentromere antibodies have been found to be associated with defects in oocyte maturation and embryonic cleavage. Women with anticentromere antibody also have a significantly reduced number of mature oocytes and a decreased embryo cleavage rate. The development of mouse embryos incubated with polyclonal anti-CENP-A antibody showed significant growth impairment or death.

4.5 Anti-Thyroid Antibodies

Anti-thyroid antibodies (ATAs) have been suggested to be independent markers of "at-risk" pregnancy.

Autoimmune thyroid disease is common, affecting approximately 1% of the population, while subclinical, focal thyroiditis, and circulating thyroid antibodies can be found in about 15% of otherwise healthy subjects who are euthyroid. Studies have shown that anti-TPOAbs are strongly associated with miscarriage and LBW irrespective of gestational age [9]. Thyroid autoimmunity is frequently present in women with APS and recurrent abortions and is often associated with either reduced fecundity or poor pregnancy outcome. Thyroid antibodies should always be evaluated in women with recurrent spontaneous abortions including those with aPL [10]. A meta-analysis showed that TPOAb(+) with normal thyroid function increases the risks of miscarriage and premature delivery [11]. The highest incidence rates for PROM and low birth weight were in the TPOAb−/TgAb+ and TPOAb+/TgAb+ subjects, respectively. TgAb positivity and TPOAb positivity were associated with PROM and low birth weight, respectively [12].

However, there is inadequate data regarding both the adverse effect of thyroid antibody positivity in euthyroid women on pregnancy outcomes and the effects of levothyroxine on these women. It seems that the results of most studies indicate adverse effects of thyroid antibody positivity in euthyroid women on pregnancy outcomes. Euthyroid women with recurrent miscarriages have increased levels of autoantibodies against either thyroglobulin (aTG) or thyroid peroxidase (TPO), while the probability of abortion in women with ATA has been shown to be greater than in controls [13]. However, in Shoenfeld et al.'s [7] large study, there was no association with recurrent miscarriage as a whole, but anti-Tg antibodies were associated with late pregnancy loss compared with controls. Therefore, the prognostic value of ATA remains uncertain. Further randomized clinical trials are needed to investigate the effects of treating pregnant euthyroid women with positive thyroid antibodies on the maternal and early/late neonatal outcomes [14].

4.6 Anti-prothrombin Antibodies

These antibodies are associated with pregnancy loss in cases with antiphospholipid antibody syndrome and are also associated with recurrent miscarriages. A trial in 2006 showed a significantly increased level of aPT in women with infertility, and in recurrent pregnancy loss [7]. These antibodies were more closely associated with secondary abortions (miscarriages after a livebirth) than primary abortions.

4.7 Anti-laminin Antibodies

Laminin-1 is an integral part of basement membranes composed of glycoprotein. IgG anti-laminin antibodies have been associated with infertility and recurrent first-trimester miscarriages in humans [15]. Active immunization of naive mice with laminin-1 followed by elevated circulating anti-laminin-1 antibodies results in reproductive failure [16].

4.8 Anti-trophoblast Antibody

During the course of a normal uncomplicated human pregnancy, the mother generates an antibody response directed against determinants present on the plasma membrane of the outer fetal layer of the term placenta, the syncytiotrophoblast. The response, measured by an ELISA that utilizes syncytiotrophoblast plasma membrane as the antigenic target, is predominantly IgG in nature, but with a minor contribution from IgM molecules, and maximum responses were observed during the first trimester and the levels gradually declined as the pregnancy progressed. Anti-trophoblast antibodies, suggested to be directed against fetal trophoblast antigens, appear early in pregnancy and participate in mediating harmful immune responses, predisposing for recurrent miscarriage.

On a population basis, this antibody response profile was mainly restricted to first and second pregnancies, although anti-trophoblast antibody responses could be detected in multiparous women but with a greatly reduced incidence compared with primipara [17]. It has been demonstrated that more than 50% of women with recurrent spontaneous abortions were positive for the IgG isotype of this antibody compared to 25% in controls [18].

4.9 Maternal Antibodies to Paternal B Lymphocytes

Apart from the harmful effects on fetus due to maternal antibodies, protective serum antibodies are also seen. In a study on 22 pregnant women with 27 pregnancies for antibodies against paternal B lymphocytes determined by the EA rosette inhibition (EAI), it was seen that 5 out of 12 successful pregnancies were associated with such detectable antibodies. However, only 1 out 15 spontaneous abortions had positive antibodies to paternal B lymphocytes. These results indicated that normal, but not abnormal, pregnancies were often associated with blocking antibody formation, with protection of fetus from abortion [19].

4.10 HLA Antibodies

Neonatal alloimmune thrombocytopenia (NAIT) generally results from platelet opsonization by maternal antibodies against fetal platelet antigens inherited from the infant's father. Newborn monochorionic twins with severe thrombocytopenia nonresponsive to platelet transfusions and intravenous immunoglobulin were evaluated in a previous study. Class I human leucocyte antigen (HLA) antibodies with broad specificity against several HLA-B antigens were detected in the maternal serum. Weak antibodies against HLA-B57 and HLA-B58 in sera from both twins supported NAIT as the most likely diagnosis. Transfusion of HLA-matched platelet concentrates was more efficacious to manage thrombocytopenia compared with platelet concentrates from random donors [20]. It also reported that pregnant women positive for anti-HLA (class I or II) antibodies may be at an increased risk of fetal damage and spontaneous preterm delivery [21] HLA-C-specific antibodies were found more often in women with recurrent miscarriages by inducing platelet activation by placental thromboxane production [22].

4.11 Anti-IgA Antibodies in Pregnancy

It is possible that maternal anti-IgA exerts a transplacental effect on the fetal immune system, causing IgA deficiency in some instances. Using an enzyme-linked immunosorbent assay (ELISA) in a study of 61 serum samples from IgA-deficient pregnant women, it was observed antibodies to IgA2 alone in 20%, as compared with 7.5% of pregnant women not deficient in IgA and no IgA-deficient blood donors. Antibodies reacting with IgA1 alone were present in occasional serum samples (2–7%) from all groups studied, and class-specific anti-IgA antibodies were present in 17% of IgA-deficient blood donors and in 16% of IgA-deficient pregnant women. The offspring of IgA-deficient mothers (but not of IgA-deficient fathers) had levels of serum IgA below the normal mean [23].

4.12 Anti-*Saccharomyces cerevisiae* Antibodies (ASCA)

In Shoenfeld et al.'s [7] series, ASCAs were found to be associated with recurrent pregnancy losses. ASCAs can predict the development of the growth restriction and preterm labor, and fetal loss [24].

4.13 Anti-Human Platelet Antigen (HPA)-1a Antibodies

Fetal and neonatal alloimmune thrombocytopenia (FNAIT) is a bleeding disorder caused by maternal antibodies against paternal human platelet antigens (HPAs) on fetal platelets. Antibodies against HPA-1a account for the majority of FNAIT cases. Maternal anti-HPA-1a antibodies present during early pregnancy may affect placental function through binding to the HPA-1a antigen epitope on invasive trophoblasts. It was found that human anti-HPA-1a mAb partially inhibits adhesion and migratory capacity of HTR8/SVneo cells, suggesting anti-HPA-1a antibodies may affect trophoblast functions crucial for normal placental development [25].

4.14 Polymyositis Anti-SRP Antibodies and Pregnancy

Anti-SRP myopathy represents 4–6% of all the inflammatory myopathies. There are two cases of anti-SRP myopathy reported with pregnancy with flare of symptoms during postpartum period. However, inactive myopathy does not seem to cause serious maternal–fetal complications. Treatment (corticosteroid) of myopathy during pregnancy is indicated, given the risk of worsening of symptoms during the postpartum period [26] (Table 4.1).

Table 4.1 Antibodies positivity in various studies with recurrent pregnancy losses

Antibody	Interpretation	Reference
Antinuclear antibody	The incidence of ANA positivity among the cases (35.3%) was significantly higher than the controls (13.3%) ($p = 0.005$)	Antinuclear antibodies predict a higher incidence of pregnancy loss in unexplained recurrent pregnancy loss [3]
	31.8%	Antinuclear autoantibodies and pregnancy outcome in women with unexplained recurrent miscarriage [5]
	25%	[7]
ASCA	19.4%	[7]
Prothrombin	33%	[7]
Combined (ASCA, aPL or anti-prothrombin)	52.3%	[7]
Anti-Annexin	16.67%	[7]
TPO	33%	[7]
Anti-trophoblast antibody	50%	[18]
Anti-HLA antibody	25–63%	[22]

4 Autoantibodies in Pregnancy

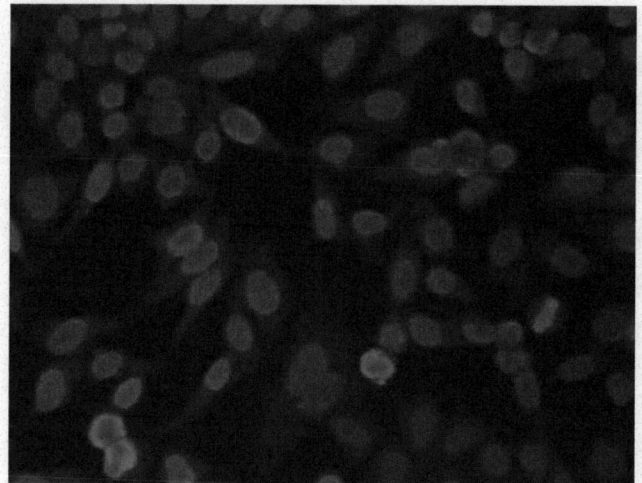

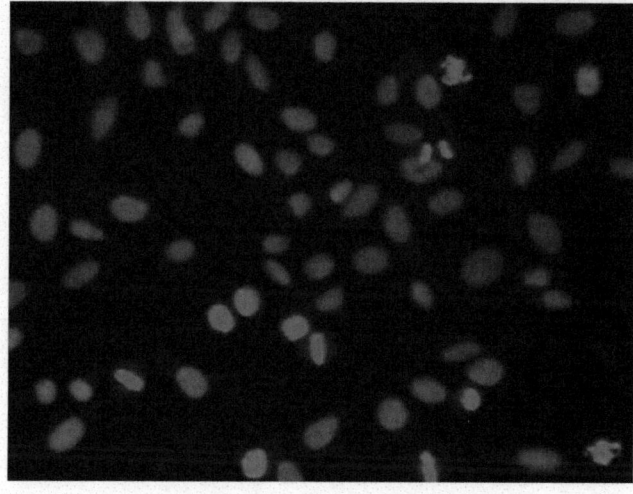

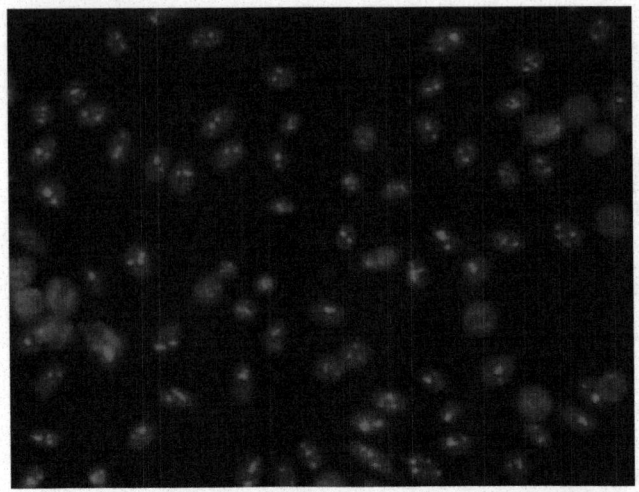
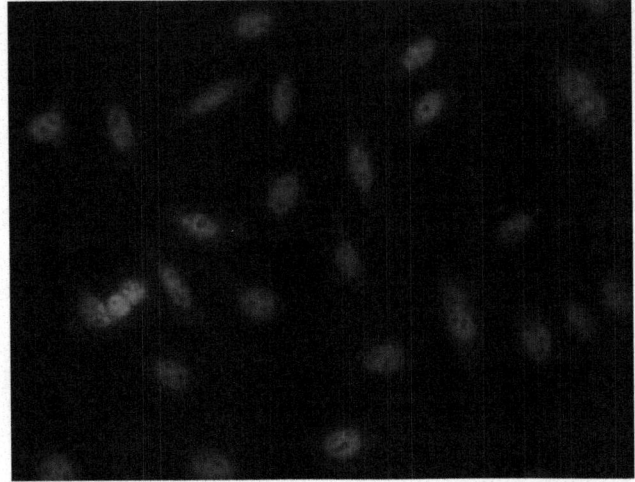

4 Autoantibodies in Pregnancy

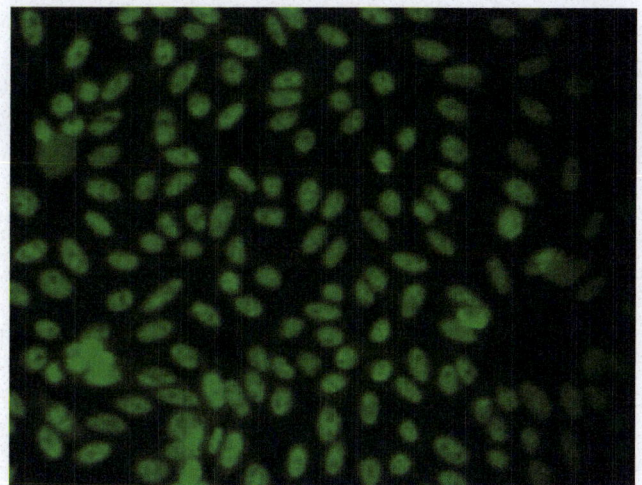

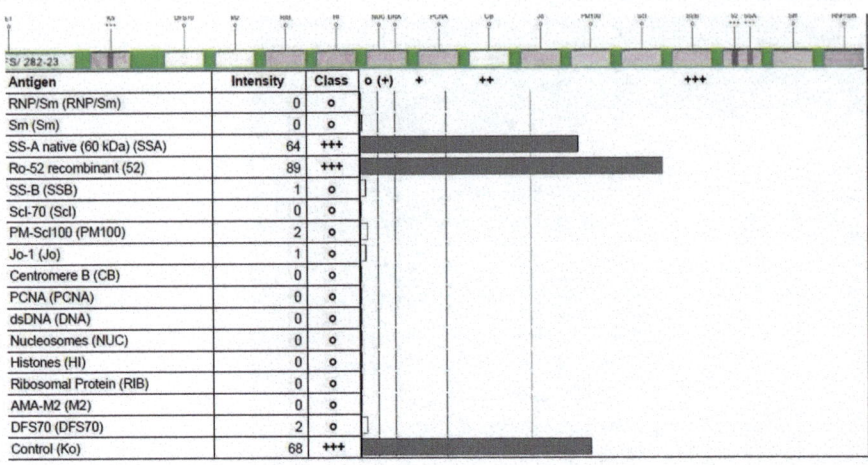

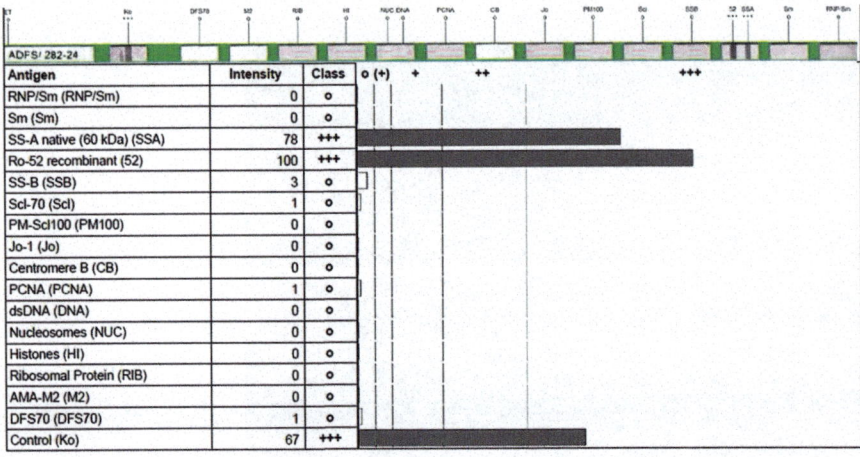

References

1. Yang X, Zhang C, Chen G, Sun C, Li J (2019) Antibodies: the major participants in maternal-fetal interaction. J Obstet Gynaecol Res 45(1):39–46
2. Panaitescu AM, Nicolaides K (2018) Maternal autoimmune disorders and fetal defects. J Matern-Fetal Neonatal Med 31(13):1798–1806
3. Sakthiswary R, Rajalingam S, Norazman MR, Hussein H (2015) Antinuclear antibodies predict a higher number of pregnancy loss in unexplained recurrent pregnancy loss. Clin Ter 166(2):e98–e101
4. Hefler-Frischmuth K, Walch K, Hefler L, Tempfer C, Grimm C (2017) Serologic markers of autoimmunity in women with recurrent pregnancy loss. Am J Reprod Immunol 77(4). https://doi.org/10.1111/aji.12635
5. Ticconi C, Pietropolli A, Borelli B, Bruno V, Piccione E, Bernardini S et al (2016) Antinuclear autoantibodies and pregnancy outcome in women with unexplained recurrent miscarriage. Am J Reprod Immunol 76(5):396–399

6. Cubillos J, Lucena A, Lucena C, Mendoza JC, Ruiz H, Arango A et al (1997) Incidence of autoantibodies in the infertile population. Early Pregnancy 3(2):119–124
7. Shoenfeld Y, Carp HJA, Molina V, Blank M, Cervera R, Balasch J et al (2006) Autoantibodies and prediction of reproductive failure. Am J Reprod Immunol 56(5–6):337–344
8. Tonello M, Hoxha A, Mattia E, Zambon A, Visentin S, Cerutti A et al (2017) Low titer, isolated anti Ro/SSA 60 kd antibodies is correlated with positive pregnancy outcomes in women at risk of congenital heart block. Clin Rheumatol 36(5):1155–1160
9. Meena A, Nagar P (2016) Pregnancy outcome in euthyroid women with anti-thyroid peroxidase antibodies. J Obstet Gynaecol India 66(3):160–165
10. De Carolis C, Greco E, Guarino MD, Perricone C, Dal Lago A, Giacomelli R et al (2004) Anti-thyroid antibodies and antiphospholipid syndrome: evidence of reduced fecundity and of poor pregnancy outcome in recurrent spontaneous aborters. Am J Reprod Immunol 52(4):263–266
11. Zhang SC, Wang SW, Zhao XD, Zhang JR (2016) [Obstetrical complications of thyroid peroxidase antibody positive during pregnancy and effects of intervention: a meta-analysis]. Zhonghua Fu Chan KeZaZhi 51(4):250–257
12. Chen L-M, Zhang Q, Si G-X, Chen Q-S, Ye E, Yu L-C et al (2015) Associations between thyroid autoantibody status and abnormal pregnancy outcomes in euthyroid women. Endocrine 48(3):924–928
13. Matalon ST, Blank M, Ornoy A, Shoenfeld Y (2001) The association between anti-thyroid antibodies and pregnancy loss. Am J Reprod Immunol 45(2):72–77
14. Nazarpour S, Ramezani Tehrani F, Simbar M, Azizi F (2016) Thyroid autoantibodies and the effect on pregnancy outcomes. J Obstet Gynaecol 36(1):3–9
15. Inagaki J, Matsuura E, Nomizu M, Sugiura-Ogasawara M, Katano K, Kaihara K et al (2001) IgG anti-laminin-1 autoantibody and recurrent miscarriages. Am J Reprod Immunol 45(4):232–238
16. Matalon ST, Blank M, Matsuura E, Inagaki J, Nomizu M, Levi Y et al (2003) Immunization of naïve mice with mouse laminin-1 affected pregnancy outcome in a mouse model. Am J Reprod Immunol 50(2):159–165
17. Davies M, Browne CM (1985) Anti-trophoblast antibody responses during normal human pregnancy. J Reprod Immunol 7(4):285–297
18. Tedesco F, Pausa M, Nardon E, Narchi G, Bulla R, Livi C et al (1997) Prevalence and biological effects of anti-trophoblast and anti-endothelial cell antibodies in patients with recurrent spontaneous abortions. Am J Reprod Immunol 38(3):205–211
19. Power DA, Mather AJ, MacLeod AM, Lind T, Catto GR (1986) Maternal antibodies to paternal B-lymphocytes in normal and abnormal pregnancy. Am J Reprod Immunol Microbiol 10(1):10–13
20. Wendel K, Akkök ÇA, Kutzsche S (2017) Neonatal alloimmune thrombocytopaenia associated with maternal HLA antibodies. BMJ Case Rep 2017. https://doi.org/10.1136/bcr-2016-218269
21. Lee J, Romero R, Xu Y, Miranda J, Yoo W, Chaemsaithong P et al (2013) Detection of anti-HLA antibodies in maternal blood in the second trimester to identify patients at risk of antibody-mediated maternal anti-fetal rejection and spontaneous preterm delivery. Am J Reprod Immunol 70(2):162–175
22. Meuleman T, Haasnoot GW, van Lith JMM, Verduijn W, Bloemenkamp KWM, Claas FHJ (2018) Paternal HLA-C is a risk factor in unexplained recurrent miscarriage. Am J Reprod Immunol 79(2). https://doi.org/10.1111/aji.12797
23. Petty RE, Sherry DD, Johannson J (1985) Anti-IgA antibodies in pregnancy. N Engl J Med 313(26):1620–1625
24. Katz JA (2004) Pregnancy and inflammatory bowel disease. Curr Opin Gastroenterol 20(4):328–332
25. Eksteen M, Heide G, Tiller H, Zhou Y, Nedberg NH, Martinez-Zubiaurre I et al (2017) Anti-human platelet antigen (HPA)-1a antibodies may affect trophoblast functions crucial for placental development: a laboratory study using an in vitro model. Reprod Biol Endocrinol 15(1):28
26. Ousmane C, Makhtar BEH, Fatoumata B, Massi GD, Lémine DSM, Soda D-SM et al (2016) Polymyositis anti-SRP antibodies and pregnancy about 2 cases. Pan Afr Med J 24:192

Laboratory Testing for the Antiphospholipid Syndrome

5

Jasmina Ahluwalia and Saniya Sharma

Abstract

Antiphospholipid syndrome (APS) is an autoimmune disorder characterized by thrombosis or recurrent pregnancy losses. It is a significant cause of pregnancy morbidity manifesting as recurrent miscarriages in young females of reproductive age-group. Classification criteria for definite APS are met when at least one clinical criterion, either thrombosis (arterial, venous or small vessel) or pregnancy morbidity, and one laboratory criterion (persistent positivity for Lupus anticoagulant, anticardiolipin or anti-beta 2 Glycoprotein 1 antibodies on two or more occasions at least 12 weeks apart) are present. For detection of Lupus anticoagulant, at least 2 assays- diluted Russell viper venom time and activated partial thromboplastin time based test using silica as an activator are recommended. Anticardiolipin and anti-beta 2 Glycoprotein 1 IgG/IgM antibodies are detected by enzyme linked immunosorbent assay, chemiluminescence or fluorescence enzyme immunoassay. Testing for lupus anticoagulant may be challenging while in acute phase of thrombosis and on anticoagulant therapy. Laboratory participation in external quality assurance exercises is highly recommended for standardization and inter-laboratory agreement of laboratory assays. In this chapter we discuss the key issues in APS pertaining to women with a focus on laboratory testing.

Keywords

Antiphospholipid antibodies · Antiphospholipid syndrome · Autoimmune diseases · Thrombosis

---

J. Ahluwalia (✉) · S. Sharma
Department of Hematology, Postgraduate Institute of Medical Education and Research, Chandigarh, India

© Springer Nature Singapore Pte Ltd. 2020
S. K. Sharma (ed.), *Women's Health in Autoimmune Diseases*,
https://doi.org/10.1007/978-981-15-0114-2_5

5.1 Antiphospholipid Antibody Syndrome (APS)

APS is an autoimmune disorder characterised by a propensity to thrombosis or recurrent pregnancy losses with persistent positivity for one or more of the antibodies—Lupus anticoagulant (LAC), anticardiolipin antibody (aCLa) and anti-beta 2 Glycoprotein 1 antibodies (aβ2GPI). It has an estimated incidence of five cases per 100,000 people per year, and is the most common cause for acquired thrombophilia manifesting as deep vein thrombosis, young stroke in patients less than 50 years and recurrent pregnancy losses. APS can manifest alone or secondary to diseases particularly systemic lupus erythematosus (SLE) and rheumatoid arthritis. Being primarily a disease of young individuals especially females in the reproductive age group, it is a significant cause of morbidity in this segment of the population.

5.1.1 APS and Other Autoimmune Disorders

APS is associated with other autoimmune disorders (AD). Perhaps the strongest association is with systemic lupus erythematosus (SLE) [1]. In fact, the antiphospholipid antibodies (aPLas) were first detected in patients with SLE [1]. According to different series, aPLas are seen in 12–44% of SLE patients [2, 3]. In a meta-analysis, the presence of lupus anticoagulant in SLE led to a sixfold risk of thrombotic events [4]. In a recent study comprising 376 patients with SLE, the prevalence of aPLas was 54%. However, APS was present in 9.3% patients [5]. Positivity for rheumatoid factor, pulmonary and cardiovascular involvement was significantly associated with APS [5]. aPLas may be present silently without changing the natural history of the disease while in some aPLas may lead to thrombotic events and increased obstetric morbidity. aPLas were found in 43% of patients with autoimmune thyroiditis, 17% of patients with systemic vasculitis and 30% of patients with primary Sjögren's syndrome [6–8]. aPLas have also been reported in Behcet's disease, though to a more variable extent with a positivity rate ranging from 13.5% to 40% [9, 10]. There is lack of clarity on the pathogenetic mechanism of aPLas in Behcet's disease (BD) [11]. In a prospective study comprising 98 patients with newly diagnosed giant cell arteritis (GCA) and/or polymyalgia rheumatica, anticardiolipin antibodies (aCLas) were detected in 20.4% of the patients [12]. Merkel et al. reported aCLa in 16% of patients with rheumatoid arthritis (RA) and SLE [13]. APS may also be associated with systemic sclerosis, systemic vasculitis, dermatopolymyositis, primary biliary cirrhosis and autoimmune hepatitis. Many autoimmune disorders are common in females and hence these antibodies are likely to test positive in a number of female patients.

5.1.2 APS in Women (Pregnancy, Infertility, Adolescence)

Pregnancy morbidity is the hallmark of APS. It is implicated as the underlying cause in 10–15% of the women with recurrent miscarriages, the most common obstetric complication of APS [14]. Approximately, 50% of the APS-associated pregnancy losses occur in the first trimester [14]. Other than foetal loss, pregnancy-related morbidity includes early delivery, oligohydramnios, neonatal prematurity, intrauterine growth restriction, foetal distress, placental insufficiency, pre-eclampsia or eclampsia and HELLP syndrome (haemolytic anaemia, elevated liver enzymes and low platelet counts, arterial or venous thrombosis). Circulating aPLas have been found as the main risk factor in 7–25% of early recurrent pregnancy loss (RPL) [15]. The risk of RPL varies with the different types of antibodies. The presence of aCLa is associated with an odds ratio (OR) of 22.6 for subsequent pregnancy losses [16]. The presence of anti-β2GPI antibodies increases the risk of RPL from 6.8% to 22.2% in comparison with women with LAC or aCLa [17].

The risk of venous thromboembolism (VTE), which is 4–5 times higher in pregnant and post-partum period, is further increased in the presence of APS [14]. Additionally, arterial thrombosis leading to cerebral ischaemia and manifesting as stroke in young women has also been found to be strongly associated with aPLas [18]. There have been several studies on the role of aPLas in infertility with conflicting results, some of which indicate that the chances of spontaneous conception and/or conception with in vitro fertilisation are reduced in the presence of aPLas [19]. Bleeding is a rare manifestation in females with aPLas. The occurrence of non-neutralising anti-prothrombin (aPT) antibodies can result in a haemorrhagic diathesis [20].

5.1.3 Pathogenetic Role of the aPLas

The aPLas are a heterogeneous group of autoantibodies with varied targets. Currently, of these, the ones that are considered of diagnostic relevance for the purpose of classification are the LAC, IgG and IgM isotypes of the aCLa and aβ2GPI antibodies. The primary targets for these antibodies are phospholipid-binding proteins which are present in many cell surfaces. The risk of a thrombotic event in asymptomatic persons positive for LAC, aCLa and aβ2GPI antibodies is 5.3% per year [21]. β2GPI acts as a cofactor that facilitates the binding between aPLa and phospholipid. β2GPI is probably a natural inhibitor of coagulation with antiangiogenic and anti-apoptotic activities. β2GPI can adopt two different conformations: a circular 'closed' conformation in plasma, and an 'activated' open conformation. On binding to anionic phospholipids, there is a conformational change from the circular to open unfolded form that exposes antigenic determinants where the antibody can bind [22]. Bound antibody–β2GPI complexes to a number of receptors on phospholipid membranes trigger intracellular signalling and inflammatory responses. The β2GPI complex comprises five domains with the pathogenic effects closely related to antibodies that target domain 1.

The role of other antibodies referred to as the 'non-criteria antibodies', such as specific antibodies against phosphatidic acid, phosphatidylserine–prothrombin complex, vimentin–cardiolipin complex, protein C-S, factor X, factor XII, Annexin A2 and Annexin A5, in the pathogenesis of APS is not yet established [23].

Although, there is a clear association between aPLa and thrombosis/pregnancy morbidity, other pathogenic processes are also involved in the development of APS—'double-hit theory'. The factors that trigger thrombosis could be genetic, endothelial injury, inflammation and infectious diseases, immune-mediated and other non-immune procoagulant factors [23]. This, probably, explains why all patients with aPLas do not develop thrombosis.

The other important mechanisms that play a role in thrombotic manifestations in APS include complement activation, generating C3a and C5a, resulting in vascular injury, activation of mTOR signalling pathway contributing to endothelial and intimal cell proliferation, which may result in peripheral ischaemia, skin ulcers, microthrombi generation, diffuse alveolar haemorrhage and nephropathy, acquired activated protein C resistance and down-regulation of the TF pathway inhibitor (TFPI) by anti-TFPI antibodies (aTFPI).

Binding of aPLas to monocytes, platelets, endothelium and plasma proteins of the coagulation cascade may cause placental thrombosis. Another proposed mechanism for aPLa-induced placental thrombosis is the disruption of protective Annexin A5 shield on placental trophoblast and endothelial cell layers. Once the aPLas bind and interfere with the function of Annexin A5 on the surface of trophoblastic cells of the placental intervillous space, the proliferation and syncytia formation are inhibited, which induces cell injury and apoptosis, decreases the human chorionic gonadotrophin production and leads to abnormal placentation [24].

5.1.4 APS Diagnostic Criteria

Classification criteria for definite APS are met when at least one clinical criterion, either thrombosis (arterial, venous or small vessel) in any tissue or pregnancy morbidity, and one laboratory criterion (LAC, aCLa or aβ2GPI antibodies) are present [25]. The pregnancy morbidity criteria include ≥3 pregnancy losses before 10 weeks of gestation, ≥1 pregnancy loss at/after 10 weeks of gestation and preterm birth before 34 weeks of gestation due to eclampsia/pre-eclampsia or placental insufficiency. Positive laboratory tests should be confirmed 12 weeks after the initial testing.

5.2 Laboratory Testing for APS

5.2.1 Who to Test?

Positive immunoassays have ranged from 3% to 20% in asymptomatic and healthy individuals in various clinical studies [26]. Based on the recommendations of 'The Antiphospholipid Antibodies Subcommittee of the International Society of Thrombosis and Hemostasis' on selecting patients for aPLa testing, three categories have been suggested (Table 5.1)

Table 5.1 Summary of recommendations of laboratory testing for APS according to 2006 International consensus statement

1. Detection of Lupus anticoagulant (LAC) in plasma on two or more occasions at least 12 weeks apart
2. Detection of β2GPI-dependent anticardiolipin antibodies (aCLa) of IgG/IgM isotype in plasma or serum, present at higher levels (>40 GPL or MPL or >99th percentile of normal controls) on two or more occasions at least 12 weeks apart, measured by solid-phase assays (ELISA or automated systems)
3. Detection of aβ2GPI-antibodies (aβ2GPI) of IgG/IgM isotype in plasma or serum, present at higher levels (>99th percentile of normal controls) on two or more occasions at least 12 weeks apart, measured by solid-phase assays (ELISA or automated systems)

(a) *low* appropriateness group includes elderly patients with venous or arterial thrombosis
(b) *moderate* appropriateness group includes young patients with recurrent spontaneous early pregnancy loss and provoked venous thromboembolism and asymptomatic healthy patients who are incidentally found to have a prolonged aPTT and
(c) *high* appropriateness group includes young patients (below 50 years of age) with unprovoked and unexplained venous thromboembolism and with arterial thrombosis, unusual site thrombosis (cerebral veins, dermal veins or abdominal veins), pregnancy loss in the late gestation and any thrombotic event or pregnancy morbidity with an underlying autoimmune disease [26].

5.2.2 What Test to Do?

For the laboratory diagnosis of APS, immunological assays (ELISA-based) or chemiluminescence (CLIA) or fluorescence enzyme immunoassays (FEIA) detecting aCLa and aβ2GPI antibodies and clot-based assays that detect LAC by measuring their effect on the coagulation system are recommended.

The standardisation for aCLa is influenced by a major challenge of defining its cut-off value. There is an inter-laboratory variation and disagreement between different assay kits and methods particularly when the antibody levels are in the lower range [27]. The current guidelines require only medium and high levels (greater than the 99th percentile or >40 units IgG or IgM antibody titre of aCLa), thereby improving the specificity of the test [27]. Though different studies have reported a lack of correlation between aCLa and thrombosis or pregnancy morbidity, testing for aCLa is still included in the diagnostic criterion as it carries a high sensitivity despite low specificity [27]. Nonspecific positivity has been reported in syphilis, Lyme disease, EBV, CMV, HIV and HCV infections.

The variation between different laboratories is relatively less for aβ2GPI than the aCLa assay. However, testing for aβ2GPI antibodies also needs standardisation of the assay components including ELISA plates, calibrators and concentration of b2GPI. The aβ2GPI antibody assay has higher specificity than aCLa for diagnosing

APS as these aPLas have a higher predilection for vascular thrombosis and pregnancy morbidity including pre-eclampsia and eclampsia. Therefore, they are of value when the aCLa and LA are negative and the clinical index of suspicion for APS is high.

For both aCLa and aβ2GPI, IgM positivity could be false positive in the lower range, particularly in the presence of rheumatoid factor (RF) and cryoglobulins.

5.2.2.1 Lupus Anticoagulant (LAC)

Lupus anticoagulant assays show a strong correlation with thrombosis, pregnancy morbidity or foetal loss and thrombosis in SLE patients when compared to aCLa. Detection of LAC is based on its in vitro functional inhibition of phospholipid-dependent steps in the coagulation cascade. Several types of phospholipids are available. The current recommendation is to perform two LAC assays as no single assay is 100% sensitive for LAC detection. The diluted Russel viper venom time (dRVVT) and aPTT-based test using silica as an activator with low concentration of phospholipids are used for screening. In a patient with LAC, the screen clotting time will be prolonged [27]. The mixing step can then be performed to exclude a factor deficiency which may also result in prolonged bleeding times. This is achieved by a 1:1 mixing of test plasma with normal pooled plasma (NPP), which will correct the prolonged clotting time due to factor deficiency. Finally, in the confirmation step, the phospholipid dependency of the LAC is confirmed by repeating the test with a reagent with a high concentration of phospholipids (preferably bilayer or hexagonal phase type). There is a poor inter-laboratory agreement and lack of standardisation for the several LAC assays available. The Sydney criteria recommends integration of the screening and confirmation steps into one assay so that it becomes less time consuming, has higher diagnostic accuracy and inter-laboratory agreement [27]. Thrombin time should also be performed before LAC assay to exclude the interference by heparin, which patients with APS are likely to be receiving at some point of management.

Performing the coagulation-based LAC assays is discouraged during the acute phase of thrombosis and also when the patient is on oral anticoagulant therapy, until the international normalised ratio (INR) falls below 1.5 [27]. Oral anticoagulant may be discontinued, bridged with low-molecular-weight heparin (LMWH), and the blood sample may be collected after 12 h of the last dose of heparin.

5.2.3 Sample Considerations

Doubly centrifuged, platelet poor (with a platelet count of <10,000/μl) citrated plasma (0.109 M sodium citrate) is the recommended sample for testing for LAC [27]. Plasma or serum may be used for aCLa or aβ2GPI antibodies. The sample may be stored at −20 °C for up to 4 weeks and at −80 °C for 6 months or more [28]. Icteric, lipemic or haemolysed samples should be avoided as bilirubin, triglycerides and haemoglobin may interfere with results of automated coagulation analysers. Cryoglobulins, rheumatoid factor, monoclonal immunoglobulins and heterophile antibodies may yield false-positive results [28].

5.2.4 Testing While on Anticoagulant Therapy

According to ISTH recommendations, LAC assay can be performed on an undiluted plasma in a patient on oral Vitamin K antagonists if the international normalised ratio (INR) is less than 1.5. However, if the INR is between 1.5 and <3.0, a 1:1 dilution of patient plasma and NPP is required to correct the interference by Vitamin K-induced factor deficiency which may prolong the screen and confirm times [28]. For the patients who are on unfractionated heparin (UFH), results should be interpreted with caution or else testing should not be done [28].

5.2.5 Effect of Directly Acting Oral Anticoagulants (DOACs) on aPLa Testing

DOACs like Dabigatran, Apixaban, Edoxaban and Rivaroxaban are currently being used in the treatment and prevention of venous thromboembolism. These drugs interfere with coagulation assays for thrombophilia including dRVVT-based LAC assay giving rise to false-positive result, particularly in the presence of C_{MAX} (peak plasma levels and anticoagulant effect of drug). Therefore, it is recommended to perform LAC assay preferably at C_{TROUGH}, i.e. 12–24 h after the last dose for twice or once daily administration, respectively [29]. ELISA-based aPLa assays are not affected by DOACs [29].

5.2.6 The Testing Algorithm

We currently perform aPLa testing on nearly 4000 patients referred annually. The algorithm in use at our centre is shown in Fig. 5.1.

5.2.7 Issues Associated with Laboratory Testing for aPLas

Improper sample collection and timing of sample may compromise the results of the LAC test. It is difficult to repeat the test at the recommended time since many patients are still on anticoagulant therapy at the end of 3 months. Studies have shown that triple positivity for all three aPLas—LAC, aCLa and aβ2GPI—at initial diagnosis has the highest likelihood of testing positive in repeat testing and may do away with the need for repeat testing in the future. In a study of 1222 patients with documented thrombosis screened for aPLas, 47 patients (3.85%) had thrombotic APS. Triple positivity was associated with the highest positive predictive value of APS (88.9%) [30].

Laboratory participation in external quality assurance exercises is recommended. Reference ranges for the antibodies in the paediatric population are not available, and most laboratories are forced to use the cut-off values defined in adults.

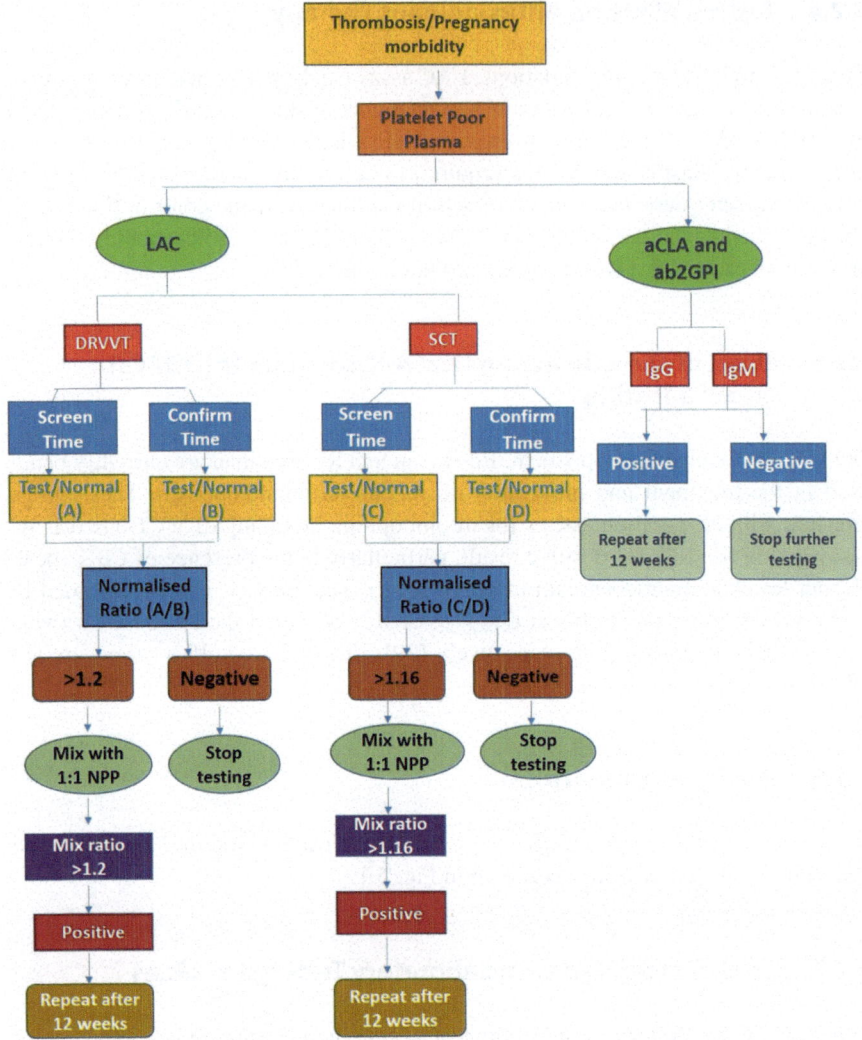

Fig. 5.1 An algorithmic approach for lab testing for APS

5.3 Treatment and Prophylaxis

Treatment of thrombotic APS in an acute episode of first venous thrombosis mandates parenteral anticoagulation with heparin (UFH or LMWH) followed by oral anticoagulation with vitamin K antagonist (VKA) with a target INR of 2–3. In a secondary venous event or arterial thrombosis, the target INR should be in the range of 2.5–3.5. After an acute event, long-term prophylaxis with oral anticoagulant is recommended. In an obstetric APS, the treatment is based on aspirin combined with heparin that is continued up to 6 weeks of delivery. Triple therapy is offered to patients with catastrophic APS (CAPS) that required anticoagulation, plasmapheresis or intravenous immunoglobulin and corticosteroids. In patients with SLE, addition of hydroxychloroquine (HCQ) to anticoagulant therapy is considered as it reduces the aPLa titres.

5.4 Conclusions

Antiphospholipid antibodies are frequently associated with autoimmune disorders. When accompanied by thrombotic events or pregnancy losses, they constitute the APS. Though a large number of antibodies have been implicated in APS, currently testing of LAC, aCLa and aβ2GP1 antibodies is recommended. Repeat testing excludes transient positivity usually associated with infections. Triple positivity of the antibodies is associated with highest positivity for APS. The clinical spectrum of APS may need to be expanded to include other manifestations. Better standardisation and harmonisation of laboratory testing and updated tests to cater for new therapeutic modalities are the need of the hour.

References

1. Sebastiani GD, Galeazzi M, Tincani A et al (1999) Anticardiolipin and anti-beta2GPI antibodies in a large series of European patients with systemic lupus erythematosus. Prevalence and clinical associations. European Concerted Action on the Immunogenetics of SLE. Scand J Rheumatol 28:344–351
2. Soltesz P, Veres K, Lakos G, Kiss E, Muszbek L, Szegedi G (2003) Evaluation of clinical and laboratory features of antiphospholipid syndrome: a retrospective study of 637 patients. Lupus 12:302–307
3. Love PE, Santoro SA (1990) Antiphospholipid antibodies: anticardiolipin and the lupus anticoagulant in systemic lupus erythematosus (SLE) and in non SLE disorders. Ann Int Med 112:682–698
4. Wahl DG, Guillemin F, de Maistre E, Perret C, Lecompte T, Thibaut G (1997) Risk for venous thrombosis related to antiphospholipid antibodies in systemic lupus erythematosus—a meta-analysis. Lupus 6:467–473
5. Franco JS, Molano-González N, Rodríguez-Jiménez M et al (2014) The coexistence of antiphospholipid syndrome and systemic lupus erythematosus in Colombians. PLoS One 9:e110242
6. Nabriski D, Ellis M, Ness-Abramof R, Shapiro M, Shenkman L (2000) Autoimmune thyroid disease and antiphospholipid antibodies. Am J Hematol 64:73–75
7. Rees JD, Lanca S, Marques PV et al (2006) Prevalence of antiphospholipid syndrome in primary systemic vasculitis. Ann Rheum Dis 65:109–111
8. Fauchais AL, Lambert M, Launay D et al (2004) Antiphospholipid antibodies in primary Sjögren's syndrome and clinical significance in a series of 74 patients. Lupus 13:245–248
9. Hull RG, Harris EN, Gharavi AE et al (1984) Anticardiolipin antibodies: occurrence in Behcet's syndrome. Ann Rheum Dis 43:746–748
10. Mader R, Ziv M, Adawi M, Mader R, Lavi I (1999) Thrombophilic factors and their relation to thromboembolic and other clinical manifestations in Behçet's disease. J Rheumatol 11:2404–2408

11. Tokay S, Direskeneli H, Yurdakul S, Akoglu T (2001) Anticardiolipin antibodies in Behcet's disease: a reassessment. Rheumatology (Oxford) 40:192–195
12. Chakravarty K, Pountain G, Merry P, Byron M, Hazleman B, Scott DG (1995) A longitudinal study of anticardiolipin antibody in polymyalgia rheumatica and giant cell arteritis. J Rheumatol 22:1694–1697
13. Merkel PA, Chang Y, Pierangeli SS, Convery K, Harris EN, Polisson RP (1996) The prevalence and clinical associations of anticardiolipin antibodies in a large inception cohort of patients with connective tissue diseases. Am J Med 101:576–583
14. Di Prima FA, Valenti O, Hyseni E, Giorgio E, Faraci M, Renda E et al (2011) Antiphospholipid syndrome during pregnancy: the state of the art. J Prenat Med 5:41–53
15. Jaslow CR, Carney JL, Kutteh WH (2010) Diagnostic factors identified in 1020 women with two versus three or more recurrent pregnancy losses. Fertil Steril 93(4):1234–1243
16. Kutten WH, Rote NS, Silver R (1999) Antiphospholipid antibodies and reproduction. Am J Reprod Immunol 4:13–152
17. Oron G, Ben-Haroush A, Goldfarb R, Molad Y, Hod M, Bar J (2011) Contribution of the addition of anti-β2-glycoprotein to the classification of antiphospholipid syndrome in predicting adverse pregnancy outcome. J Matern Fetal Neonatal Med 24:606–609
18. Brey RL, Stallworth CL, McGlasson DL, Wozniak MA, Wityk RJ, Stern BJ et al (2002) Antiphospholipid antibodies and stroke in young women. Stroke 33:2396–2400
19. Ulcova-Gallova Z (2014) The role of antiphospholipid antibodies (aPls) in infertile women: the long-lasting experience. Reprod Med Biol 14:49–55
20. Forastiero R (2012) Bleeding in the antiphospholipid syndrome. Hematology 17(Suppl 1):S153–S155
21. Lockshin MD, Kim M, Laskin CA et al (2012) Prediction of adverse pregnancy outcome by the presence of lupus anticoagulant, but not anticardiolipin antibody, in patients with antiphospholipid antibodies. Arthritis Rheum 64:2311–2318
22. Agar C, van Os GM, Morgelin M et al (2010) Beta2-glycoprotein I can exist in 2 conformations: implications for our understanding of the antiphospholipid syndrome. Blood 116:1336–1343
23. Arachchillage DRJ, Laffan M (2017) Pathogenesis and management of antiphospholipid syndrome. Br J Haematol 178:181–195
24. Rand JH, Wu XX, Andree HA et al (1997) Pregnancy loss in the antiphospholipid-antibody syndrome—a possible thrombogenic mechanism. N Engl J Med 337:154–160
25. Miyakis S, Lockshin MD, Atsumi T et al (2006) International consensus statement on an update of the classification criteria for definite antiphospholipid syndrome (APS). J Thromb Haemost 4:295–306
26. Rand JH, Wolgast LR (2012) Dos and don'ts in diagnosing antiphospholipid syndrome. Hematology Am Soc Hematol Educ Program 2012:455–459
27. Devreese K, Hoylaerts M (2010) Challenges in the diagnosis of the antiphospholipid syndrome. Clin Chem 56:930–940
28. An GD, Lim HH, Han JY (2017) Laboratory diagnosis of antiphospholipid syndrome. Clin Exp Thromb Hemost 3:2–7
29. Douxfils J, Ageno W, Samama CM, Lessire S, Ten Cate H, Verhamme PJ et al (2018) Laboratory testing in patients treated with direct oral anticoagulants: a practical guide for clinicians. Thromb Haemost 16:209–219
30. Ahluwalia J, Sreedharanunni S, Kumar N, Masih J, Bose SK, Varma N et al (2016) Thrombotic primary antiphospholipid syndrome: the profile of antibody positivity in patients from North India. Int J Rheum Dis 19:903–912

Fertility and Pregnancy in Autoimmune Diseases

6

Susheel Kumar

Abstract

Autoimmune diseases usually affect females in their reproductive years of age. Fertility, fecundity and the foetal outcome are affected by these disorders. Conversely, the course of these diseases might be affected by the pregnant state. Clinicians dealing with these patients should be well versed with the interaction between autoimmune disease and pregnancy. Previously pregnancy in these women used to be discouraged as there was fear of worsening of autoimmune disorder besides the possibility of a poor obstetric outcome. The approach and outlook to pregnancy in these patients have changed considerably now. Preconception counselling, maintaining disease in stable remission state, withdrawal of potentially teratogenic medications, availability and substitution with safe drugs to maintain remission besides close anti-natal follow-up of these patients have tremendously improved the maternal and foetal outcome. We here review some of the important autoimmune disorder with special emphasis on fertility and pregnancy in them.

Keywords

Autoimmune disorder · Fertility · Pregnancy · Outcome

A major chunk of patients with autoimmune diseases is composed of women in their reproductive years of age. There is sufficient epidemiological, clinical and immunological proof emphasizing the important role of female sex hormones in etiopathogenesis of many autoimmune disorders. These diseases affect the fertility, fecundity, pregnancy course and perinatal outcome. Conversely, pregnancy might affect the disease course in these patients.

S. Kumar (✉)
Nehru Hospital, Postgraduate Institute of Medical Education and Research, Chandigarh, India

6.1 Fertility and Pregnancy in Rheumatoid Arthritis

Rheumatoid arthritis (RA) is a chronic autoimmune systemic disorder with predominant joint involvement. The prevalence of this chronic inflammatory disorder varies from 0.5% to 1%. It affects fertility and pregnancy outcome [1]. Fertility is basically the ability to procreate within a year of regular sexual intercourse. Many studies have documented reduced fertility in females harbouring these disorders. Reduced fertility may be secondary to the primary autoimmune disease process itself. Pain, reduced libido, malnutrition, depression, medical therapies, informed decisions by patients on family size and genital disorders may contribute to lower fertility. Production of various antibodies targeted against corpus luteum, endometrium and dysfunction of hypothalamic–pituitary–adrenal axis also contributes to reduced fertility. In an observational population-based study from Norway, a comparison was undertaken of fertility rates in patients with chronic inflammatory arthritides including RA with age-matched women selected from the national population registry. Among 338 RA patients, higher percentages of women were found nulliparous as compared to women from matched reference population (28.4% vs 24.5%). These patients of chronic inflammatory arthritides also had a smaller family size [2]. Studies both prospective and retrospective observational across various regions have uniformly noted an improvement in disease activity during pregnancy in RA patients. The earliest documentation of substantial improvement in disease activity was made by Hench [3]. Studies reported from 1950 to 2000 had shown spontaneous improvement of disease activity which ranged from 54% to as high as 95%. But later reported studies especially prospective observational studies have shown improvement rate to be lower [1]. In a nationwide prospective study from the Netherlands over a period of 4 years, 84 patients and their pregnancies were prospectively assessed using validated tools of objective disease activity assessment. There was an improvement in 48% of patients having DAS28 >3.2 in the first trimester of pregnancy. There was an increase in the percentage of patients attaining disease remission from 17% in the first trimester to 27% in the third trimester. From preconception to the third-trimester visit, mean DAS28 dropped 0.4 points [4]. In another large prospective nationwide study from Britain, 140 pregnant females with RA were assessed. The health assessment questionnaire score showed improvement during pregnancy. The improvement in joint pain and swelling was reported in almost two-thirds of patients. 23 (16%) patients were in complete remission [5]. The subgroup of patients negative both for rheumatoid factor and anti-citrullinated peptide antibodies show improvement in disease activity. The effect of rheumatoid arthritis on obstetric outcome has been reported in various retrospective and prospective studies. Many studies in past though smaller in size have not shown greater risk of spontaneous abortions. In a large study reported from Norway, a total of 1578 women with RA were analysed in terms of numbers of early and late miscarriages. Compared to the reference population, higher risk of miscarriage both early and late was noted in RA patients [6]. Studies have uniformly shown an increased rate of preterm delivery in women with RA. In a retrospective observational study, the largest US inpatient care database, Nationwide Inpatient Sample of Healthcare

Cost and Utilization Project database, with 31,439 RA women with pregnancy was analysed. It showed a substantially higher rate of hypertensive disorders, preterm delivery, intrauterine growth restriction and caesarean section delivery after adjusting for potential confounders in pregnant women with RA as compared to the reference population [7]. In another large retrospective cohort study from the USA analysed 6068 pregnant patients with rheumatoid arthritis. A higher percentage of patients with RA developed pre-eclampsia/eclampsia, had preterm delivery and small for gestational age (SGA) babies [8]. In a prospective cohort study, over a period of 9 years, 440 pregnant women with RA were enrolled. This study showed a higher risk of preterm delivery and SGA babies with increasing disease activity scores. The adjusted relative risk of preterm delivery increased by 58% with each unit increase in health assessment questionnaire disability index [9]. A prevalence study from 1994 to 2006 studied combined Swedish and Danish population of 1199 women with RA. It showed a higher prevalence of preterm delivery and SGA babies [10]. There was lower birth weight in the offsprings documented in the subgroup of RA patients with disease activity in a study reported by de Man et al. [4]

6.2 Fertility and Pregnancy in Systemic Lupus Erythematosus

SLE is an autoimmune disorder which might involve multiple organ systems with chronic disease course punctuated by relapses and remissions. Female in reproductive age groups are primarily involved by this inflammatory disorder, underlining the importance of knowing the course of pregnancy and maternal/foetal outcome in these patients [11, 12]. In a multicentre study enrolling patients from SLICC inception cohort, a total of 339 patients with SLE were recruited. A large number of patients (42%) never reported being pregnant [13]. There are various reasons postulated for suboptimal fertility in these patients. Some of them are as follows: production of anticorpus luteum antibodies, autoimmune oophoritis leading to diminished ovarian reserve, prolonged inflammatory state producing dysfunction of the hypothalamic–pituitary–ovarian axis, gonadotoxic chemotherapy agents such as cyclophosphamide, lupus nephritis causing renal failure, antiphospholipid syndrome and psychosocial issues. As compared to RA, the effect of pregnancy on SLE disease course is conflicting. There are studies reporting both increased rates of flare and no increase in disease activity during pregnancy. Overall scrutiny of studies though reveals a higher rate of disease flare, but most of these are of mild to moderate severity. Disease flares are more common in patients with lupus nephritis. Past history of a lupus flare, discontinuation of hydroxyl-chloroquine and serological activity at the time of conception are important predictors of lupus flare during pregnancy [11, 12]. Disease activity assessment sometimes becomes tricky during pregnancy as some of the physiological changes occurring during pregnancy and few of pregnancy-related complications closely mimic symptoms and signs elicited by lupus flare. One important issue pertains to differentiating active lupus nephritis from pre-eclampsia. A nationwide study reported by Clowse et al. compared maternal and pregnancy outcomes among pregnant patients with SLE and a reference population. The study showed higher rates of pre-eclampsia, preterm labour and caesarean sections in lupus patients [14]. In a systematic review and meta-analysis, 37 studies with 1842 SLE patients and 2751 pregnancies were analysed. Various forms of maternal complications noted were lupus flare (25.6%), hypertension (16.3%), pre-eclampsia (7.6%) and eclampsia (0.8%). Two important factors contributing to maternal complications were active nephritis and the presence of antiphospholipid antibodies [15]. There has been a progressive drop in the rate of adverse foetal outcome in these patients over the years. A study from the USA reported a substantial decrease in SLE pregnancy loss from a mean of 43% in 1960–1965 to 17% in 2000–2003 [16]. This report of improvement in foetal outcome is the result of good planning of pregnancy, better control of lupus activity preconceptionally, close monitoring of patients and availability of better medications for control of lupus flare during pregnancy. Despite remarkable improvement in foetal outcome, still, pregnancy in SLE carries a higher risk of complications than the normal population. A systematic review and meta-analysis of 1842 pregnant patients of SLE reported wide spectrum of foetal complications including spontaneous abortion (16.0%), stillbirth (3.6%), neonatal deaths (2.5%) and intrauterine growth retardations (12.7%) [15]. A meta-analysis undertaken of 11 studies published between 2001 and 2016 analysed 3395 pregnant women with SLE. It showed significantly higher rate of spontaneous abortion, premature delivery and small for gestational age babies. Besides, higher number of infants delivered by SLE patients required neonatal intensive care unit care and had congenital defects [17]. One of the most important predictors of pregnancy outcome in these patients is the severity of disease activity. Greater disease activity months prior to conception and during pregnancy significantly worsens foetal outcome. Active lupus nephritis, elevated dsDNA and low complement predict bad outcome. Another important parameter associated uniformly with poor pregnancy outcome is the presence of antiphospholipid antibodies. The positivity rate for antiphospholipid antibodies in SLE patients has ranged from 34% to 44% in some of the bigger studies. Recently some of the novel predictors of poor pregnancy outcomes reported are serum ferritin, uric acid, oestradiol and uterine artery Doppler findings. Larger studies are required before these could be incorporated in the routine investigative armamentarium. Entity termed neonatal lupus syndrome results from transplacental transfer of Anti-Ro/La antibodies. It manifests in the form of spontaneously resolving skin rash or more dramatically in the form of congenital heart block (CHB). Other manifestations noted are thrombocytopenia and liver function test abnormalities. The risk of developing CHB is 2% but rises substantially to 15–20% in patients with a past history of a similarly affected pregnancy. Close monitoring is advised with foetal cardiac ultrasound from 16–20 week of gestation. Studies have shown a significant reduction in the occurrence of neonatal lupus in offspring of anti-Ro/La positive SLE patients who continued to take hydroxychloroquine throughout their pregnancy [11, 12].

6.3 Fertility and Pregnancy in Systemic Sclerosis

Systemic sclerosis (SSc) is an autoimmune disorder involving skin, lungs, gastrointestinal, pulmonary cardiovascular and renal system. Females are involved more frequently and almost half of these patients have disease onset before age 40. Fertility rates are noted to be lower in these patients in some studies while other studies have reported otherwise [18]. In a retrospective single centre observational study, 214 scleroderma patients were analysed to determine fertility and pregnancy outcome. The study showed that 79% of the SSc patients had been pregnant at least once compared with 88% of the healthy controls. The rate of infertility in patients with SSc was 15% [19]. In the 1970s and 1980s pregnancy used to be discouraged in these patients. Studies off late have shown that these patients can have successful pregnancies though maternal and foetal morbidity/mortality remains high. In a study of 214 women with SSc by Steen et al., adverse pregnancy outcome including the rate of premature births and small full-term infants was found to be significantly higher in patients with SSc, particularly after the onset of their rheumatic disease [19]. In a US study of nationwide inpatient sample from 2002 to 2004, out of 11.2 million deliveries, 504 deliveries in SSc patients were analysed. Higher rates of hypertensive disease, pre-eclampsia, IUGR and longer duration of hospital stay were noted in pregnant SSc patients [20]. The effect of pregnancy on disease course is variable. Disease course remains stable in 60% of the patients, improves in around 20% and worsens in 20% of patients [21]. Disease progression has been reported primarily in patients with Scl 70-positivity. Some of the symptoms like Reynaud's phenomenon show spontaneous improvement. This positive impact is related to vasodilatation and increased cardiac output during pregnancy. Clinical parameters which might worsen are gastro-oesophageal reflux, skin thickening and arthritis. These patients also develop rising pressures in the pulmonary circulation because of the increase in blood volume and hyperdynamic circulation leading to worsening of pulmonary arterial hypertension (PAH). It is recommended that patients with PAH should not become pregnant as it leads to severe hemodynamic complications and even maternal death. There is though no evidence of increased risk of renal crisis during pregnancy, but closer and frequent scrutiny of renal function is recommended. Scleroderma renal crisis can be confused with pre-eclampsia and haemolysis, elevated liver enzymes and a low platelet count (HELLP) syndrome. Progressive increase in serum creatinine level without significant proteinuria initially supports the possibility of scleroderma renal crisis. In contrast, jaundice/transaminitis and proteinuria with oedema favour the diagnostic possibility of pre-eclampsia and HELLP syndrome. This renal complication is primarily seen in patients with early diffuse disease. Antihypertensive medications, angiotensin-converting enzyme (ACE) inhibitors, are essential to manage renal crisis in this situation.

6.4 Fertility and Pregnancy in Primary Sjogren's Syndrome

Primary Sjogren's syndrome (pSS) is a chronic autoimmune disorder primarily manifesting as dryness of eyes and mouth. It may also involve other organs besides mucosal surfaces. It is one of the most common autoimmune disorders, prevalence varying from 0.1% to 4.8%. It primarily affects female (female:male ratio of 9:1). Majority of patients present with symptoms in the fourth or fifth decade of life. Because of the advanced age of disease onset, lesser data is available regarding fertility and pregnancy in these patients. Studies though small have shown similar fertility rate in these patients as noted in the general population. A systematic review and meta-analysis were undertaken to assess the rate of complications during pregnancy in pSS patients and compare them with healthy controls. From the date of inception of MEDLINE and EMBASE till March 2016, the search yielded seven studies involving 544 patients and 1586 pregnancies. Rate of premature delivery, spontaneous abortion, artificial abortion and stillbirth were not significantly higher in pSS patients as compared to reference population in this study [22]. In a case-control study reported by Ballester et al., 19 women with pSS (54 pregnancies) matched by age and BMI to 216 controls were analysed to find out the impact of pSS in pregnant women on foetal and pregnancy outcomes. Significantly higher rates of preterm delivery, spontaneous abortions and lower birthweight were found in pSS patients [23].

6.5 Fertility and Pregnancy in Vasculitis

The primary systemic vasculitides (SV) are a group of autoimmune inflammatory diseases manifesting as vessel wall inflammation. The vessel involvement leads to stenosis, aneurysm, infarction and/or haemorrhage. This disease can affect the reproductive organs directly leading to decreased fertility. One of the pillars of induction treatment in these patients, cyclophosphamide is also a very potent gonadotoxic drug. The course of pregnancy is not adversely affected in these patients, if the disease is well controlled before pregnancy [24]. A retrospective observational study evaluated maternal/neonatal outcome in 65 pregnancies in 50 women with SV. Rate of preterm, particularly early preterm (before 34 weeks) deliveries, was significantly higher in SV patients. SV patients also delivered more infants which were small for gestational age and had very low birth weight [25]. In another retrospective study, 51 pregnancies in 29 SV patients were analysed. It found lower median gestational age and median birth weight in SV patients as compared to healthy pregnant controls [26]. Takayasu arteritis (TAK) is one of the important primary systemic vasculitides in context of pregnant female patients as young women in the reproductive age group are mainly affected. A study analysed 240 pregnancies in 96 patients with TAK (142 pregnancies in 52 patients preceding the diagnosis of TAK and 98 pregnancies in 52 patients, pregnancies either concomitant with or after diagnosis of TAK). Later cohort of patients had a 13-fold higher rate of maternal/foetal adverse outcomes in the form of pre-eclampsia/

eclampsia, premature delivery and intrauterine foetal growth restriction or death [27]. Literature does suggest that the course of systemic vasculitis is not adversely impacted by pregnancy. Some of the pregnancy-related complications might mimic vasculitic disease flare. As the management of these two conditions is markedly different, careful attention to clinical details and thoughtful laboratory investigations are warranted to differentiate these two conditions. Managing disease flare during pregnancy is also tricky as many immunosuppressive agents are contraindicated. Corticosteroids are the mainstay of treatment. Another agent rituximab can be used during the second and third trimester if a careful assessment shows that benefits outweigh risks.

6.6 Fertility and Pregnancy in Mixed Connective Tissue Disease

Mixed connective tissue disease (MCTD) is a multisystem autoimmune disease presenting with a combination of some of the clinical manifestations of systemic sclerosis, poly/dermatomyositis and systemic lupus erythematosus. These patients also have high titres of antibodies targeting the U1 small nuclear ribonucleoprotein particle (U1 snRNP). Studies indicate that fertility rate is not diminished in these patients but the same is not the case regarding the foetal and maternal outcome. Tardif and Mahone evaluated 12 pregnancies in MCTD patients managed in their centre from 1986 to 2015 and also analysed data of previously published 68 pregnancies collected from a systematic literature review for medical and obstetric complications. The foetal outcome assessed in the form of prematurity, IUGR and perinatal mortality was higher in MCTD patients as compared to the healthy general population. Higher rates of these complications were seen in patients with active disease. Neonatal lupus was seen in as high as 28.6% of live births [28].

6.7 Fertility and Pregnancy in Myositis

There are no large studies regarding fertility in myositis patient, but it seems to be decreased as compared to the general population. In a study by Váncsa et al., 144 female patients of idiopathic inflammatory myopathy (IIM) with 186 pregnancies were analysed. Only nine of them became pregnant after disease onset with 14 gravidities. Out of 14 pregnancies, six ended in abortions and two ended in prematurity. The foetal outcome was much worse in the case of active disease during pregnancy [29]. The Nationwide Inpatient Sample over 1993–2007 was used, and data of 853 deliveries occurring in women with dermatomyositis/polymyositis (DM/PM) was analysed. DM/PM patients had an increased risk of hypertensive disorders and longer duration of hospital stay. As compared to reference general population, there were though no increased rates of PROM, IUGR or caesarean section noted in PM/DM patients [30]. In a retrospective observational study by Gupta et al., 81 IIM patients were analysed. Two hundred and five pregnancies in 63 patients were conceived before disease onset. Seven women had 24 pregnancies after disease onset. More frequent obstetric and foetal complications were noted in pregnancies after the onset of myositis [31].

6.8 Preconceptional Counselling and Management of High-Risk Pregnancies

An informed decision needs to be taken regarding the decision to get pregnant. As obvious in the studies quoted above, maternal and foetal complications can be brought down to a minimum if pregnancy is planned properly. Preconception counselling is thus must in patients with such autoimmune disorders. As maternal and foetal outcome are universally worse in cases of active disease during pregnancy, every effort must be made to bring the disease under control before deciding regarding pregnancy. The ideal time to conceive is during the stage of remission or minimal disease activity and the patient should be on stable medication. A multidisciplinary team consisting of qualified rheumatologist and obstetrician should manage such cases. Patients with chronic heart failure, advanced restrictive pulmonary disease, moderate to severe symptomatic pulmonary hypertension, chronic renal failure, recent disease flare and arterial thrombosis should be strongly discouraged and advised not to conceive. In every autoimmune disorder, there are some disease-related parameters and laboratory findings which put them at higher risk for maternal as well as foetal complications. Some of the important predictors of higher complication rates are any past history of complicated pregnancies, chronic visceral organ damage, anti-SSA/SSB positivity and persisting antiphospholipid antibody, especially lupus anticoagulant positivity. Medications safe during pregnancy is low-dose glucocorticoids, hydroxychloroquine and azathioprine. In case of organ and life-threatening flares in lupus, myositis and systemic vasculitides patients, high-dose pulse steroids can be used.

Autoimmune disorders are an important group of diseases involving multiple organ systems. As many of them affect female in the reproductive age group, it becomes pertinent to know their effect on fertility and obstetric outcomes. It is also of great importance to know the effect of pregnancy on the course of these diseases. Majority of rheumatoid arthritis patients experience improvement of joint symptoms post conception. The obstetric outcome is relatively poorer especially in cases with active disease. Systemic lupus erythematosus patients behave more heterogeneously during pregnancy as in some the disease remains quiescent but in the small majority can have a flare of disease activity. But in the majority, these flares are of mild to moderate severity. Patients with lupus nephritis and antiphospholipid antibody positivity need proactive management and careful monitoring as the foetal outcome has been found to be poorer in these subsets of patients. SSc patients with advanced ILD/PAH should avoid pregnancy. Neonatal lupus and congenital heart block are the important and well-documented complications in newborns of pSS requiring careful antenatal monitoring and management. Pregnancy generally does not affect the course of systemic vasculitis. The obstetric outcome is guarded especially in cases of Takayasu Arteritis though planned pregnancy results in better maternal and foetal outcome in the majority of these patients. Both in myositis and MCTD obstetric outcome are good if the disease is in remission before conception. Overall, a comprehensive preconception counselling is mandatory to minimise the adverse maternal and foetal outcome. Planning pregnancy during remission or low disease activity, the substitution of potentially teratogenic medications with safe ones, close anti-natal monitoring of mother and multidisciplinary management of these patients have tremendously improved both maternal and foetal outcome.

References

1. Ince-Askan H, Dolhain RJ (2015) Pregnancy and rheumatoid arthritis. Best Pract Res Clin Rheumatol 29:580–596
2. Wallenius M, Skomsvoll JF, Irgens LM, Salvesen KÅ, Nordvåg BY, Koldingsnes W, Mikkelsen K, Kaufmann C, Kvien TK (2011) Fertility in women with chronic inflammatory arthritides. Rheumatology 50:1162–1167
3. Hench PS (1938) The ameliorating effect of pregnancy on chronic atrophic (infectious rheumatoid) arthritis, fibrositis and intermittent hydrarthritis. Mayo Clin Proc 13:161–167
4. de Man YA, Dolhain RJ, van de Geijn FE, Willemsen SP, Hazes JM (2008) Disease activity of rheumatoid arthritis during pregnancy: results from a nationwide prospective study. Arthritis Rheum 15(59):1241–1248
5. Barrett JH, Brennan P, Fiddler M, Silman AJ (1999) Does rheumatoid arthritis remit during pregnancy and relapse postpartum? Results from a nationwide study in the United Kingdom performed prospectively from late pregnancy. Arthritis Rheum 42:1219–1227
6. Wallenius M, Salvesen KÅ, Daltveit AK, Skomsvoll JF (2015) Miscarriage and stillbirth in women with rheumatoid arthritis. J Rheumatol 42:1570–1572
7. Kishore S, Mittal V, Majithia V (2019) Obstetric outcomes in women with rheumatoid arthritis: results from Nationwide Inpatient Sample Database 2003–2011. Semin Arthritis Rheum 49:236–240. pii: S0049-0172(18)30633-4
8. Aljary H, Czuzoj-Shulman N, Spence AR, Abenhaim HA (2018) Pregnancy outcomes in women with rheumatoid arthritis: a retrospective population-based cohort study. J Matern Fetal Neonatal Med 1–7. https://doi.org/10.1080/14767058.2018.1498835
9. Bharti B, Lee SJ, Lindsay SP, Wingard DL, Jones KL, Lemus H, Chambers CD (2015) Disease severity and pregnancy outcomes in women with rheumatoid arthritis: results from the organization of teratology information specialists autoimmune diseases in pregnancy project. J Rheumatol 42:1376–1382
10. Nørgaard M, Larsson H, Pedersen L, Granath F, Askling J, Kieler H et al (2010) Rheumatoid arthritis and birth outcomes: a Danish and Swedish nationwide prevalence study. J Intern Med 268:329–337
11. Jones A, Giles I (2016) Fertility and pregnancy in systemic lupus erythematosus. Indian J Rheumatol 11:128–134
12. Lazzaroni MG, Dall'Ara F, Fredi M, Nalli C, Reggia R, Lojacono A, Ramazzotto F, Zatti S, Andreoli L, Tincani A (2016) A comprehensive review of the clinical approach to pregnancy and systemic lupus erythematosus. J Autoimmun 74:106–117
13. Vinet E, Clarke AE, Gordon C, Urowitz MB, Hanly JG, Pineau CA et al (2011) Decreased live births in women with systemic lupus erythematosus. Arthritis Care Res (Hoboken) 63:1068–1072
14. Clowse ME, Jamison M, Myers E, James AH (2008) A national study of the complications of lupus in pregnancy. Am J Obstet Gynecol 199:127.e1–127.e6

15. Smyth A, Oliveira GH, Lahr BD, Bailey KR, Norby SM, Garovic VD (2010) A systematic review and meta-analysis of pregnancy outcomes in patients with systemic lupus erythematosus and lupus nephritis. Clin J Am Soc Nephrol 5:2060–2068
16. Clark CA, Spitzer KA, Laskin CA (2005) Decrease in pregnancy loss rates in patients with systemic lupus erythematosus over a 40-year period. J Rheumatol 32:1709–1712
17. Bundhun PK, Soogund MZ, Huang F (2017) Impact of systemic lupus erythematosus on maternal and fetal outcomes following pregnancy: a meta-analysis of studies published between years 2001-2016. J Autoimmun 79:17–27
18. Rao VKR (2016) Fertility and pregnancy in systemic sclerosis and other autoimmune rheumatic diseases. Indian J Rheumatol 11:150–155
19. Steen VD, Medsger TA Jr (1999) Fertility and pregnancy outcome in women with systemic sclerosis. Arthritis Rheum 42:763–768
20. Chakravarty EF, Khanna D, Chung L (2008) Pregnancy outcomes in systemic sclerosis, primary pulmonary hypertension, and sickle cell disease. Obstet Gynecol 111:927–934
21. Kumar S, Suri V, Wanchu A (2010) Pregnancy and rheumatic disorders. Indian J Rheumatol 5:35–41
22. Upala S, Yong WC, Sanguankeo A (2016) Association between primary Sjögren's syndrome and pregnancy complications: a systematic review and meta-analysis. Clin Rheumatol 35:1949–1955
23. Ballester C, Grobost V, Roblot P, Pourrat O, Pierre F, Laurichesse-Delmas H, Gallot D, Aubard Y, Bezanahary H, Fauchais AL (2017) Pregnancy and primary Sjögren's syndrome: management and outcomes in a multicentre retrospective study of 54 pregnancies. Scand J Rheumatol 46:56–63
24. Pathak H, Mukhtyar C (2016) Pregnancy and systemic vasculitis. Indian J Rheumatol 11:145–149
25. Fredi M, Lazzaroni MG, Tani C, Ramoni V, Gerosa M, Inverardi F et al (2015) Systemic vasculitis and pregnancy: a multicenter study on the maternal and neonatal outcome of 65 prospectively followed pregnancies. Autoimmun Rev 14:686–691
26. Sangle SR, Vounotrypidis P, Briley A, Nel L, Lutalo PM, Sanchez-Fernandez S et al (2015) Pregnancy outcome in patients with systemic vasculitis: a single-Centre matched case-control study. Rheumatology (Oxford) 54:1582–1586
27. Comarmond C, Mirault T, Biard L, Nizard J, Lambert M, Wechsler B, Hachulla E, Chiche L, Koskas F, Gaudric J, Cluzel P, Messas E, Resche-Rigon M, Piette JC, Cacoub P, Saadoun D (2015) Takayasu arteritis and pregnancy. Arthritis Rheumatol 67:3262–3269
28. Tardif ML, Mahone M (2019) Mixed connective tissue disease in pregnancy: a case series and systematic literature review. Obstet Med 12(1):31–37. https://doi.org/10.1177/1753495X18793484
29. Váncsa A, Ponyi A, Constantin T, Zeher M, Dankó K (2007) Pregnancy outcome in idiopathic inflammatory myopathy. Rheumatol Int 27:435–439
30. Kolstad KD, Fiorentino D, Li S, Chakravarty EF, Chung L (2018) Pregnancy outcomes in adult patients with dermatomyositis and polymyositis. Semin Arthritis Rheum 47:865–869
31. Gupta L, Zanwar A, Ahmed S, Aggarwal A (2019) Outcomes of pregnancy in women with inflammatory myositis: a retrospective cohort from India. J Clin Rheumatol. https://doi.org/10.1097/RHU.0000000000000996

Update on Use of Biologic and Targeted Synthetic Drugs in Pregnancy

Hanh Nguyen and Ian Giles

Abstract

The availability of biologic disease modifying anti-rheumatic drugs (bDMARDs) and the development of targeted synthetic (ts)DMARDs has led to a new treatment era for patients with inflammatory rheumatic disease (IRD). The advent of these therapies has multiplied the number of therapeutic options available to induce remission and thus improved opportunities for women with previously poorly controlled disease activity to consider pregnancy during low disease activity states. These IRDs include systemic lupus erythematosus (SLE), rheumatoid arthritis (RA), psoriatic arthritis (PsA) and axial spondyloarthritis. Many of these conditions occur in women of reproductive age, and require use of traditional DMARDs and/or targeted biologic drugs to control and suppress active disease. Numerous studies have identified that women with IRD, particularly SLE, have an increased risk of experiencing adverse pregnancy outcomes (APOs), such as miscarriages, premature delivery, maternal hypertension or intrauterine growth restriction. The management of pregnancy in women with IRD is complicated by factors relating to disease, pregnancy, medication and patient concerns. Therefore, appropriate pre-pregnancy counselling and monitoring by a multidisciplinary team of obstetric and rheumatology specialists during pregnancy is essential to ensure that optimal control of maternal disease activity is achieved by appropriate use of compatible DMARDs before and during pregnancy, to enhance the chance for women with IRD to have successful pregnancy

---

H. Nguyen
Centre for Rheumatology Research, Rayne Institute, University College London (UCL), London, UK

I. Giles (✉)
Centre for Rheumatology Research, Rayne Institute, University College London (UCL), London, UK

Department of Rheumatology, University College London Hospital, London, UK
e-mail: i.giles@ucl.ac.uk

outcomes. In this chapter we aim to summarise and update current British and European evidence-based guidance on prescribing of bDMARDs and tsDMARDs during pregnancy and breastfeeding.

Keywords

Rheumatic disease · Pregnancy · Biologic · Targeted synthetic · Disease modifying anti-rheumatic drugs · Breast feeding

7.1 Introduction

The management of inflammatory rheumatic diseases (IRD), such as systemic lupus erythematosus (SLE), rheumatoid arthritis (RA), psoriatic arthritis (PsA) and axial spondyloarthritis, in women who are considering pregnancy is complicated and demands consideration of multiple factors, particularly safe use of disease modifying anti-rheumatic drugs (DMARDs). It is paramount for clinicians to ensure that adequate control of disease activity is achieved with use of traditional, biologic (b) DMARDs and/or newer targeted synthetic (ts)DMARDs. A multidisciplinary approach involving healthcare professionals (HCPs) with experience in management of obstetric and rheumatic disease in pregnancy is essential to provide close monitoring and individualised management and therapeutic plans for IRD patients during pregnancy as they are known to have an increased risk of experiencing adverse pregnancy outcomes (APOs). These APOs are associated with increased disease activity, so HCPs must discuss with patients how to maintain disease control through use of anti-rheumatic drugs that are compatible with pregnancy.

In an era where many different bDMARDs and now tsDMARDs options exist to treat various IRDs, such as SLE and RA, women with these diseases are increasingly likely to be achieving disease control and thus considering pregnancy whilst taking these drugs. There are many safety concerns however, surrounding use of certain DMARDs in pregnancy with well-defined risks identified for some DMARDs and uncertainty surrounding the use of others, particularly bDMARDs and tsDMARDs. Consequently, HCPs are required to discuss an increasing array of medication where clarity is still required for many drugs as to whether they can safely be given in pregnancy and breastfeeding.

Therefore, this chapter will summarise the current evidence-based recommendations from British Society of Rheumatology (BSR) and European League Against Rheumatism (EULAR) guidance and review more recent evidence regarding the use of bDMARDs and tsDMARDs in pregnancy and during lactation period [1, 2].

7.1.1 Adverse Pregnancy Outcomes Associated with Active Rheumatic Disease

It has been established that IRDs, particularly SLE, have an increased burden of adverse pregnancy outcomes (APO) including maternal hypertensive disorders in pregnancy (13–23%) and foetal growth restriction (5%), higher rates of pregnancy loss, premature delivery and caesarean section delivery in comparison to a healthy population [3–5].

There is also a direct link between severe/active disease immediately before and during pregnancy, and APO in RA [6] and SLE [7] cohorts. Additionally, IRD patients with certain auto-antibody profiles are associated with increased chance of experiencing APO, particularly anti-phospholipid antibodies (aPL) in anti-phospholipid syndrome and anti-SSA/Ro or anti-SSB/La antibodies in neonatal lupus [4]. Further consideration of these issues is beyond the scope of this article, and readers are referred to a recent review [8].

7.1.2 Biologic Drugs

Biologic DMARDs are complex molecules, frequently composed of varying amounts of immunoglobulin (Ig) G, such as whole IgG, antigen-binding (Fab) fragments, or the Fc portion of IgG joined to receptor blocking proteins, that all bind to target molecules to neutralise their effect (Fig. 7.1). These drugs are used in patients

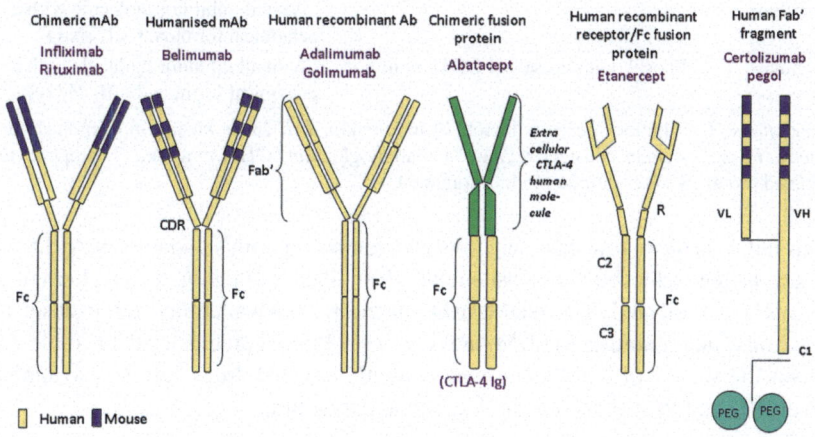

Abbreviations: Fab'-Antigen-binding fragment; mAb– monoclonal anti-body; CDR– Complementarity-determining region; Fc—heavy-chain constant region; CTLA-4 -cytotoxic T-lymphocyte-associated protein 4; PEG– Polyethylene glycol; C– Constant region; R– Region; VH—variable heavy chain domain of Ab; VL– variable light chain domain of Ab

Fig. 7.1 Structures of various biologics. *Abbreviations*: *Fab'* antigen-binding fragment, *mAb* monoclonal antibody, *CDR* complementarity-determining region, *Fc* heavy-chain constant region, *CTLA-4* cytotoxic T-lymphocyte-associated protein 4, *PEG* polyethylene glycol, *C* constant region, *R* region, *VH* variable heavy-chain domain of Ab, *VL* variable light chain. (Adapted from [9])

Table 7.1 Biologic and tsDMARDs used for treatment of rheumatic diseases classified by mode of action [1, 2, 10–15]

Drug	Mode of action	Structure
Infliximab	TNF inhibition	A chimeric (human-murine) mAb
Adalimumab Golimumab		A fully humanised recombinant mAb
Etanercept		A human recombinant receptor/Fc fusion protein
Certolizumab pegol		A PEGylated humanised Fab′ fragment
Rituximab	B-cell depletion/inhibition	A chimeric (human-murine) mAb
Belimumab		A fully humanised mAb
Abatacept	Inhibits co-stimulatory signalling pathways required for T cell activation	A chimeric CTLA 4-Ig fusion protein
Anakinra	IL-1 inhibition	A recombinant human form of IL-1 receptor
Canakinumab		A recombinant humanised mAb
Rilonacept		An anti-IL-1 fusion protein
Tocilizumab Sarilumab	IL6-inhibition	A recombinant humanised mAb that inhibits IL-6 receptor
Ixekizumab	IL17-inhibition	An anti-IL-17-A hinge-modified humanised IgG subclass-4 (IgG-4)
Secukinumab		A fully humanised mAb
Ustekinumab	IL-12/23 inhibition	A fully humanised mAb
Baricitinib	JAK inhibition	A small inhibitor molecule with a chemical formula: $C_{16}H_{17}N_7O_2S$
Tofacitinib		A small inhibitor molecule with a chemical formula: $C_{16}H_{20}N_6O$
Apremilast	Phosphodiesterase 4 (PDE4) inhibition	A small inhibitor molecule with a chemical formula: $C_{22}H_{24}N_2O_7S$

Abbreviations: *TNF* tumour necrosis factor, *IL* interleukin, *JAK* Janus kinase, *mAb* monoclonal antibody, *Fc* heavy-chain constant region, *Ig* immunoglobulin, *CTLA* cytotoxic T-lymphocyte-associated protein 4, *Fab′* antigen-binding fragment

whom fail to achieve low disease activity or remission with standard DMARDs. If efficacy is not achieved, or subsequently lost, then switching to an alternative bDMARD is indicated. The tsDMARDs have oral bioavailability, rapid onset of action and efficacy similar to bDMARDs but very limited pregnancy data. Table 7.1 displays the variety of bDMARDs and synthetic targeted drugs currently available to treat IRD and their mechanism of action and structure.

7.1.3 Transplacental Passage of bDMARD in Pregnancy

The passage of maternal IgG into foetal circulation occurs by active transplacental transfer involving the binding of maternal IgG to neonatal Fc receptor (FcRn) expressed by syncytiotrophoblast cells to form an IgG-FcRn complex that crosses

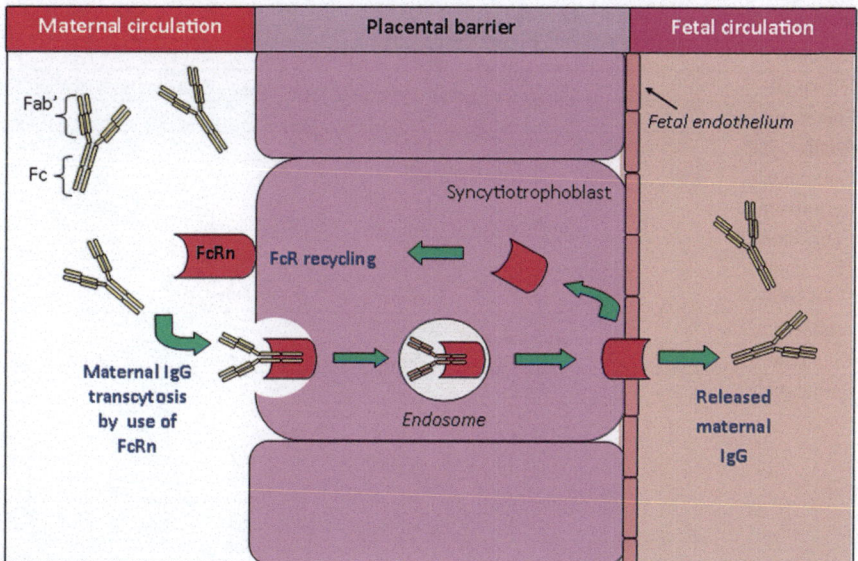

Abbreviations: Fc—heavy-chain constant region; Fab'-Antigen-binding fragment; IgG-Immunoglobulin G; FcRn— neonatal Fc receptor

Fig. 7.2 Schematic diagram illustrating the transplacental transfer of maternal IgG across the placental barrier from maternal blood circulation into foetal circulation. *Abbreviations*: *Fc* heavy-chain constant region, *Fab'* antigen-binding fragment, *IgG* immunoglobulin, *FcRn* neonatal Fc receptor. (Adapted from [9])

the placental barrier into foetal blood circulation [16]. This transplacental transfer accelerates from the 16th week of pregnancy (Fig. 7.2). Of the four IgG (1–4) subclasses, placental transfer of IgG1 and IgG4 has been shown to be more efficient from mother to foetus compared with IgG2 and IgG3 subclasses [17].

The Biologics with mAb structure listed in Table 7.1 are large recombinant protein structures (~150 kDa) that share similar characteristics to maternal IgG [18, 19], including the ability to actively cross the placental barrier. The bDMARDs that are mAbs or fusion proteins comprising the Fc portion of IgG1 (Fig. 7.1) are unlikely to be transferred at high levels across the placental barrier [20, 21] within the first trimester (up to 12 weeks of gestation) because foetal trophoblast cells do not express Fc receptors that facilitate active transportation of mAbs, until the end of the first trimester [16].

Current evidence-based guidance from BSR and EULAR covers the use of various drugs in pregnancy including bDMARDs with either limited or no information on tsDMARDs. They consider various factors that influence transplacental passage and thus levels of bDMARD in foetal circulation during pregnancy and in neonatal/cord blood at time of delivery. These factors include drug half-life, gestational age during drug administration and bDMARD structure that influence advice given to patients on when to stop the drug in relation to pregnancy so that the infant can have a normal vaccination schedule [1, 2].

Table 7.2 Half-life of biologic DMARDs [1, 2, 22–24]

Biologic	Half-life (days)
Infliximab	8–10
Etanercept	3
Adalimumab	14
Golimumab	12
Certolizumab	14
Canakinumab	22
Tocilizumab	8–14
Ustekinumab	15–32
Abatacept	8–25
Rituximab	18–22
Belimumab	19–20

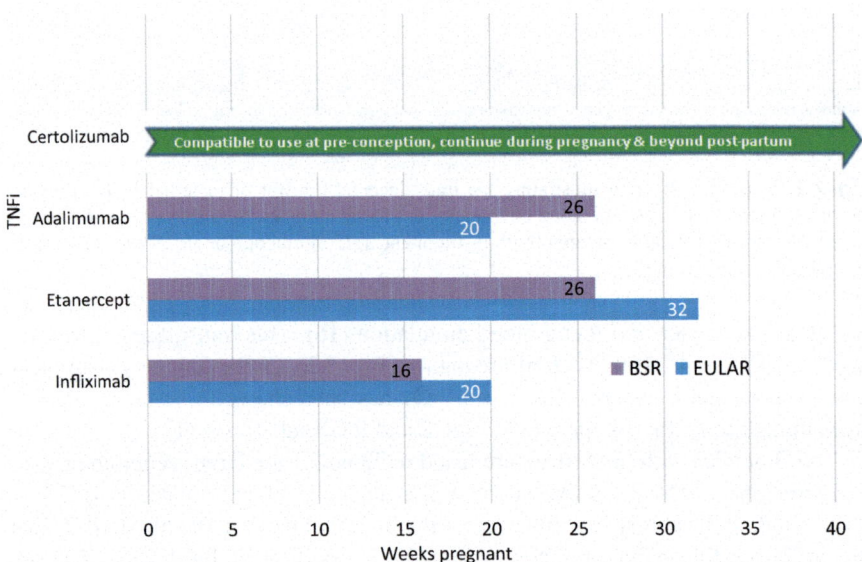

Fig. 7.3 Chart summarising EULAR and BSR 2016 guidelines recommended time points for stopping TNFi during pregnancy [1, 2]

For instance, if infliximab a bDMARD with mAb structure that has a long half-life (Table 7.2) and bioavailability is given in mid to late pregnancy, it has been shown to be present in infant circulation for up to 7 months post-partum. In contrast, bDMARDs that contain altered Fc regions (etanercept) or completely lack an Fc region (certolizumab) have been shown to have markedly reduced (etanercept) or minimal (certolizumab) placental transfer into foetal circulation [10, 25, 26].This information regarding placental transfer informs current BSR and EULAR advice on when to stop a TNFi in pregnancy (Fig. 7.3) to ensure low/no detectable levels of drug levels in infant at delivery, although the guidance from both organisations states

Table 7.3 Summary of EULAR and BSR 2016 guidelines recommendations and points to consider for use of biologic DMARDs at conception/in early pregnancy [1, 2]

Drug	EULAR	BSR
Infliximab	Yes	Yes
Etanercept	Yes	Yes
Adalimumab	Yes	Yes
Certolizumab	Yes	Yes
Golimumab	No increased risk of malformations (insufficient evidence)	No
Anakinra	Yes	No (insufficient data available to recommend drug)
Tocilizumab	Insufficient evidence	Recommend stopping drug 3 months prior conception (insufficient data to recommend drug)
Ustekinumab	No increased risk of malformations (insufficient evidence)	–
Abatacept	Insufficient evidence	No
Rituximab	Yes—can be considered to be used in exceptional situations	Recommend stopping 6 months prior to conception (insufficient data to recommend drug)
Belimumab	No increased risk of malformations (insufficient evidence)	No (insufficient data to recommend drug)

Abbreviations: *EULAR* European League Against Rheumatism, *BSR* British Society of Rheumatology

that certain drugs may be continued throughout pregnancy if required to maintain control of disease activity. Similarly, a consensus statement for the management of inflammatory bowel disease in pregnancy recommends continuation of bDMARDs that are tumour necrosis factor inhibitor (TNFi) maintenance therapy throughout pregnancy to avoid the risk of disease flare and its associated harmful effects on pregnancy outcomes [27]. All documents agree that if TNFi are given beyond mid-second trimester, then live vaccines should be avoided until the infant is 6–7 months old, although routine inactivated immunisations should be given as normal.

7.1.4 Biologics in Early Pregnancy and During Pregnancy

The current EULAR and BSR recommendations and points to be considered for bDMARDs and tsDMARDs use in early pregnancy are summarised in Table 7.3.

7.1.5 Biologics Use in Lactation Period

Certain bDMARDs are deemed to be compatible for use during breastfeeding by BSR and EULAR documents (Table 7.4), although this guidance was based on

Table 7.4 Summary of EULAR and BSR 2016 guidelines recommendations/points to consider for use biologic DMARDs during breastfeeding/lactation period [1, 2]

Drug	EULAR	BSR
Infliximab	Yes	Yes
Etanercept	Yes	Yes
Adalimumab	Yes	Yes
Certolizumab	Yes	No data available
Golimumab	Yes	No data available
Anakinra	No (no data available)	No data available
Tocilizumab	No (no data available)	No data available
Ustekinumab	No (no data available)	–
Abatacept	No (no data available)	No data available
Rituximab	No (no data available)	No data available
Belimumab	No (no data available)	No data available

limited evidence [1, 2]. Subsequent studies have confirmed minimal transfer of various biologics into breast milk of mothers with mostly rheumatic [20] and/or IBD [28]. There is a consensus that the use of biologics should not influence the decision to breastfeed, and breastfeeding should not influence the decision to use these medications, reviewed in publication [29].

7.1.6 Updates on Use of bDMARDs and tsDMARDs in Pregnancy

7.1.6.1 Tumour Necrosis Factor Inhibitors

The use of various TNFi in pregnancy is supported by BSR and EULAR documents (Table 7.4). More recent published studies have reported largely reassuring pregnancy outcomes. The majority of these studies are retrospective studies, case reports of inadvertent exposures to TNFi, pharma-covigilence databases or observational registry/database studies. The largest body of evidence relates primarily to maternal cases exposed to adalimumab, infliximab and etanercept, in the first and second trimesters of pregnancy, whilst fewer studies have addressed the effects of TNFi exposure throughout pregnancy.

A systematic review and meta-analysis that comprehensively reviews all studies on TNFi use in pregnancy including several published after the end-dates of BSR and EULAR evidence reviews has assessed the risk of TNFi used during pregnancy in female patients with RA, inflammatory bowel disease (IBD) and other various immune-mediated diseases (i.e. PsA, Behcet's disease and others). A total of 13 studies were identified, reporting on $n = 1390$ TNFi-exposed pregnancies, $n = 1173$ non-exposed to TNFi pregnancies and $n = 3051$ pregnancies from the general population. They found that although TNFi-exposed patients had a higher risk of preterm delivery, spontaneous abortion and low-birth weight in comparison to pregnancies from the general population, their outcomes were comparable to those of non-TNFi-exposed patients, thus common to underlying disease rather than TNFi exposure. Furthermore, no increased risk of congenital anomalies was identified in TNFi-exposed pregnancies [30].

7.1.6.2 Belimumab and Rituximab: B Cell Depletion Therapies

A large number of publications (registry, case series and case reports) have reported on pregnancy outcomes for belimumab and rituximab since the EULAR and BSR guidelines were published. It is beyond the scope of this article to list all studies but a total of $n = 51$ studies (belimumab $n = 6$ and rituximab $n = 45$) have reported $n = 62$ maternal exposures to belimumab and $n = 78$ maternal exposures to rituximab (at pre-conception and/or during pregnancy and/or at post-partum period).

Pregnancy outcomes reported for belimumab-exposed pregnancy cases included the following: $n = 61$ live births, $n = 26$ spontaneous abortions, $n = 3$ still births and $n = 10$ elective terminations. It was not clear if adverse pregnancy outcomes were associated with any exposure to any other concomitant drugs as these were not reported [31–36].

Pregnancy outcomes reported for rituximab included the following: $n = 73$ live births, $n = 4$ miscarriages/foetal deaths ($n = 1$ at 21 weeks—placental histology review showed severe hypotrophy with marked vascular lesions and diffuse infarcts), $n = 2$ stillbirths, $n = 3$ elective terminations and no congenital anomalies were reported. Maternal complications included one maternal death occurring due to hypertensive crisis and heamorrhagic stroke. In another case, the mother experienced complications with pericardial effusion and pleuritic chest pain during pregnancy. Additionally, few foetal complications were reported for $n = 2$ neonates, where one neonate spent 10 weeks in the neonatal intensive care unit before being discharged in healthy condition due to neonatal CD19+ cell levels being depleted at birth (associated transient lymphopenia without infectious complications). The second neonate had abnormal heart sounds [36–42].

7.1.6.3 Ustekinumab

Sixteen studies ($n = 2$ cohort studies, $n = 7$ case series and $n = 7$ case reports) have been published since the EULAR and BSR guidelines were released. A total of $n = 39$ maternal cases were exposed to drug in early-late stages of pregnancies, and patient studies had a mixture of diagnoses, i.e. RA, IBD, psoriasis and other autoimmune diseases. Overall, a total of $n = 18$ live births were reported, with no malformations and only one case of miscarriage [22, 28, 43–52].

7.1.6.4 Anakinra, Canakinumab and Rilonacept: IL1 Inhibitors

Safety data on IL1 inhibitors anakinra (a recombinant, non-glycosylated human IL1 receptor (IL1-R) antagonist) and canakinumab (an anti-human IL1β IgG1) remain very limited, but evidence is building that would support their use in pregnancy when no other pregnancy suitable drugs can effectively control maternal disease. An International Society for Systemic Auto-inflammatory diseases conducted a retrospective study of $n = 23$ mothers exposed to anakinra and $n = 8$ exposed to canakinumab, as well as 11 paternal exposures to ($n = 6$) anakinra and ($n = 5$) canakinumab [53]. Of $n = 23$ anakinra-exposed pregnancies, $n = 21$ healthy deliveries were reported, one infant was born with unilateral renal agenesis and ectopic neuro-hypophysis and one early first trimester miscarriage occurred in a mother with Cogan's syndrome. Eight pregnancies from $n = 7$ women exposed to canakinumab resulted in $n = 7$ live births and $n = 1$ miscarriage. A total of 14 infants ($n = 10$ exposed to anakinra and $n = 4$ exposed to canakinumab) were breastfed without any complications/adverse effects. There were no serious infections in any infants/mothers and on follow-up ranging from 1 week to 10 years (median $n = 18$ months), no developmental problems were observed in any children [53].

Other small case series ($n = 7$ pregnancies) in mothers with adult onset still's disease (AOSD) treated with anakinra during pregnancy have reported largely reassuring outcomes with complications linked to active disease ($n = 2$ mothers developed oligo-hydramnios, $n = 1$ mother developed pregnancy-induced hypertension). Infants were born full term (range: 36–40 weeks of gestation) and no adverse outcomes or major complications were reported. Three out of seven mothers breastfed their newborns successfully, where two mothers chose to breastfeed whilst continuing anakinra treatment [54, 55].

To date there are no controlled data on human pregnancy cases exposed to rilonacept, a dimeric fusion protein consisting of portions of IL1-R and the IL1-R accessory protein linked to the Fc portion of IgG1.

7.1.6.5 Tocilizumab and Sarilumab: IL6 Inhibitors

Several publications on use of IL6 inhibitors in pregnancy have been published since EULAR and BSR guidelines were released, including registry data reported from a manufacturer's (Roche) global safety database [56–61].

Overall this data describes maternal exposure to tocilizumab (TOC) an anti-human IL6 IgG1 molecule occurring prior to and/or during pregnancy for $n = 483$ women for the treatment of RA, JIA and various other rheumatic indications (included AOSD, systemic sclerosis, Takayasu's arthritis and PsA). A total of $n = 204$ pregnancy outcomes were reported in studies, which included $n = 127$ prospectively reported pregnancies and $n = 67$ retrospectively reported pregnancies with a sum of $n = 204$ live births, $n = 80$ miscarriages/spontaneous abortions, $n = 1$ post-neonatal death (neonatal asphyxia) and $n = 54$ elective terminations. Although the global safety database reported an increased risk of preterm birth from 399 pregnancy exposures to TOC compared to the general population [60], the likely influence of underlying disease upon this finding cannot be assessed because a non-TOC exposed disease comparator was lacking. Overall, no other increase in adverse event was identified in pregnancy, in particular no increase in congenital malformation was observed.

To date there are no publications reporting on human pregnancy exposures to Sarilumab, a fully human anti-IL6 IgG1 molecule.

7.1.6.6 Secukinumab and Ixekizumab: IL17A-Inhibitors

The Novartis global safety database has reported on $n = 292$ pregnancy outcomes from maternal or paternal exposure to secukinumab, an IgG1 molecule that selectively targets IL-17A [62]. The majority of patients were exposed in the first trimester only and 50% of pregnancy outcomes from maternal exposure were unknown. Overall, no adverse safety signals were observed and adverse pregnancy outcome rates were in line with those of the general population.

Regarding Ixekizumab, another IgG1 that blocks IL-17A, only one study has been published that reported integrated data obtained from $n = 7$ randomised controlled trials (RCTs) on $n = 4209$ psoriasis cases exposed to this drug. Although this study included $n = 3$ cases who had treatment withdrawn due to maternal exposure during pregnancy, it did not report any related feto-maternal outcomes [63].

7.1.6.7 Abatacept

There was insufficient evidence at time of evidence review for the EULAR and BSR documents to recommend use of abatacept (a soluble fusion protein, linking the extracellular domain of human cytotoxic T-lymphocyte-associated antigen 4 to the modified Fc portion of human IgG1) in pregnancy. Further publications have studied abatacept exposure in pregnancy [37, 43, 64, 65]. A total of $n = 157$ maternal exposures were reported in these studies with pregnancy outcomes including $n = 87$ live births. One large study published included autoimmune disease patients, with data on pregnancy outcomes following maternal or paternal exposure from the Bristol-Myers Squibb safety database. Data was collected from clinical trials (prospective) and post-marketing reports (prospective and retrospective data). Of the $n = 151$ maternal exposure pregnancies with known outcomes, $n = 68$ were from the clinical trials, $n = 80$ were reported as post-marketing reports and $n = 3$ were from the ongoing Organization of Teratology Information Services (OTIS) registry. Pregnancy outcome data reported there were $n = 7$ congenital anomalies (includes $n = 1$ of each: cleft lip/cleft palate, down's syndrome, congenital aortic anomaly, meningocele, pyloric stenosis, skull malformation, ventricular septal defect; congenital arterial malformation), where a total of $n = 20$ mothers were exposed to teratogenic concomitant drug methotrexate [64]. Furthermore, one case report of an active RA mother exposed to abatacept who was treated with methotrexate prior to conception had $n = 1$ live birth at 40 weeks, with no maternal or foetal complications were observed. The healthy newborn was followed up for 3.5 years, and infant was reported to have a healthy outcome [65].

7.1.6.8 Tofacitinib

Of the tsDMARDs human pregnancy data is currently only available for tofacitinib. One recent large study has extracted pregnancy outcomes data obtained from a tofacitinib safety database for patients with RA or psoriasis cases [11]. A total of $n = 9815$ patients were included and $n = 1821$ female patients of child-bearing age were enrolled in the RA/psoriasis RCTs. A total of $n = 47$ women became pregnant (RA $n = 31$ cases and psoriasis $n = 16$ cases), including $n = 33$ who received tofacitinib monotherapy, $n = 13$ who received combination therapy with methotrexate (RA patients only) and $n = 1$ patient whose therapy was still blinded. All cases were exposed to drug during the first trimester period and no foetal deaths were reported. Only $n = 1$ congenital pulmonary valve stenosis (monotherapy, $n = 1$), $n = 7$ spontaneous abortions ($n = 4$ monotherapy; $n = 3$ combination therapy) and $n = 8$ medical terminations ($n = 4$ monotherapy; $n = 3$ combination therapy; $n = 1$ blinded therapy) were identified [11]. This limited data set did not reveal any differences in tofacitinib-exposed pregnancy outcomes compared to the general population.

7.1.6.9 Summary of Emerging Evidence on bDMARDs and tsDMARDs in Pregnancy

Of bDMARDs the TNFi remain the most studied drugs that have a growing and reassuring safety profile in pregnancy and lactation. Despite additional, largely reassuring pregnancy outcomes to date for non-TNFi bDMARDs, the overall number of pregnancy exposures for each drug remains relatively small, so the general advice for these drugs remains that they should be withdrawn before conception but may be considered for use during pregnancy when no other pregnancy compatible drug can effectively control maternal disease. Information on tsDMARDs remain very limited, so these drugs are best avoided in pregnancy and breastfeeding until further evidence is available. In the case of accidental exposure to non-TNFi bDMARDs and tsDMARDS, outcomes to date are reassuring, particularly first trimester exposure to drugs with IgG1, IgG4 or Fc segments structure that will have minimal placental transfer during this period.

7.2 Conclusion

It is essential for women with an IRD whom have the desire to start a family to seek advice and be managed by a multidisciplinary team of rheumatologists and obstetric physicians as active disease is associated with adverse pregnancy outcomes. It is important that IRD activity is closely monitored by clinicians to ensure disease can be suppressed and well controlled from the pre-conception period and then throughout pregnancy to optimise the chances of a successful pregnancy outcome. The increasing use of bDMARDs and tsDMARDs to control active disease means these drugs may impact upon management of IRD during pregnancy. There is increasing evidence to support the compatibility of TNFi bDMARDs in pregnancy. A growing body of evidence on outcomes of non-TNFi bDMARDs- or tsDMARDs-exposed pregnancies are reassuring but remain limited, so routine use of these drugs should currently be avoided in pregnancy. This evidence is invaluable for healthcare professionals when counselling and managing patients with IRD during pregnancy to enable more informed conversations around compatibility of these drugs in pregnancy and thus avoid stopping certain drugs unnecessarily in pregnancy.

References

1. Flint J, Panchal S, Hurrell A, van de Venne M, Gayed M, Schreiber K et al (2016) BSR and BHPR guideline on prescribing drugs in pregnancy and breastfeeding-part I: standard and biologic disease modifying anti-rheumatic drugs and corticosteroids. In: Rheumatology (Oxford), vol 55, p 1693
2. Skorpen CG, Hoeltzenbein M, Tincani A, Fischer-Betz R, Elefant E, Chambers C et al (2016) The EULAR points to consider for use of antirheumatic drugs before pregnancy, and during pregnancy and lactation. Ann Rheum Dis 75:795–810

3. Borella E, Lojacono A, Gatto M, Andreoli L, Taglietti M, Iaccarino L et al (2014) Predictors of maternal and fetal complications in SLE patients: a prospective study. Immunol Res 60(2–3):170–176
4. Andreoli L, Chighizola CB, Banzato A, Pons-Estel GJ, De Jesus GR, Erkan D (2013) Estimated frequency of antiphospholipid antibodies in patients with pregnancy morbidity, stroke, myocardial infarction, and deep vein thrombosis: a critical review of the literature. Arthritis Care Res 65(11):1869–1873
5. Chakravarty EF, Nelson L, Krishnan E (2006) Obstetric hospitalizations in the United States for women with systemic lupus erythematosus and rheumatoid arthritis. Arthritis Rheum 54:899
6. De Man YA, Dolhain RJEM, Van De Geijn FE, Willemsen SP, Hazes JMW (2008) Disease activity of rheumatoid arthritis during pregnancy: results from a nationwide prospective study. Arthritis Care Res 59:1241–1248
7. Clowse MEB, Magder LS, Witter F, Petri M (2005) The impact of increased lupus activity on obstetric outcomes. Arthritis Rheum 52(2):514–521
8. Giles I, Yee C-S, Gordon C (2019) Stratifying management of rheumatic disease for pregnancy and breastfeeding. Nat Rev Rheumatol 15:391
9. Nguyen H, Giles I (2016) Biologic disease modifying anti-rheumatic drugs in pregnancy and breast-feeding period. In: Ciurtin C, Isenberg DA (eds) Biologics in rheumatology: new developments, clinical uses and health implication. Nova Science Publisher, New York, pp 377–403
10. Mariette X, Förger F, Abraham B, Flynn AD, Moltó A, Flipo RM et al (2018) Lack of placental transfer of certolizumab pegol during pregnancy: results from CRIB, a prospective, postmarketing, pharmacokinetic study. Ann Rheum Dis 77(2):228–233
11. Clowse MEB, Feldman SR, Isaacs JD, Kimball AB, Strand V, Warren RB et al (2016) Pregnancy outcomes in the tofacitinib safety databases for rheumatoid arthritis and psoriasis. Drug Saf 39(8):755–762
12. Ostensen M, Lockshin M, Doria A, Valesini G, Meroni P, Gordon C et al (2008) Update on safety during pregnancy of biological agents and some immunosuppressive anti-rheumatic drugs. Rheumatology 47(Suppl 3):iii28–iii31
13. Rawla P, Sunkara T, Raj JP (2018) Role of biologics and biosimilars in inflammatory bowel disease: current trends and future perspectives. J Inflamm Res 11:215–226
14. Lovell DJ, Giannini EH, Reiff AO, Kimura Y, Li S, Hashkes PJ et al (2013) Long-term safety and efficacy of rilonacept in patients with systemic juvenile idiopathic arthritis. Arthritis Rheum 65(9):2486–2496
15. Giunta A, Ventura A, Chimenti MS, Bianchi L, Esposito M (2017) Spotlight on ixekizumab for the treatment of moderate-to-severe plaque psoriasis: design, development, and use in therapy. Drug Des Devel Ther 11:1643–1651
16. Hyrich KL, Verstappen SMM (2014) Biologic therapies and pregnancy: the story so far. Rheumatology (Oxford) 53(8):1377–1385
17. Garty BZ, Ludomirsky A, Danin YL, Peter JB, Douglas SD (1994) Placental transfer of immunoglobulin G subclasses. Clin Diagn Lab Immunol 1(6):667–669
18. Palmeira P, Quinello C, Silveira-Lessa AL, Zago CA, Carneiro-Sampaio M (2012) IgG placental transfer in healthy and pathological pregnancies. Clin Dev Immunol 2012:1
19. Nesbitt A, Kevorkian L, Baker T (2014) Lack of FcRn binding in vitro and no measurable levels of ex vivo placental transfer of certolizumab pegol. Hum Reprod 29:i127
20. Clowse ME, Förger F, Hwang C, Thorp J, Dolhain RJ, Van Tubergen A et al (2017) Minimal to no transfer of certolizumab pegol into breast milk: results from CRADLE, a prospective, postmarketing, multicentre, pharmacokinetic study. Ann Rheum Dis 76(11):1890–1896
21. Porter C, Armstrong-Fisher S, Kopotsha T, Smith B, Baker T, Kevorkian L et al (2016) Certolizumab pegol does not bind the neonatal Fc receptor (FcRn): consequences for FcRn-mediated in vitro transcytosis and ex vivo human placental transfer. J Reprod Immunol 116:7–12

22. Rowan CR, Cullen G, Mulcahy HE, Keegan D, Byrne K, Murphy DJ et al (2018) Ustekinumab drug levels in maternal and cord blood in a woman with Crohn's disease treated until 33 weeks of gestation. J Crohns Colitis 12(3):376–378
23. Friedrichs B, Tiemann M, Salwender H, Verpoort K, Wenger MK, Schmitz N (2006) The effects of rituximab treatment during pregnancy on a neonate. Haematologica 91:1426–1427
24. Egawa M, Imai K, Mori M, Miyasaka N, Kubota T (2017) Placental transfer of canakinumab in a patient with muckle-wells syndrome. J Clin Immunol 37(4):339–341
25. Murashima A, Watanabe N, Ozawa N, Saito H, Yamaguchi K (2009) Etanercept during pregnancy and lactation in a patient with rheumatoid arthritis: drug levels in maternal serum, cord blood, breast milk and the infant's serum. Ann Rheum Dis 68(11):1791–1793
26. Berthelsen BG, Fjeldsøe-Nielsen H, Nielsen CT, Hellmuth E (2010) Etanercept concentrations in maternal serum, umbilical cord serum, breast milk and child serum during breastfeeding. Rheumatology 49(11):2225–2227
27. Nguyen GC, Seow CH, Maxwell C, Huang V, Leung Y, Jones J et al (2016) The Toronto Consensus Statements for the management of inflammatory bowel disease in pregnancy. Gastroenterology 150(3):734–757.e1
28. Matro R, Martin CF, Wolf D, Shah SA, Mahadevan U (2018) Exposure concentrations of infants breastfed by women receiving biologic therapies for inflammatory bowel diseases and effects of breastfeeding on infections and development. Gastroenterology 155(3):696–704
29. Pham-Huy A, Sadarangani M, Huang V, Ostensen M, Castillo E, Troster SM et al (2019) From mother to baby: antenatal exposure to monoclonal antibody biologics. Expert Rev Clin Immunol 15(3):221–229
30. Komaki F, Komaki Y, Micic D, Ido A, Sakuraba A (2017) Outcome of pregnancy and neonatal complications with anti-tumor necrosis factor-α use in females with immune mediated diseases; a systematic review and meta-analysis. J Autoimmun 76:38–52
31. Bitter H, Bendvold AN, Østensen ME (2018) Lymphocyte changes and vaccination response in a child exposed to belimumab during pregnancy. Ann Rheum Dis 77(11):1692–1693
32. Kumthekar A, Abhijeet D, Deodhar A (2013) Use of belimumab throughout 2 consecutive pregnancies in a patient with systemic lupus erythematosus. J Rheumatol 40(6):1–3
33. Danve A, Perry L, Deodhar A (2015) Use of belimumab throughout pregnancy to treat active systemic lupus erythematosus—a case report. Semin Arthritis Rheum 44(2):195–197
34. Wallace DJ, Navarra S, Petri MA, Gallacher A, Thomas M, Furie R et al (2013) Safety profile of belimumab: pooled data from placebo-controlled phase 2 and 3 studies in patients with systemic lupus erythematosus. Lupus 22(2):144–154
35. Emmi G, Silvestri E, Squatrito D, Mecacci F, Ciampalini A, Emmi L et al (2016) Favorable pregnancy outcome in a patient with systemic lupus erythematosus treated with belimumab: a confirmation report. Semin Arthritis Rheum 45(6):e26–e27
36. Sandhu VK, Wallace DJ, Weisman MH (2015) Monoclonal antibodies, systemic lupus erythematosus, and pregnancy: insights from an open-label study. J Rheumatol 42(4):4–6
37. Bazzani C, Scrivo R, Andreoli L, Baldissera E, Biggioggero M, Canti V et al (2015) Prospectively-followed pregnancies in patients with inflammatory arthritis taking biological drugs: an Italian multicentre study. Clin Exp Rheumatol 33(5):688–693
38. Abisror N, Mekinian A, Brechignac S, Ruffatti A, Carbillon L, Fain O (2015) Inefficacy of plasma exchanges associated to rituximab in refractory obstetrical antiphospholipid syndrome. Press Med 44(1):100–102
39. Tsao NW, Lynd LD, Sadatsafavi M, Hanley G, De Vera MA (2018) Patterns of biologics utilization and discontinuation before and during pregnancy in women with autoimmune diseases: a population-based cohort study. Arthritis Care Res 70(7):979–986
40. Andreoli L, Bazzani C, Taraborelli M, Reggia R, Lojacono A, Brucato A et al (2010) Pregnancy in autoimmune rheumatic diseases: the importance of counselling for old and new challenges. Autoimmun Rev 10(1):51–54
41. Conduit C, Yew S, Jose S, Jayne J, Kirkland G (2017) A case of de novo diagnosis antineutrophil cytoplasmic antibody negative pauci-immune necrotising glomerulonephritis in pregnancy. Intern Med J 47(5):593–600

42. Arce-Salinas CA, Rodríguez-García F, Gómez-Vargas JI (2012) Long-term efficacy of anti-CD20 antibodies in refractory lupus nephritis. Rheumatol Int 32(5):1245–1249
43. Bröms G, Haerskjold A, Granath F, Kieler H, Pedersen L, Berglind IA (2018) Effect of maternal psoriasis on pregnancy and birth outcomes: a population-based cohort study from Denmark and Sweden. Acta Derm Venereol 98(8):728–734
44. Fotiadou C, Lazaridou E, Sotiriou E, Ioannides D (2012) Spontaneous abortion during ustekinumab therapy. J Dermatol Case Rep 6(4):105–107
45. Lund T, Thomsen SF (2017) Use of TNF-inhibitors and ustekinumab for psoriasis during pregnancy: a patient series. Dermatol Ther 30(3):1–5
46. Cortes X, Borrás-Blasco J, Antequera B, Fernandez-Martinez S, Casterá E, Martin S et al (2017) Ustekinumab therapy for Crohn's disease during pregnancy: a case report and review of the literature. J Clin Pharm Ther 42(2):234–236
47. Echeverría-García B, Nuño-González A, Dauden E, Vanaclocha F, Torrado R, Belinchón I et al (2017) A case series of patients with psoriasis exposed to biologic therapy during pregnancy: the BIOBADADERM Register and a review of the literature. Actas Dermosifiliogr 108(2):168–170
48. Beaulieu DB, Ananthakrishnan AN, Martin C, Cohen RD, Kane SV, Mahadevan U (2018) Use of biologic therapy by pregnant women with inflammatory bowel disease does not affect infant response to vaccines. Clin Gastroenterol Hepatol 16(1):99–105
49. Alsenaid A, Prinz JC (2016) Inadvertent pregnancy during ustekinumab therapy in a patient with plaque psoriasis and impetigo herpetiformis. J Eur Acad Dermatol Venereol. 30(3):488–490
50. Galli-Novak E, Mook S-C, Buning J, Schmidt E, Zillikens D, Thaci D et al (2016) Successful pregnancy outcome under prolonged ustekinumab treatment in a patient with Crohn's disease and paradoxical psoriasis. J Eur Acad Dermatol Venereol 30(12):e189–e191
51. Da Rocha K, Piccinin MC, Kalache LF, Reichert-Faria A, Silva De Castro CC (2015) Pregnancy during ustekinumab treatment for severe psoriasis. Dermatology 231(2):103–104
52. Sheeran C, Nicolopoulos J (2014) Pregnancy outcomes of two patients exposed to ustekinumab in the first trimester. Australas J Dermatol 55(3):235–236
53. Youngstein T, Hoffmann P, Gül A, Lane T, Williams R, Rowczenio DM et al (2017) International multi-centre study of pregnancy outcomes with interleukin-1 inhibitors. Rheumatology (Oxford) 56(12):2102–2108
54. Smith CJF, Chambers CD (2018) Five successful pregnancies with antenatal anakinra exposure. Rheumatology (Oxford) 57(7):1271–1275
55. Fischer-Betz R, Specker C, Schneide M (2011) Successful outcome of two pregnancies in patients with adult-onset Still's disease treated with IL-1 receptor antagonist (anakinra). Clin Exp Rheumatol 29(6):1021–1023
56. Saito J, Yakuwa N, Takai C, Nakajima K, Kaneko K, Goto M et al (2018) Tocilizumab concentrations in maternal serum and breast milk during breastfeeding and a safety assessment in infants: a case study. Rheumatology (Oxford) 57(8):1499–1500
57. Weber-Schoendorfer C, Schaefer C (2016) Pregnancy outcome after tocilizumab therapy in early pregnancy-case series from the German Embryotox Pharmacovigilance Center. Reprod Toxicol 60:29–32
58. Tan BE, Lim AL, Kan SL, Lim CH, Tsang EEL, Ch'ng SS et al (2017) Real-world clinical experience of biological disease modifying anti-rheumatic drugs in Malaysia rheumatoid arthritis patients. Rheumatol Int 37(10):1719–1725
59. Kaneko K, Sugitani M, Goto M, Murashima A (2016) Tocilizumab and pregnancy: four cases of pregnancy in young women with rheumatoid arthritis refractory to anti-TNF biologics with exposure to tocilizumab. Mod Rheumatol 26(5):672–675
60. Hoeltzenbein M, Beck E, Rajwanshi R, Gøtestam Skorpen C, Berber E, Schaefer C et al (2016) Tocilizumab use in pregnancy: analysis of a global safety database including data from clinical trials and post-marketing data. Semin Arthritis Rheum 46(2):238–245

61. Nakajima K, Watanabe O, Mochizuki M, Nakasone A, Ishizuka N, Murashima A (2016) Pregnancy outcomes after exposure to tocilizumab: a retrospective analysis of 61 patients in Japan. Mod Rheumatol 26(5):667–671
62. Warren RB, Reich K, Langley RG, Strober B, Gladman D, Deodhar A et al (2018) Secukinumab in pregnancy: outcomes in psoriasis, psoriatic arthritis and ankylosing spondylitis from the global safety database. Br J Dermatol 179(5):1205–1207
63. Strober B, Leonardi C, Papp KA, Mrowietz U, Ohtsuki M, Bissonnette R et al (2017) Short- and long-term safety outcomes with ixekizumab from 7 clinical trials in psoriasis: etanercept comparisons and integrated data. J Am Acad Dermatol 76:432
64. Kumar M, Ray L, Vemuri S, Simon TA (2015) Pregnancy outcomes following exposure to abatacept during pregnancy. Semin Arthritis Rheum 45(3):351–356
65. Ojeda-Uribe M, Afif N, Dahan E, Sparsa L, Haby C, Sibilia J et al (2013) Exposure to abatacept or rituximab in the first trimester of pregnancy in three women with autoimmune diseases. Clin Rheumatol 32(5):695–700
66. Flint J, Panchal S, Hurrell A, van de Venne M, Gayed M, Schreiber K et al (2016) BSR and BHPR guideline on prescribing drugs in pregnancy and breastfeeding-part II: analgesics and other drugs used in rheumatology practice. Rheumatology (Oxford) 55:1698

Managing Menstrual Irregularities in AID

Rama Walia and Anshita Aggarwal

Abstract

Autoimmune rheumatological diseases (AIDs) can have a detrimental effect on a woman's menstrual health and fertility prospects. The underlying pathophysiology is multi-factorial. The inflammatory milieu can suppress the hypothalamic-pituitary-gonadal axis, the co-existence of other autoimmune conditions such as primary hypothyroidism can play a role and the drugs used for the treatment of AIDs such as steroids and cyclophosphamide also have adverse effects pertaining to reproductive health. The work-up involves hormonal assessment and tests for ovarian reserve. Oral contraceptive pills can be used for restoring regularity of menstrual cycles, while steroid-sparing regimens and GnRH analogs have been used for ovarian function preservation.

Keywords

Autoimmune diseases · Menstrual irregularities · Hypothalamic-pituitary-gonadal axis · Steroids · Cyclophosphamide · GnRH analogs

8.1 Introduction and Background

Autoimmune rheumatological disorders can have a remarkable effect on a woman's menstrual cycles and thus fertility prospects. This is of concern considering that most such diseases are more common in women in the reproductive age group. However, due to the plethora of other systemic problems that these diseases encompass, this aspect often remains neglected. Both disease-related factors and the

R. Walia (✉) · A. Aggarwal
Post Graduate Institute of Medical Education and Research, Chandigarh, India

treatment offered for the disease can have implications on menstrual health. Strictly coordinated functions of the hypothalamus, pituitary, ovaries, and endometrium are essential for cyclic, predictable menses that are indicative of regular ovulation. Pulsatile release of GnRH from the hypothalamus, within a critical range of frequencies, is required for cyclical menses.

8.2   Epidemiology and Pathophysiology

According to previous studies, the prevalence of menstrual irregularities in patients with rheumatological disorders varies from 15% to 40% [1]. In one study, oligomenorrhea was reported to be the most common menstrual abnormality (54%) in systemic lupus erythematosus (SLE) patients. Those patients who had menstrual irregularities had higher prolactin (PRL) levels, more active disease, and lower progesterone levels [2]. Menorrhagia, which may be multi-factorial, has been observed in 12–15% of patients [3, 4]. Thrombocytopenia, antiphospholipid antibodies, and the use of drugs like glucocorticoids and/or nonsteroidal anti-inflammatory drugs (NSAIDs) may be contributory. Inflammatory cytokines, which are increased in autoimmune rheumatological disorders, can have an inhibitory effect on gonadotropin-releasing hormone (GnRH) secretion. Interleukin-1 beta (IL-1 beta) has been established as the most powerful inhibitor of GnRH secretion in animal studies [5, 6]. In vivo studies have demonstrated inhibition of the GnRH-LH systems after central infusion of TNFα [6–9]. However, these findings could not be reproduced in in vitro studies where TNFα had no effect on the release of GnRH in hypothalamic explants of male rats or proestrus female rats [10]. The inhibition of GnRH secretion leads to secondary amenorrhea and chronic anovulation. SLE activity, which is expected to correlate with the levels of inflammatory cytokines, is known to be the main risk factor for amenorrhea in patients not receiving alkylating drugs [11]. Secondary amenorrhea has been observed in 17–25% of patients.

Apart from this, autoimmune endocrine disorders may coexist with an autoimmune rheumatological disorder, which can lead to menstrual abnormalities. Studies have shown that the prevalence of autoimmune hypothyroidism, but not hyperthyroidism, is greater in SLE patients as compared to the prevalence in the general population. Both autoimmune thyroid disease and SLE share a Th1 immune predominance which could be the immune-pathogenic base of the association of these two disorders [12]. Hypothyroidism can lead to anovulation, which in turn leads to low levels of progesterone. A hyperestrogenic state ensues, leading to persistent and unchecked endometrial proliferation, resulting in excessive, irregular, and unpredictable breakthrough menstrual bleeding. These changes may be due to deficient secretion of LH and altered pulse frequency and amplitude because of untreated hypothyroidism.

Previous studies have also reported antibodies capable of increasing PRL levels in SLE patients [13]. This could theoretically lead to secondary hypogonadism and thus secondary amenorrhea or secondary polycystic ovary syndrome (PCOS) and oligomenorrhea. Hyperprolactinemia may not be only antibody-mediated but may also be secondary to intake of certain over-the-counter drugs like domperidone or proton-pump inhibitors, which have D2 receptor agonist activity.

In the general population, most cases of menstrual irregularities can be attributed to PCOS. As such, there have not been many large-scale studies on the prevalence of PCOS in rheumatological disorders. In a small retrospective cross-sectional study, among women aged 10–50 years, the prevalence of PCOS in rheumatic diseases paralleled that of the general population. However, the prevalence was much higher in those with psoriatic arthritis, psoriasis, and ankylosing spondylitis [14].

The levels of anti-Mullerian hormone (AMH), which is a marker of ovarian reserve, have been shown to be lower in treatment-naive SLE women compared with healthy women. This could be due to autoimmune oophoritis, which is seen commonly in SLE [15, 16]. Elevated levels of anti-corpus luteum antibody have been linked to ovarian dysfunction in patients with lupus [17]. Presence of comorbid conditions like chronic renal failure [18] and hypothalamic amenorrhea may also culminate in amenorrhea.

Another major concern with respect to menstrual cycles in patients of autoimmune rheumatological diseases is the adverse effect of the various therapeutic agents used which include steroids, chemotherapeutic and immunomodulatory/immunosuppressive agents. Exogenous steroids inhibit the hypothalamic–pituitary–gonadal (HPG) axis and hence the GnRH pulsatility and LH/FSH secretion, thus leading to menstrual irregularities and eventually secondary amenorrhea. Though this inhibition is reversible, since most of the patients receiving steroids are in the reproductive age group, it has many implications with respect to fertility prospects. Not only this, long-term steroid therapy has various other systemic side effects as well. This makes it imperative to opt for a "steroid-sparing regimen" for certain patients. Usually, in patients with moderate-to-severe disease who require 10 mg prednisolone/day or higher doses to maintain disease remission, other immunosuppressive agents should be added so as to enable one to reduce the steroid doses. Azathioprine is commonly used as a steroid-sparing agent in mild-to-moderate disease. The advent of newer biological drugs such as rituximab, epratuzumab, and abatacept has shown promise in reducing the cumulative steroid burden in such patients.

Cyclophosphamide (CYC) is another commonly used agent for treating active rheumatological disease. Studies of patients of SLE have shown a high prevalence of ovarian failure varying from 10–83% in women treated with CYC. The prevalence of ovarian insufficiency may vary depending on the subject's age at initiation of treatment and the cumulative dose of CYC received [19–21].

CYC crosslinks DNA, which damages the chromosomes of rapidly dividing cells, leading to permanent damage to the limited population of germ cells present in ovaries [20, 21]. The larger follicles, as well as antral and pre-ovulatory follicles, bear the largest brunt as they are more sensitive to toxicity. Studies have shown that the total dose of CYC required to produce amenorrhea goes on decreasing steeply as the age advances, which is due to physiological age-related decline in ovarian function. The culprit dose is 20.4 g in women aged 20–29 years; 9.3 g between 30 and 39 years, and 5.2 g between 40 and 49 years [22]. A retrospective review of women treated for SLE showcased the importance of total drug exposure with CYC

[23]. Persistent early amenorrhea developed in none of the 16 women who had been treated only with pulse glucocorticoids, in 2 of the 16 treated with seven monthly pulses of CYC, and in 9 of the 23 treated with 15 or more monthly pulses of CYC. One-half of the affected patients who had amenorrhea developed it within the first 7 months, occurring earlier in women over the age of 25. The amenorrhea was permanent in the majority of the cases, with recovery occurring only in those women who had received the shorter pulse CYC regimen. Among the other drugs, methotrexate is generally not considered gonadotoxic, but recent studies have shown an association with reduced ovarian function [24, 25].

The two main determinants of risk for ovarian failure are age at the time of initiation of CYC therapy and the cumulate dose of the drug received, with the risk sharply increasing over the age of 30 years and with doses over 10 g [20, 21]. In a meta-analysis comparing low-dose CYC v/s high-dose CYC regimens, it was seen that there was a lower risk of menstrual disturbances with the low-dose CYC induction therapy as compared to the high-dose therapy for lupus nephritis (RR = 0.46, 95% CI, 0.31–0.69). The venous pulse doses were 500–1000 mg/m^2 and 400–500 mg/m^2 in the high- and low-dose groups, respectively.

Among the newer drugs for rheumatological disorders, mycophenolate mofetil (MMF) has shown promise. It is thought to be more feasible and acceptable as compared to CYC in women in the reproductive age group, as it does not have a toxic effect on the gonadal cells. However, it is teratogenic and thus patients must be counseled to refrain from getting pregnant while they are on treatment with MMF.

8.3 Management of Menstrual Irregularities

8.3.1 Hormonal Evaluation

Evaluation of menstrual abnormalities in autoimmune rheumatological disorders entails measurement of gonadotropins (LH, FSH) in the follicular phase (day 2 or 3 of the menstrual cycle). Apart from these, serum estradiol, di-hydro-epiandrosterone (DHEAS), testosterone, prolactin, AMH, and thyroid function test should also be done. AMH is a noninvasive and a fairly reliable marker of ovarian reserve. A profile of elevated gonadotropin levels, with low estradiol and/or low AMH (at an age of <40 years), is consistent with premature ovarian failure, likely due to autoimmune oophoritis/cyclophosphamide toxicity. On the other hand, if gonadotropin levels are low or "inappropriately normal" for low estradiol, then secondary hypogonadism is diagnosed. Secondary hypogonadism may be related to disease activity per se. Apart from these, mild hyperprolactinemia may also be seen.

8.3.2 Role of Hormonal Replacement

Irrespective of the cause, long-standing secondary amenorrhea can have a detrimental effect on the bone mineral density. Moreover, anovulation would eventually lead to infertility.

Remission of disease activity may lead to an improvement in menstrual function. However, in long-standing amenorrhea, hormone replacement may have to be considered, but owing to the concerns about increasing disease activity and elevated risk of thrombotic events, clinicians rarely prescribe combined estrogen-progestin oral contraceptive pills (COCs) to women with this disease. Women with SLE are at higher risk for ischemic heart disease, stroke, and venous thromboembolism, especially in the presence of antiphospholipid antibodies (APLA).

Data have shown that COCs are safe in women with SLE provided they have a stable, mild disease, are seronegative for antiphospholipid antibodies, and have no prior history of thrombosis. It is recommended that COCs can be used in SLE patients who have no other cardiovascular risk factors [26]. For women with SLE and antiphospholipid antibodies, COCs are contraindicated (category 4). Thus, prior to initiating contraceptives in women with SLE, the level of disease activity, the presence of APLA and thrombocytopenia should be established.

8.3.3 Role of GnRH Agonists

GnRH agonists (GnRH-a) may attenuate the depletion of ovarian reserve in women treated with CYC. GnRH-a bind to the GnRH receptors located on the pituitary, initially leading to a spike in gonadotropin release, but eventually leading to down-regulation of receptors and thus a decline in both gonadotropin and estrogen levels. These hormonal changes may arrest the rate of follicular maturation such that the follicles do not develop to the point of becoming vulnerable to the toxicity of CYC [19]. A meta-analysis of nine studies of adjunctive GnRH-a therapy during chemotherapy illustrated that co-therapy with GnRH-a during CYC treatment resulted in a significant increase of 68% in the continuation of regular menstruation over chemotherapy alone [27]. Dosing was fairly standard between studies, with most women receiving 3.75 mg of GnRH-a every 4 weeks throughout chemotherapy administration. Most studies described starting treatment about 2 weeks prior to the commencement of chemotherapy or treatment with short-acting GnRH-a to avoid chemotherapy during the period of expected ovarian flare that follows GnRH-a therapy by 5–10 days. In one study, many women received their first leuprolide dose following their initial CYC dose to avoid treatment during the ovarian flare.

The decline in AMH levels has been shown to be of lesser magnitude in patients who received GnRH-a co-therapy as compared to those who received chemotherapy alone. However, it may not directly translate into improved pregnancy outcomes, as pregnancy has been seen to be far less frequent than ovarian function preservation in all studies.

Apart from this, treatment of associated comorbidities like hypothyroidism and renal failure should be optimized and that may lead to an improvement in menstrual irregularities.

References

1. Fatnoon NNA, Azarisman SMS, Zainal D (2008) Prevalence and risk factor for menstrual disorders among systemic lupus erythematosus patients. Singapore Med 49:413–418
2. Shabanova SS, Ananieva LP, Alekberova ZS, Guzov II (2008) Ovarian function and disease activity in patients with systemic lupus erythematosus. Clin Exp Rheumatol 26:436
3. Harvey AM, Shulman LE, Tumulty PA et al (1954) Systemic lupus erythematosus: review of the literature and clinical analysis of 138 cases. Medicine (Baltimore) 33:291
4. Wallace DJ, Dubois EL (eds) (1987) Dubois' lupus erythematosus, 3rd edn. Lea & Febiger, Philadelphia, PA
5. Rivest S, Rivier C (1993) Central mechanisms and sites of action involved in the inhibitory effects of CRF and cytokines on LHRH neuronal activity. Ann N Y Acad Sci 697:117–141
6. Kalra PS, Edwards TG, Xu B, Jain M, Kalra SP (1998) The antigonadotropic effects of cytokines: the role of neuropeptides. Domest Anim Endocrinol. 15:321–332
7. Rivier C, Vale W (1990) Cytokines act within the brain to inhibit luteinizing hormone secretion and ovulation in the rat. Endocrinology 127:849–856
8. Watanobe H, Hayakawa Y (2003) Hypothalamic interleukin-1 beta and tumor necrosis factor-alpha, but not interleukin-6, mediate the endotoxin-induced suppression of the reproductive axis in rats. Endocrinology 144:4868–4875
9. Yoo MJ, Nishihara M, Takahashi M (1997) Tumor necrosis factor-alpha mediates endotoxin induced suppression of gonadotropin-releasing hormone pulse generator activity in the rat. Endocr J 44:141–148
10. Russell SH, Small CJ, Stanley SA, Franks S, Ghatei MA, Bloom SR (2001) The in vitro role of tumour necrosis factor-alpha and interleukin-6 in the hypothalamic–pituitary gonadal axis. J Neuroendocrinol 13:296–301
11. Pasoto SG, Mendonça BB, Bonfá EF (2002) Menstrual disturbances in patients with systemic lupus erythematosus without alkylating therapy: clinical, hormonal and therapeutic associations. Lupus 11:175–180
12. Ferrari SM, Elia G, Virili C, Centanni M, Antonelli A, Fallahi P (2017) Systemic lupus erythematosus and thyroid autoimmunity. Front Endocrinol (Lausanne) 8:138. Published 19 Jun 2017. https://doi.org/10.3389/fendo.2017.00138
13. Blanco-Favela F, Quintal MG, Chavez-Rueda AK, Leanos-Miranda A, Berron-Peres R, Baca-Ruiz V, Lavalle-Montalvo C (2001) Anti-prolactin autoantibodies in paediatric systemic lupus erythematosus patients. Lupus 10:803–808
14. Edens C, Antonelli M (2017) Polycystic ovarian syndrome in rheumatic disease [Internet]. ACR Meeting Abstracts. Available from: https://acrabstracts.org/abstract/polycystic-ovarian-syndrome-in-rheumatic-disease/
15. Ma W, Zhan Z, Liang X et al (2013) Subclinical impairment of ovarian reserve in systemic lupus erythematosus patients with normal menstruation not using alkylating therapy. J Womens Health 22:1023–1027
16. Ulug P, Oner G, Kasap B et al (2014) Evaluation of ovarian reserve tests in women with systemic lupus erythematosus. Am J Reprod Immunol 72:85–88
17. Pasoto SG, Viana VS, Mendonca BB et al (1999) Anti-corpus luteum antibody: a novel serological marker for ovarian dysfunction in systemic lupus erythematosus? J Rheumatol 26:1087–1093
18. Holley JL, Schmidt RJ (2013) Changes in fertility and hormone replacement therapy in kidney disease. Adv Chronic Kidney Dis 20:240–245
19. Blumenfeld Z, Shapiro D, Shteinberg M, Avivi I, Nahir M (2000) Preservation of fertility and ovarian function and minimizing gonadotoxicity in young women with systemic lupus erythematosus treated by chemotherapy. Lupus 9:401–405
20. Huong DL, Amoura Z, Duhaut P et al (2002) Risk of ovarian failure and fertility after intravenous cyclophosphamide. A study in 84 patients. J Rheumatol 29:2571–2576. Epub 5 Dec 2002

21. Park MC, Park YB, Jung SY, Chung IH, Choi KH, Lee SK (2004) Risk of ovarian failure and pregnancy outcome in patients with lupus nephritis treated with intravenous cyclophosphamide pulse therapy. Lupus 13:569–574
22. Mattinson DR, Nightingale MS, Shiromizu K (1983) Effects of toxic substances on female reproduction. Environ Health Perspect 48:43–52
23. Boumpas DT, Austin HA 3rd, Vaughan EM et al (1993) Risk for sustained amenorrhea in patients with systemic lupus erythematosus receiving intermittent pulse cyclophosphamide therapy. Ann Intern Med 119:366
24. de Araujo DB, Yamakami LY, Aikawa NE et al (2014) Ovarian reserve in adult patients with childhood-onset lupus: a possible deleterious effect of methotrexate? Scand J Rheumatol 43:503–511
25. McLaren JF, Burney RO, Milki AA et al (2009) Effect of methotrexate exposure on subsequent fertility in women undergoing controlled ovarian stimulation. Fertil Steril 92:515–519
26. Centers for Disease Control and Prevention (2010) U.S. medical eligibility criteria for contraceptive use, 2010. MMWR Morb Mortal Wkly Rep 59:1–86
27. Clowse ME, Behera MA, Anders CK et al (2009) Ovarian preservation by GnRH agonists during chemotherapy: a meta-analysis. J Womens Health (Larchmt) 18:311–319. Epub 14 Mar 2009

Fertility Preservation in Women with Autoimmune Diseases Treated with Gonadotoxic Agents

9

Aashima Arora

Abstract

Auto-immune diseases commonly affect women of reproductive age group. These women most often need chemotherapeutic agents which may cause significant gonado-toxicity. Therefore, fertility preservation techniques must be offered to women undergoing treatment for auto-immune diseases before starting such therapy. This chapter discusses in detail the various fertility preservation techniques available with their merits and de-merits.

Keywords

Auto-immune diseases · Gonadotoxic drugs · Fertility preservation options

Autoimmune diseases are common in women of reproductive age and are commonly treated with gonadotoxic agents like cyclophosphamide. However, the aspect of fertility preservation treatment has not received much importance in these women. As the survival rates of these patients have improved, long-term aspects including fertility preservation are gaining significance [1].

9.1 Risk and Mechanism of Gonadotoxicity

Significant number of young women with SARDs is exposed to gonadotoxic drugs, which may lead to premature ovarian failure and infertility. The most commonly used such drug is cyclophosphamide, which is mainly used for life or organ threatening autoimmune disorders such as SLE with renal involvement or ANCA-associated systemic vasculitis [2]. CYC is toxic to both male and female gonads. The risks and benefits of these immunosuppressive agents must be explained to the

A. Arora (✉)
Post Graduate Institute of Medical Education and Research, Chandigarh, India

© Springer Nature Singapore Pte Ltd. 2020
S. K. Sharma (ed.), *Women's Health in Autoimmune Diseases*,
https://doi.org/10.1007/978-981-15-0114-2_9

young patients prior to treatment as issues related to fertility may be an important concern to many of them.

Cyclophosphamide is an alkylating agent which exerts its action by preventing cell division via covalent binding and cross-linking of a variety of macromolecules [3]. Alkylating agents have potentially severe side effects like bone marrow suppression, gonadal toxicity and increased chances of infections and malignancies. The damage induced is usually reversible in tissues with rapidly dividing cells such as bone marrow, gastrointestinal tract and thymus. However, the toxicity to ovaries is progressive and irreversible, where the number of germ cells is determined since foetal life and cannot be regenerated. Alkylating agents are not cell-cycle specific, and it is believed that they act on undeveloped oocytes and pregranulosa cells of primordial follicles. This toxicity is mediated by metabolite phosphoramide mustard [4].

The gonadotoxicity of CYC is dependent mainly on the following:

1. Age at exposure
2. Cumulative dose.

The risk of premature ovarian failure and infertility is directly proportional to age at exposure. Before menarche, CYC does not seem to cause significant ovarian toxicity. In patients <30 years of age, studies have shown the risk of amenorrhoea to be around 10% as compared to >50% in women above 40 years. In general, greater the ovarian reserve at the time of exposure, lesser is the damage caused. Data suggests that women <20 years of age at drug exposure have <5% chance of ovarian failure with initial course of CYC as compared to women >30 years (25–50%) and >40 years (75%) [5–8].

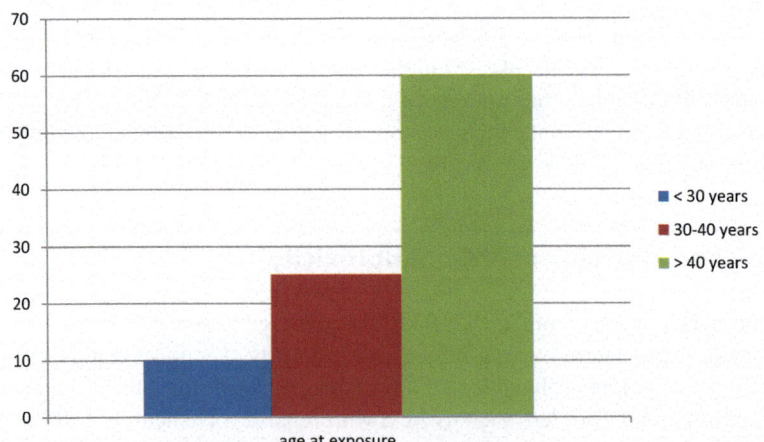

The level of gonadal dysfunction is also dependent on the dose of CYC that the lady receives. The cumulative CYC dose is an independent risk factor for ovarian toxicity, regardless of how the medication is used. Cumulative dose of 12 g/m^2 or higher has been shown to be significantly more gonadotoxic than 8 g/m^2 [9]. The evidence regarding the effect of duration of CYC treatment and baseline severity of disease on gonadotoxicity is less convincing.

9.2 Measures for Fertility Preservation

Various fertility preservation strategies are available for women exposed to chemotherapy, including the following:

1. Administration of GnRH agonist
2. Embryo cryopreservation
3. Ovarian tissue cryopreservation
4. Unfertilized ovum cryopreservation.

Each method has its own advantages and disadvantages in terms of availability, efficacy, cost, need for male partner and effect on primary disease, hence shall be discussed subsequently.

9.2.1 Administration of GnRH Agonist

The use of GnRH agonist to protect ovaries from the toxicity of chemotherapeutic agents has been considered for over two decades. Several possible mechanisms have been postulated through which GnRH analogues may exert this protective action. These include the following:

(a) Decreased levels of circulating gonadotropins, thereby putting the ovaries in an artificial pre-pubertal state. This hypogonadotropic milieu decreases the number of primordial follicles entering the vulnerable differentiation stage.
(b) Decreased blood supply to ovaries leading to lesser concentration of chemotherapeutic agents in the ovarian tissue.
(c) Up regulation of an intragonadal anti-apoptotic molecule such as sphingosine-1-phosphate by GnRH agonist.

The efficacy of GnRH agonist in fertility preservation has remained controversial for many years. Until the previous decade, most of the data was from observation studies carried out in young pre-menopausal women with breast cancer or lymphoma and was considered to be non-conclusive due to lack of randomized controlled trials. However, over the last 10 years, multiple RCTs have been conducted worldwide on the use of GnRH agonists concurrently with chemotherapy both for malignancy and for SLE. Meta-analysis of these studies has proven the efficacy of this pharmacological intervention in preserving ovarian function [10]. Though the earlier literature appeared stronger for prevention of POF and less convincing in terms of pregnancy rates, the recent POEMS/S0230 trial which was an international, phase 3, randomized study extended this benefit to increased pregnancy rates (21% vs. 11%) [11]. Also, a recent systematic review and meta-analysis of data from premenstrual women with early breast cancer concluded POF rates of 14% vs. 30% and pregnancy rates of 10% vs. 5% in women receiving chemotherapy with or without GnRH agonist co-treatment, respectively [12]. Cochrane Database Systematic Review in March 2019 concluded that GnRH agonist appears to be effective in protecting the ovaries during chemotherapy, in terms of maintenance and resumption of menstruation, treatment-related premature ovarian failure and ovulation. Evidence for protection of fertility was insufficient and needs further investigation as per the authors [13].

It needs to be emphasized that the use of GnRH agonist has not been associated with any significant effect on the course of SLE. Also, the preservation of ovarian function in itself is highly significant in women with SLE as POF leads to premature atherosclerosis which is the leading cause of death in SLE. The odds ratio for preservation of cyclic ovarian function vs. POF has been reported to be as high as 6.8 in women receiving GnRH agonist treatment before and during gonadotoxic chemotherapy [14].

9.2.2 Embryo Cryopreservation

Ovarian stimulation followed by in vitro fertilization and embryo cryopreservation is considered to be the gold standard technique for fertility preservation in young women desirous of future fertility prior to chemotherapy for malignancies. However, in case of women with SLE, the path physiology of the disease per se may alter this decision. Though the exact aetiology of SLE is unknown, the role of female hormones has been suggested for many years as 90% of affected patients are females. Increased flares have been reported in post-menopausal women who receive hormone replacement therapy with E+P. Males with SLE also have been proven to have altered sex hormones with higher oestrogen to androgen ratio, all suggesting a role of oestrogen in disease pathogenesis. Therefore, the safety of IVF procedures where ovarian hyperstimulation leads to markedly increased oestradiol levels has been questioned [15].

It has been recommended that ovarian hyperstimulation must be discouraged in women with SLE during active flare (and 6–12 months thereafter) and in SLE patients with major previous thrombotic events, uncontrolled hypertension, pulmonary hypertension, advanced renal disease and severe valvulopathy/heart disease [16]. If the disease is stable, IVF may be performed but only in expert hands and after detailed couple counselling. These women need to be under close and continuous monitoring during IVF procedures. The most threatening condition associated with ovarian stimulation in women with SLE is thrombosis. At present, no specific type of gonadotropins has been shown to offer a clear advantage in the prevention of thrombosis. However, as most cases of thrombosis have been associated to OHSS, the main aim in these women is to avoid OHSS by using all preventable strategies such as mild stimulation protocols, coasting, use of GnRH agonist as trigger for ovulation, embryo freezing, etc.

9.2.3 Ovarian Tissue Cryopreservation

Ovarian tissue cryopreservation is a possible fertility preservation technique especially for young unmarried girls who do not have a male partner and hence cannot opt for embryo freezing [17]. It provides additional benefit of restoring oestrogen activity in the body following ovarian tissue autotransplantation though the survival of this tissue may be limited in time. However, this technique requires two surgical procedures: one to excise the ovarian tissue and second for auto-grafting. It is not widely available for poor patients in a country like India.

9.2.4 Unfertilized Ovum Cryopreservation

Aspiration and preservation of both mature and immature oocytes have been proven to be efficient alternative techniques for fertility preservation in women scheduled for gonadotoxic chemotherapy. While the aspiration of mature oocytes generally requires ovarian stimulation with gonadotropins (like IVF procedures), immature oocytes can be aspirated during a natural menstrual cycle without any hormonal stimulation. This in vitro maturation of immature oocytes (IVM) provides a hope for the patients who are in flare and in whom use of chemotherapy is imminent where other techniques that lead to increased oestradiol levels cannot be used. Though the success of these procedures is in the form of case reports and small case series till now, they appear to offer good opportunity. Literature reports clinical pregnancy rates of 25–45% per cycle with in vitro and in vivo matured oocytes with cryopreservation/vitrification [18, 19].

9.3 Comparison of Fertility Preservation Techniques

	Option	Advantages	Disadvantages
1	GnRH agonist	Simple to use Inexpensive No need of male partner Minimal side effects No risk of SLE flare Efficient Potential to preserve ovarian function	Symptoms of hypo-oestrogenism during treatment Not effective in all women
2	IVF and embryo freezing	Efficient Available at many centres Not very costly	Need for male partner May cause disease aggravation
3	Ovarian tissue cryopreservation	High potential Restores hormonal function in addition to fertility	Need for surgical procedure Not easily available Expensive
4	Oocytes preservation	High potential	Investigational Expensive Not widely available

In summary, fertility preservation options must be seriously considered and discussed in all young patients prior to starting gonadotoxic chemotherapy. Such techniques help young women to cope better emotionally with their chemotherapy, as there is a hope of being able to have a biological child in the future.

References

1. Katsifis GE, Tzioufas AG (2004) Ovarian failure in systemic lupus erythematosus patients treated with pulsed intravenous cyclophosphamide. Lupus 13(9):673–678
2. Austin HA, Klippel JH, Balow JE et al (1986) Therapy of lupus nephritis. Controlled trial of prednisone and cytotoxic drugs. N Engl J Med 314:614–619
3. Hall AG, Tilby MJ (1992) Mechanisms of action of, and modes of resistance to, alkylating agents used in the treatment of haematological malignancies. Blood Rev 6(3):163–173
4. Bines J, Oleske DM, Cobleigh MA (1996) Ovarian function in premenopausal women treated with adjuvant chemotherapy for breast cancer. J Clin Oncol 14(5):1718–1729
5. Huong DLT, Amoura Z, Duhaut P et al (2002) Risk of ovarian failure and fertility after intravenous cyclophosphamide. A study in 84 patients. J Rheumatol 29:2571–2576
6. Mok CC, Ho CTK, Chan KW, Lau CS, Wong RWS (2002) Outcome and prognostic indicators of diffuse proliferative lupus glomerulonephritis treated with sequential oral cyclophosphamide and azathioprine. Arthritis Rheum 46:1003–1013
7. Mok CC, Lau CS, Wong RWS (1998) Risk factors for ovarian failure in patients with systemic lupus erythematosus receiving cyclophosphamide therapy. Arthritis Rheum 41:831–837
8. Wetzels JFM (2004) Cyclophosphamide induced gonadal toxicity: a treatment dilemma in patients with lupus nephritis? Neth J Med 62(10):347–352
9. Ioannidis JPA, Katsifis GE, Tzioufas AG, Moutsopoulos HM (2002) Predictors of sustained amenorrhoea from pulsed intravenous cyclophosphamide in premenopausal women with systemic lupus erythematosus. J Rheumatol 29:2129–2135
10. Ben-Aharon I, Gafter-Gvili A, Leibovici L, Stemmer SM (2010) Pharmacological interventions for fertility preservation during chemotherapy: a systematic review and meta-analysis. Breast Cancer Res Treat 122(3):803–811
11. Moore HCF, Unger JM, Phillips K-A et al (2015) Goserelin for ovarian protection during breast-cancer adjuvant chemotherapy. N Engl J Med 372:923–932
12. Lambertini M, Moore HCF, Robert CF et al (2018) Gonadotropin-releasing hormone agonists during chemotherapy for preservation of ovarian function and fertility in premenopausal patients with early breast cancer: a systematic review and meta-analysis of individual patient-level data. J Clin Oncol 36:1981–1990
13. Chen H, Xiao L, Li J, Cui L, Huang W (2019) Adjuvant gonadotropin-releasing hormone analogues for the prevention of chemotherapy-induced premature ovarian failure in premenopausal women. Cochrane Database Syst Rev 3:CD008018
14. Blumenfeld Z, Zur H, Dann EJ (2015) Gonadotropin-releasing hormone agonist cotreatment during chemotherapy may increase pregnancy rate in survivors. Oncologist 20(11):1283–1289
15. Askanase AD, Buyon JP (2002) Reproductive health in SLE. Best Pract Res Clin Rheumatol 16:265–280
16. Bellver J, Pellicer A (2009) Ovarian stimulation for ovulation induction and in vitro fertilization in patients with systemic lupus erythematosus and antiphospholipid syndrome. Fertil Steril 92(6):1803–1810
17. Meirow D, Levron J, Eldar-Geva T et al (2005) Pregnancy after transplantation of cryopreserved ovarian tissue in a patient with ovarian failure after chemotherapy. N Engl J Med 353:318–321
18. Oktay K, Cil AP, Bang H (2006) Efficiency of oocytes cryopreservation: a meta-analysis. Fertil Steril 86:70–80
19. Chian RC, Huang JY, Gilbert L et al (2009) Obstetric outcomes following vitrification of in vitro and in vivo matured oocytes. Fertil Steril 91(6):2391–2398

Preconception Care and Counseling in Autoimmune Disorders

10

Bharti Sharma and Shinjini Narang

Abstract

Preconception care is an opportunity to identify the risk factors and to optimize the preexisting conditions for better perinatal outcome. This chapter reviews the preconception care and counseling for commonly encountered autoimmune diseases.

Keywords

Preconception care · Preconception counseling · Systemic lupus erythematosus

Preconception care is the provision of any form of medical, behavioral, and social health interventions to a women and her husband before the couple plans conception. It provides an opportunity to optimize the outcome of pregnancy in women with chronic medical illness, and autoimmune disorder is one of them. The common autoimmune rheumatic diseases encountered in clinical practice are systemic lupus erythematosus (SLE), systemic sclerosis, rheumatoid arthritis, scleroderma, and antiphospholipid syndrome (APS). The main concerns with these women and pregnancy are as follows:

1. Risk of maternal disease flare.
2. Adverse fetal outcome in terms of miscarriage, preterm labor, stillbirth, congenital malformations, neonatal mortality, and morbidity.
3. Risk of teratogenicity.
4. Availability of multidisciplinary team for management during pregnancy.
5. Providing effective contraception.

B. Sharma (✉) · S. Narang
Department of Obstetrics and Gynaecology, Post Graduate Institute of Medical Education and Research, Chandigarh, India

Ideally these women require multidisciplinary care since the onset of diagnosis, not just during pregnancy to ensure best obstetric outcome of both mother and fetus. So an obstetrician should always be involved in the care of women with autoimmune disorders as they have special needs like contraception advice, preconception counseling.

10.1 SLE

SLE is not a contraindication for pregnancy, but underlying chronic hypertension, interstitial lung disease, pulmonary hypertension, and renal involvement are independent risks toward maternal morbidity and mortality.

It is important to discuss the potential complications and risks involved and establish a management plan in a multidisciplinary setting. SLE is associated with increased risk of spontaneous abortions, intrauterine fetal death, preeclampsia, intrauterine growth restriction (IUGR), and preterm delivery.

Lupus flares are reported in 13.5–65% of pregnant women with SLE. Active disease in the last 6 months prior to conception is associated with an increased risk of lupus flare and poor pregnancy outcome, and these women should be advised to avoid pregnancy.

There is no evidence suggesting that SLE or other connective tissue disorders affect fertility. Though treatment with cyclophosphamide is a risk factor for infertility. Ovulation induction seems to increase the chance of flare and thrombosis, especially in cases of antiphospholipid antibodies. The preconceptional evaluation of women with SLE should always include clinical examinations along with blood investigations (Table 10.1).

Unless potential maternal benefits outweigh fetal risks, the woman should be instructed to avoid FDA pregnancy X and D drugs. Drugs safe to be used in pregnancy include prednisolone, azathioprine, cyclosporine A, and hydrochloroquine. Methotrexate, mycophenolate mofetil, and cyclophosphamide are contraindicated in pregnancy due to their teratogenic effect. Women on any of these drugs should be switched over to safer alternatives 3–6 months prior to conception as sudden withdrawal may precipitate lupus flare. Antihypertensives should also be switched over

Table 10.1 Preconceptional evaluation of women with SLE

Clinical evaluation/history	Laboratory investigations
• Cutaneous manifestation of SLE like malar rash, photosensitivity, discoid rash, Raynaud's phenomenon, urticaria, and vasculitis. • Blood pressure. • Urine output. • Details of current medications.	• Lupus serology (dsDNA and antinuclear antibodies). • Anti-Ro and anti-La antibody titers. • Antiphospholipid antibody titers. • Serum complement levels (less useful in pregnancy). • Renal function tests (creatinine, creatinine clearance, 24 h urine protein (*Serum creatinine >2.8 mg/dL have less than 30% chance of a successful pregnancy*)).

from angiotensis converting enzyme (ACE) inhibitors and angiotensin receptor blockers (ARB) to safer alternatives like labetalol and nifedipine due to the associated risk of fetal renal dysfunction and IUGR in case of second and third trimester exposure.

Thromboprophylaxis should be started if the woman is at risk for thromboembolic events, like antiphospholipid syndrome. Low dose aspirin before conception may be added for prophylaxis against preeclampsia and thrombosis.

Rate of complications in women with SLE approaches that of general population in absence of active disease, hypertension, renal involvement, or antiphospholipid antibodies.

These women should also be made aware of the risk of neonatal lupus erythematous especially congenital heart block (CHB) which is an irreversible and life threatening complication. The risk of CHB is 1–2% in women with anti-SSA/Ro antibodies and increases up to 5% when anti-SSB/La is also present along with anti-SSA/Ro. The risk of recurrence of CHB is also very high, ranges from 5% to 50% in subsequent births. That is why serial echocardiography and obstetric ultrasound to look for fetal heart rate are recommended from 16 to 18 weeks of gestation in anti-Ro/SSA and anti-La/SSB antibody-positive women.

10.2 Rheumatoid Arthritis

Disease activity usually improves in RA with up to 60% women reporting improvement in symptoms. Preconceptional counseling is important to allow for conversion to safer pharmacological drugs when possible. Potentially harmful drugs may be safely discontinued in pregnancy in case of disease improvement. Methotrexate should be stopped 3–4 months before conception to prevent fetal exposure. Leflunomide may persist in the body for 2 years and should be eliminated from the body using cholestyramine, 3 months before trying for pregnancy. Drugs safe in pregnancy are hydroxychloroquine, sulfonamide, corticosteroids, and anti-TNF (tumor necrosis factor) agents. NSAIDs are safe in pregnancy but should be avoided after 32 weeks of pregnancy as they can lead to oligohydramnios due to their effect on fetal kidney. They also carry the risk of premature closure of ductus arteriosus.

Though RA doesn't directly affect fertility but subfertility is seen in the affected women which can be attributed to the psychological effects of the disease and child bearing choices. Some studies have reported increased incidence of hypertensive disorders of pregnancy, preterm delivery, cesarean delivery, and IUGR. Relapse of RA is common in the first 6 months postpartum.

10.3 Systemic Sclerosis

In systemic sclerosis, a well-timed and planned pregnancy with proper monitoring can maximize the likelihood of a favorable outcome. The mean age of onset of systemic sclerosis is mid-40s, therefore it is not commonly seen in pregnancy and data pertaining to pregnancy in the disease is limited. The incidence of serious complications like renal crisis, severe cardiomyopathy (ejection fraction <30%), pulmonary hypertension, and severe restrictive lung disease is more common in woman who conceive within 4 years of developing systemic sclerosis, therefore women are counseled to go for pregnancy after this period.

Raynaud's phenomenon improves during pregnancy but esophageal reflux, shortness of breath (due to increased pulmonary volume), and renal function worsen during pregnancy, especially in third trimester. Mallory-Weiss tears can be present in women with esophageal involvement due to vomiting. Histamine blockers and proton pump inhibitors may be safely used in pregnancy for treatment of esophageal reflux, nausea, and vomiting. Some studies report higher incidence of miscarriages, preterm births, IUGR, and hypertensive disorders of pregnancy in these women. For treatment during pregnancy, hydroxychloroquine and corticosteroids are safe, whereas cyclophosphamide is contraindicated.

10.4 Antiphospholipid Syndrome

Antiphospholipid syndrome (APS) is an acquired autoimmune thrombophilia diagnosed by characteristic clinical features including vascular thrombosis, obstetric complications, and specified levels of circulating aPL antibodies.

Obstetric complications included recurrent early fetal loss and late second or third trimester fetal deaths, preeclampsia, IUGR, and preterm delivery. In APS, the prothrombotic risks (of both arterial and venous thromboembolism) associated with pregnancy are aggravated. In addition to risk of deep vein thrombosis, risks of pulmonary emboli, stroke, and hepatic infarction have been reported in women with APS in pregnancy and puerperium.

Treatment of APLA syndrome is LMWH or unfractionated heparin in combination with low-dose aspirin throughout pregnancy and postpartum period. Low-dose aspirin starting from the preconceptional period is recommended. In women with history of thrombosis or cerebral events with APS who are maintained on warfarin derivatives, switch over to heparin (LMWH or unfractionated heparin) is recommended preconceptionally or with positive early pregnancy test. Warfarin derivatives are then begun in postpartum period.

10.5 Conclusion

Autoimmune disorders are common in women of childbearing age, and pregnancy in these women is at high risk of maternal and perinatal (fetal, neonatal) complications. Multidisciplinary approach is required to obtain an optimal obstetric outcome with coordination between obstetrician, rheumatologist, and nephrologist. Via preconceptional counseling, a prepregnancy plan should be established to anticipate possible complications and treat them when they develop.

Further Reading

American College of Obstetricians and Gynecologists (2018) Group prenatal care. ACOG Committee Opinion No. 731. Obstet Gynecol 131:e104–e108

Brucato A, Frassi M, Franceschini F, Cimaz R, Faden D, Pisoni MP et al (2001) Risk of congenital complete heart block in newborns of mothers with anti-Ro/SSA antibodies detected by counter immunoelectrophoresis: a prospective study of 100 women. Arthritis Rheum 44:1832–1835

Buyon JP, Waltock J, Kleinman C, Copel J (1995) In utero identification and therapy of congenital heart block. Lupus 4:116–121

Chakravarty EF, Colon I, Langen ES et al (2005) Factors that predict prematurity and preeclampsiain pregnancies that are complicated by systemic lupus erythematosus. Am J Obstet Gynecol 192:1897–1890

Chung L, Flyckt RL, Colon I, Shah AA, Druzin M, Chakravarty EF (2006) Outcome of pregnancies complicated by systemic sclerosis and mixed connective tissue disease. Lupus 15:595–599

Friedman DM, Rupel A, Buyon JP (2007) Epidemiology, etiology, detection, and treatment of autoantibody associated congenital heart block in neonatal lupus. Curr Rheumatol Rep 9:101–108

Friedman DM, Kim MY, Copel JA, Davis C, Phoon CK, Glickstein JS et al, For the PRIDE Investigators (2008) Utility of cardiac monitoring in fetuses at risk for congenital heart block. The PR Interval and Dexamethasone Evaluation (PRIDE) prospective study. Circulation 117:485–493

Golding A, Haque UJ, Giles JT (2007) Rheumatoid arthritis and reproduction. Rheum Dis Clin N Am 33:319–343, vi–vii

Heit JA, Kobbervig CE, James AH, Petterson TM, Bailey KR, Melton LJ 3rd (2005) Trends in the incidence of venous thromboembolism during pregnancy or postpartum: a 30-year population-based study. Ann Intern Med 143:697–706

Khamashta MA (2006) Systemic lupus erythematosus and pregnancy. Best Pract Res Clin Rheumatol 20:685–694

Nassar AH, Uthman I, Khamashta MA (2012) Autoimmune and connective tissue disorders

Opatrny L, David M, Kahn SR, Shrier I, Rey E (2006) Association between antiphospholipid antibodies and recurrent fetal loss in women without autoimmune disease: a metaanalysis. J Rheumatol 33:2214–2221

Petri M (2007) The Hopkins Lupus Pregnancy Center: ten key issues in management. Rheum Dis Clin N Am 33:227–235 v

Reed SD, Vollan TA, Svec MA (2006) Pregnancy outcomes in women with rheumatoid arthritis in Washington State. Matern Child Health J 10:361–366

Steen VD (2007) Pregnancy in scleroderma. Rheum Dis Clin N Am 33:345–358, vii

Effect of Pregnancy on Autoimmune Rheumatic Diseases

11

Hafis Muhammed and Amita Aggarwal

Abstract

Pregnancy is associated with significant physiological changes in multiple organ systems including immune system. Due to the need to maintain the fetus, the immune responses are blunted or skewed to prevent rejection of the fetus. These changes include inhibition of uterine NK cells, increase in immunoregulatory macrophages, dendritic cells, and T cells. These changes are probably mediated by the hormonal changes present in pregnancy. Pregnancy has variable effect on disease activity of different autoimmune disease with decrease in RA and some increase in risk of flares in SLE, while data on other diseases is scant.

Keywords

Pregnancy · Autoimmune rheumatic disease · Immunoregulation

11.1 Introduction

Pregnancy is a physiological state where an allogenic fetus stays in utero for 9 months without evoking an immune response. Thus multiple immunologic changes occur in pregnancy which allows the fetus to be protected from immune reactions. At least three interrelated mechanisms are proposed:

1. Physical separation of the fetus and immune system
2. Reduced antigenicity of the fetus
3. Maternal immune suppression

H. Muhammed · A. Aggarwal (✉)
Department of Clinical Immunology and Rheumatology, Sanjay Gandhi Postgraduate Institute of Medical Sciences, Lucknow, India
e-mail: amita@sgpgi.ac.in

© Springer Nature Singapore Pte Ltd. 2020
S. K. Sharma (ed.), *Women's Health in Autoimmune Diseases*,
https://doi.org/10.1007/978-981-15-0114-2_11

It is conceivable that autoimmune disorders, which occur due to enhanced immune activation, behave differently during pregnancy owing to the immunologic changes occurring during this period. This chapter reviews the immune changes occurring during the pregnancy which brings about fetomaternal tolerance and their consequential effect on various rheumatic diseases.

11.2 Immune Changes in Pregnancy

11.2.1 Cytokines and Immune Cells

During preimplantation period, a number of cytokines influence the growth of the embryo. These cytokines include GM-CSF, heparin-binding epidermal growth factor (HB-EGF), insulin-like growth factor-I (IGF-I), and IGF-II. In contrast, TNF and IFNγ impair embryonal growth [1, 2]. HLA-G expression on embryo is an important factor during this period.

Implantation occurs approximately 1 week after conception. Complex molecular interactions occur between primed uterus and developing embryo under the influence of various hormones to bring about successful implantation. Syncytiotrophoblasts have numerous microvilli at its apical surface which interdigitates with similar protrusions of uterine epithelium called pinopodes. Apart from hormones various cytokines, chemokines, adhesion molecules, and cells of innate and adaptive immunity take part in orchestrating implantation.

Uterine natural killer (NK) cells are one of the most abundant immune cells in human decidua. Even though these cells are morphologically similar to circulating NK cells, they express a different pattern of cell surface markers and distinct set of granules. Uterine NK cells are CD56 bright CD16− in contrast to CD56 dim CD16+ circulating NK cells. Inhibition of uterine NK cells through receptors like NK2GDR plays an important role in maintaining pregnancy. Uterine NK cells also have angiogenic functions resulting in decidual vasculature that accompanies placental development [3, 4].

Decidual macrophages are the predominant antigen-presenting cells in decidua and account for 20–25% of total decidual leukocytes. During pregnancy the decidual macrophages have an M2 phenotype; that is, they are alternatively activated macrophages. M2 macrophages produce inhibitory cytokines like IL-10 and TGFβ1 resulting in immune tolerance to allogeneic fetus. These cells also have some role in trophoblastic invasion [5].

Compared to other dendritic cells (DC), decidual DCs have increased expression of CD80/86 and IDO and decreased expression of IL-12. Thus, these DCs behave as immunoregulatory DCs and lead to proliferation of regulatory T cells [6].

T cells account for 10% of the leukocytes in the decidual tissue of early pregnancy. They differ from peripheral T cells by expression of activation markers such as CD45RO, CD69, HLA-DR, and CD25, but their function and mechanism of fetus-specific immune recognition remain unclear [7]. The classical "Th1/Th2" hypothesis suggests that a predominance of Th2 immunity over Th1 immunity occurs during pregnancy which is responsible for maternal tolerance. However, Th1/Th2 paradigm was found to be insufficient to explain various pregnancy complications in systemic autoimmune disorders. Th17 cells produce IL-17 and mediate the induction of inflammation. Higher levels of Th17 cells are associated with miscarriages and prematurity. Activation of regulatory T cells is essential for successful completion of pregnancy and fetomaternal tolerance. Pregnancy complications like recurrent miscarriage and preeclampsia were found to be associated with lower numbers of T regulatory cells. Together a tightly regulated balance between Th1, Th2, Th17, and Treg cells is required for maintenance of pregnancy [8]. Role of antibodies and B cells in maintenance of pregnancy is not very clear. IL-10-producing regulatory B cells are probably important in pregnancy maintenance [9].

The mechanism behind these changes in immune system is probably the changes in the hormone levels during pregnancy. Most immune cells have receptors for female sex hormones. HCG ensures a continual supply of ovarian progesterone and helps in maintenance of pregnancy. Progesterone initially produced by the corpus luteum and later by the placenta is the most important factor in the maintenance of pregnancy. Along with estrogen, HCG plays an important role in immune cell trafficking and regulatory T-cell development.

11.2.2 Fetoplacental Factors Contributing to Tolerance

Placental and early fetal tissues lack classical HLA molecules. Instead they express HLA-G, -E, and -C [10]. These HLA molecules interact with inhibitory receptors on uterine NK cells and inhibit their cytotoxicity. In addition, placenta expresses high level of inhibitory receptor PDL1 which inhibits T-cell proliferation and activation, thus helping in the maintenance of fetal tolerance [11].

11.2.3 Microchimerism

During pregnancy there can be bidirectional transfer of cells across placental barrier. This can lead to presence of genetically distinct population of non-host cell surviving and proliferating in host. This is called microchimerism. Role of microchimerism is suggested in pathogenesis of many autoimmune diseases and may partly explain the behavior of some of the connective tissue disorders in pregnancy [12].

11.3 Pregnancy and Rheumatic Diseases

11.3.1 Rheumatoid Arthritis

Rheumatoid arthritis is a disease that has a moderate female bias and occurs in reproductive-age group. Thus, a fair number of pregnancies occur in patients with

RA. Patients with RA typically show improvement in arthritis during pregnancy. As much as 48–62% have some improvement in arthritis while 16–27% undergo complete remission during pregnancy [13, 14]. At least a half of patients experience relief in first trimester which lasts throughout pregnancy. Improvement in arthritis is more in seronegative patients (75%) than patients with seropositive RA (RF or ACPA positivity) [15]. In seropositive patients, there is no correlation of clinical improvement of arthritis with levels of RF or CCP. It was also shown that the higher the degree of class II HLA disparity between mother and fetus, the more the chance of improvement [16].

In postpartum period there is increased risk of flare of arthritis. This flare can occur over next 3–6 months and nearly 90% of patients will have clinical worsening. Risk of development of RA is also increased after pregnancy, with maximum risk in first 12 months postpartum. Presence of RF during pregnancy predicts the development of new-onset RA postpartum.

11.3.2 Seronegative Spondyloarthritis

Spondyloarthritis (SpA) are a group of diseases that are more common and severe in men. They are characterized by lower limb arthritis and inflammatory back pain. As they are believed to occur due to innate immune system activation, effect of pregnancy is minimal.

There is no significant improvement or worsening of arthritis during pregnancy in patients with SpA. There is no data on the onset of SpA during pregnancy. In patients with active arthritis, disease continues to be active in first and second trimesters with some improvement in third trimester [17]. In patients with long-standing disease, changes in the pelvic dimension may affect the mechanism of labor necessitating caesarean section.

There can be dramatic improvement in skin lesions of psoriasis during pregnancy. Skin lesions improve in 40–60% of women, worsen in 10–20%, and remain stable in the remainder during pregnancy [18]. Skin flare can occur in postpartum period Behavior of psoriatic arthritis in relation to various stages of pregnancy is not well characterized.

11.3.3 Systemic Lupus Erythematosus

Data on the behavior of SLE in pregnancy is confusing and remains controversial. Lack of uniformity in defining flare, heterogeneity in populations, and multiple confounders in various studies have contributed to confusion. Often differentiating lupus disease activity from clinical features of preeclampsia can be difficult. Based on recent studies, there is two- to threefold increase in SLE activity during pregnancy [19–21]. Risk of any flare in pregnancy is 35–70% with 15–30% risk of moderate-to-severe flare. Renal flares are more common than other manifestations

(43% of all flare) [20, 21]. Flare of arthritis is less common. Factors predicting flare in pregnancy are

(a) Active disease during the 6 months prior to conception
(b) Nephritis in past
(c) Discontinuation of hydroxychloroquine
(d) Primigravida

Prolonged remission period before pregnancy decreases the likelihood of flare. Decreased flare rate in third trimester has been reported in a recent study presumably because of blunted IL-6 response due to lower levels of estrogen. One-third of patients experience flares in postpartum period.

11.3.4 Mixed Connective Tissue Disorder

Mixed connective tissue disease (MCTD) is a rare disorder that affects young females and presents with Raynaud's phenomenon, sclerodactyly, interstitial lung disease, pulmonary artery hypertension, arthritis, and myositis. In a series of ten patients with MCTD, three had flare during pregnancy [22]. There are reports of clinical flare with proteinuria, myositis, and synovitis in patients with MCTD. However large-scale data is not available to make a definitive conclusion. Patients with ILD and PAH may have worsening of symptoms due to increase demand during pregnancy as well as restriction of lung movements due to growing fetus.

11.3.5 Sjogren's Syndrome

Sjogren's syndrome (SS) presents with dry eyes, dry mouth, and extra-glandular manifestations. There are only case reports of new-onset renal disease and pericarditis in women with SS during pregnancy. Studies involving larger population and validated tools to measure disease activity are required to see the actual effect of pregnancy on Sjogren's disease.

11.3.6 Antiphospholipid Syndrome

Obstetric APS, eclampsia, and HELLP are discussed elsewhere in the book. Catastrophic antiphospholipid syndrome, vascular thrombosis, and severe thrombocytopenia are reported in pregnant patients with antiphospholipid syndrome. Whether pregnancy increases these manifestations is still unclear.

11.3.7 Systemic Sclerosis

Unlike other connective tissue disorders, it is difficult to assess the disease activity of systemic sclerosis in pregnancy. Monitoring tools including mRSS are less sensitive to changes occurring over short duration. Many symptoms like arthralgia, reflux, and puffiness of extremities can occur in normal pregnancy and thus it is difficult to attribute these to disease flare.

In general, there is no exacerbation of SSc in pregnancy. In one large study that involved 99 pregnant women with SSc disease remained stable in most patients. Four patients, all of whom were Scl-70 positive, had disease progression within 1 year of delivery [23]. Ten-year cumulative survival for women who had scleroderma with and without pregnancy is similar [24].

Raynaud's symptoms generally improve in pregnancy presumably due to increased blood flow. Gastric reflux symptoms tend to worsen. Significant PAH is a contraindication for pregnancy as these patients may not tolerate fluid shifts during pregnancy.

There is no increased incidence of renal crisis in pregnancy. However, scleroderma renal crisis in pregnancy is associated with adverse maternal outcomes. It is often difficult to clinically differentiate between preeclampsia and scleroderma renal crisis.

11.3.8 Idiopathic Inflammatory Myositis

In general, risk of flare in quiescent disease is low. However, disease onset during pregnancy is associated with a severe course with complications including rhabdomyolysis and myoglobinuria described in literature [25].

11.3.9 Vasculitis

Pregnancy in ANCA vasculitis as such is a rare event owing to rarity of disease and age group in which the disease is more common. Hence, large-scale data on pregnancy and outcomes is not available in GPA, MPA, or EGPA. Twenty to forty percent of patients can have flare of disease during pregnancy [26]. Pregnancy is usually uneventful in well-controlled ANCA vasculitis with a significant duration of remission. Those conceiving with active disease remain active.

Monitoring disease activity can be a real challenge in pregnancy because acute-phase reactants can be affected by physiological changes in pregnancy. Imaging for pulmonary lesions can also be difficult in the setting of pregnancy.

Effect of pregnancy on PAN is unclear. However, PAN has a natural course with minimal relapse and is unlikely that PAN in remission flares during pregnancy.

Takayasu arteritis is a disease of young females. It is therefore important to understand the natural history of disease during pregnancy. Pregnancy does not seem to have a significant effect on disease activity in large-vessel vasculitis. <5% of Takayasu arteritis patients flare in pregnancy [26]. However, in Takayasu arteritis, hemodynamic changes in various stages of pregnancy can have effect on already damaged vascular areas. Congestive cardiac failure, acute kidney injury, ruptured aneurysm, and cerebral hemorrhage have been described. Complication mostly occurs during parturition when fluid shift and cardiovascular load are maximum.

In contrast to other vasculitides, up to 60% Behcet's remain stable or improve during pregnancy [26]. There are reports of thrombotic episodes developing during pregnancy. However attributable risk of developing thrombosis in Behcet's is not clear as pregnancy in itself is a hypercoagulable state.

11.4 Summary

Immune changes in pregnancy seem to have a beneficial effect on disease activity in RA which is probably related to skewing of immune response towards Th2 and regulatory T cells. In contrast, SLE patients generally have increased disease activity during pregnancy. For most of the connective tissue disorders there is insufficient data on the course of disease during pregnancy (Table 11.1).

Table 11.1 Effect of pregnancy on common rheumatic diseases

Disease	Activity during pregnancy	Comments
Rheumatoid arthritis	50–60% have improvement in arthritic symptoms	Remission more in seronegative patients Postpartum worsening of disease activity in up to 90% 10% may start RA in postpartum period
Spondyloarthropathy	No significant change in disease	
Psoriasis	Skin lesions improve in up to 60%	No large data on activity of arthritis
Lupus	Flares in about 10–30% of patients	Increased risk with active disease at conception, lupus nephritis, stoppage of HCQ One-third may flare in postpartum phase
Systemic sclerosis	No exacerbation in pregnancy No increased incidence of renal crisis	GE reflux may worsen SRC associated with poor pregnancy outcome
ANCA-associated vasculitis	20–40% can flare	–
Takayasu arteritis	<5% flare	Increased incidence of complication in pregnancy

References

1. Yockey LJ, Interferons IA (2018) Proinflammatory cytokines in pregnancy and fetal development. Immunity 49(3):397–412
2. Leach RE, Khalifa R, Ramirez ND et al (1999) Multiple roles for heparin-binding epidermal growth factor-like growth factor are suggested by its cell-specific expression during the human endometrial cycle and early placentation. J Clin Endocrinol Metab 84(9):3355–3363
3. Moffett-King A (2002) Natural killer cells and pregnancy. Nat Rev Immunol 2(9):656–663
4. Rätsep MT, Felker AM, Kay VR, Tolusso L, Hofmann AP, Croy BA (2015) Uterine natural killer cells: supervisors of vasculature construction in early decidua basalis. Reproduction 149(2):R91–R102
5. Ning F, Liu H, Lash GE (2016) The role of decidual macrophages during normal and pathological pregnancy. Am J Reprod Immunol 75(3):298–309
6. Gardner L, Moffett A (2003) Dendritic cells in the human decidua. Biol Reprod 69(4):1438–1446
7. Saito S, Nishikawa K, Morii T, Narita N, Enomoto M, Ichijo M (1992) Expression of activation antigens CD69, HLA-DR, interleukin-2 receptor-alpha (IL-2R alpha) and IL-2R beta on T cells of human decidua at an early stage of pregnancy. Immunology 75(4):710–712
8. Feyaerts D, Benner M, van Cranenbroek B, van der Heijden OWH, Joosten I, van der Molen RG (2017) Human uterine lymphocytes acquire a more experienced and tolerogenic phenotype during pregnancy. Sci Rep 7(1):2884
9. Guzman-Genuino RM, Diener KR (2017) Regulatory B cells in pregnancy: lessons from autoimmunity, graft tolerance, and cancer. Front Immunol 8:172
10. Hunt JS, Langat DK, McIntire RH, Morales PJ (2006) The role of HLA-G in human pregnancy. Reprod Biol Endocrinol 4(Suppl 1):S10
11. Petroff MG, Kharatyan E, Torry DS, Holets L (2005) The immunomodulatory proteins B7-DC, B7-H2, and B7-H3 are differentially expressed across gestation in the human placenta. Am J Pathol 167(2):465–473
12. Kinder JM, Stelzer IA, Arck PC, Way SS (2017) Immunological implications of pregnancy-induced microchimerism. Nat Rev Immunol 17(8):483–494
13. Ince-Askan H, Hazes JMW, Dolhain RJEM (2017) Identifying clinical factors associated with low disease activity and remission of rheumatoid arthritis during pregnancy. Arthritis Care Res (Hoboken) 69(9):1297–1303
14. Barrett JH, Brennan P, Fiddler M, Silman AJ (1999) Does rheumatoid arthritis remit during pregnancy and relapse postpartum? Results from a nationwide study in the United Kingdom performed prospectively from late pregnancy. Arthritis Rheum 42(6):1219–1227
15. de Man YA, Bakker-Jonges LE, Goorbergh CM et al (2010) Women with rheumatoid arthritis negative for anti-cyclic citrullinated peptide and rheumatoid factor are more likely to improve during pregnancy, whereas in autoantibody-positive women autoantibody levels are not influenced by pregnancy. Ann Rheum Dis 69(2):420–423
16. Zrour SH, Boumiza R, Sakly N et al (2010) The impact of pregnancy on rheumatoid arthritis outcome: the role of maternofetal HLA class II disparity. Joint Bone Spine 77(1):36–40
17. Østensen M, Villiger PM, Förger F (2012) Interaction of pregnancy and autoimmune rheumatic disease. Autoimmun Rev 11(6–7):A437–A446
18. Murase JE, Chan KK, Garite TJ, Cooper DM, Weinstein GD (2005) Hormonal effect on psoriasis in pregnancy and postpartum. Arch Dermatol 141(5):601–606
19. Clowse MEB, Magder LS, Witter F, Petri M (2005) The impact of increased lupus activity on obstetric outcomes. Arthritis Rheum 52(2):514–521
20. Doria A, Ghiradello A, Iaccarino L et al (2004) Pregnancy, cytokines, and disease activity in systemic lupus erythematosus. Arthritis Rheum 51:989–995
21. Petri M (2007) The Hopkins Lupus Pregnancy Center: ten key issues in management. Rheum Dis Clin North Am 33(2):227–235, v
22. Kitridou RC (2005) Pregnancy in mixed connective tissue disease. Rheum Dis Clin N Am 31(3):497–508

23. Taraborelli M, Ramoni V, Brucato A et al (2012 Jun) Brief report: successful pregnancies but a higher risk of preterm births in patients with systemic sclerosis: an Italian multicenter study. Arthritis Rheum 64(6):1970–1977
24. Steen VD, Conte C, Day N et al (1989) Pregnancy in women with systemic sclerosis. Arthritis Rheum 32(2):151–157
25. Kofteridis DP, Malliotakis PI, Sotsiou F, Vardakis NK, Vamvakas LN, Emmanouel DS (1999) Acute onset of dermatomyositis presenting in pregnancy with rhabdomyolysis and fetal loss. Scand J Rheumatol 28(3):192–194
26. Gatto M, Iaccarino L, Canova M, Zen M et al (2012) Pregnancy and vasculitis: a systematic review of the literature. Autoimmun Rev 11(6–7):A447–A459

Management of Lupus Flare During Pregnancy

12

Rajeswari Sankaralingam

Abstract

Systemic lupus erythematosus (SLE)/lupus continues to be the ten-headed monster posing challenges in diagnosis and management during all periods of life especially during pregnancy, when associated with a flare. The flare may be mild, moderate, or severe. Usually there would be at least consideration of a change or increase in treatment. Many disease activity indices are present, and some of them are used in pregnancy after suitable modifications. Lupus being a great masquerader has to be differentiated when it flares from other conditions which have been lucidly presented in tables in this chapter. The poor prognostic markers and pregnancy planning have been discussed. Management of different types and difficult flares have been dealt with for easy reading and understanding.

Keywords

Lupus flare · Pregnancy · Outcome measures · APLA · Mimics

Systemic lupus erythematosus (SLE)/lupus continues to be the ten headed monster posing challenges in diagnosis and management during all periods of life especially during pregnancy, when associated with a flare. The flare may be mild, moderate, or severe. A flare has been defined and described differently. In simple term it means "a measurable increase in disease activity in one or more organ systems involving new, worsening clinical signs, symptoms and laboratory measurements." It must be considered clinically significant by the assessor. Usually there would be at least consideration of a change or increase in treatment. This definition was framed by the Lupus foundation of America in 2006 [1]. A pragmatic definition of a "major" flare defined by Fortin and colleagues includes new or increased use of

R. Sankaralingam (✉)
Sri Ramachandra Institute of Higher Education and Research, Chennai, India

© Springer Nature Singapore Pte Ltd. 2020
S. K. Sharma (ed.), *Women's Health in Autoimmune Diseases*,
https://doi.org/10.1007/978-981-15-0114-2_12

immunosuppressive therapy, new or increased use of corticosteroids greater than 0.5 mg/kg/day, and hospitalization or death because of SLE disease activity [2, 3].

Many disease activity indices (DAI), responder indices (RIs), and health-related quality of life (HRQOL) have been adapted after a period of time.

Among these, the SLE disease activity index (SLEDAI) has been validated. It has modified versions.

Like the SELENA-SLEDAI and SLEDAI, which measure disease activity over the past 28–30 days to assess improvement, the SLEDAI 2K Responder Index 50 (52K RI 50) indicates a 50% improvement in the 24 descriptors [4].

The SLICC (Systemic Lupus International Collaborating Clinic) developed the SLE damage index (SDI) which calculates damage from disease activity, medications, and comorbid conditions for a duration of 6 months.

The indices used in pregnancy are SLEPDAI (Systemic Lupus Erythematosus Pregnancy Disease Activity Index), LAI-P (Lupus Activity Index in Pregnancy), and MSLAM (Modified Systemic Lupus Activity Measure). The SLEDAI has 24 descriptors and 15 are modified. LAI-P has a sensitivity and specificity of >90%. Here the physician's Global Assessment and asthenia have been eliminated. Asthenia has been replaced by fever, a CNS score of 3, anti-dsDNA and complement, scoring a maximum of 2.

As SLE is a disease of relapses, damage can occur. Early accrual of damage reflects poor prognosis with increased mortality. Different organs have different SLEDAI and SDI (Table 12.1) [5].

However ultimately an exhaustive history, meticulous physical examination, along with the respective laboratory investigations, will help in the identification of the type of organ flare and also to assess the disease activity. The rate of lupus flares at conception increases to 60% in active disease (Table 12.2).

In this chapter the key points will be:

1a. Identification of a flare in lupus pregnancy.
1b. Preconception counselling.
1c. Contraindications.
2a. Differences between normal and lupus pregnancy.
2b. Poor prognostic factors.
3a. Types of organ flares in pregnancy.
3b. Types of adverse outcomes.
4. Types of flares based on severity, in pregnancy.
5. Differentiation between lupus pregnancy flares and associations, e.g., TTP, eclampsia, lupus nephritis flare, fatty liver of pregnancy, HELLP, catastropic antiphospholipid syndrome.
6. How to identify flares.
7. Management of flares.
8. Maternal and fetal complications.
9. Postpartum management.
10. Recent advances.

Table 12.1 SLEPDAI [5]

Score	Descriptor	Modified for pregnancy	Considerations
8	Seizure	Yes	r/o Eclampsia
8	Psychosis	No	
8	Organic brain syndrome	No	
8	Visual disturbance	No	Hypertension is already considered an exclusion in SELENA-SLEDAI and SLEDAI
8	Cranial nerve disorder	Yes	r/o Bell palsy
8	Lupus headache	Yes	
8	CVA	Yes	r/o Eclampsia
8	Vasculitis	Yes	Consider palmar erythema
4	Arthritis	Yes	Consider bland knee effusions
4	Myositis	No	
4	Urinary casts	No	
4	Hematuria	Yes	r/o Cystitis and vaginal RBC reflective of placental problems
4	Proteinuria	Yes	r/o Eclampsia
4	Pyuria	Yes	r/o Infection
2	Rash	Yes	Consider chloasma
2	Alopecia	Yes	Consider normal postpartum alopecia
2	Mucosal ulcers	No	
2	Pleurisy	Yes	Hyperventilation may be secondary to progesterone, dyspnea secondary to enlarging uterus
2	Pericarditis	No	
2	Low complement	Yes	Complements normally rise during pregnancy
2	Increased DNA binding	No	
1	Thrombocytopenia	Yes	r/o Preeclampsia, HELLP syndrome, incidental thrombocytopenia of pregnancy
1	Leukopenia	Yes	Consider normal rise of leukocyte count during pregnancy
1	Fever	No	

SLE pregnancy losses in stable disease have reduced to 17% [7]. As per the PROMISSE study, 80% of 333 women had a favorable pregnancy outcome (defined as the absence of fetal/neonatal death). Flares can occur in pregnancy in the postpartum period too. The frequency is lowest in the third trimester.

The rate of flares is 13.5–65%. Validated measures of disease activity have been found to have a two- to threefold increase in disease activity during pregnancy. The most common organs involved are the skin, kidneys, blood, and joints among which renal and hematological flares are the commonest.

Table 12.2 LUPUS ACTIVITY INDEX - PREGNANCY [6]

Group	Parameter	Point values				Values to calculate LAI-P
1	Fever	0	1			(a) Mean
	Rash	0		2		
	Arthritis	0		2	3	
	Serositis	0	1	2	3	
2	Neurologic	0			3	(b) Maximum
	Renal	0		2	3	
	Lung	0			3	
	Hematologic	0	1	2	3	
	Vasculitis	0			3	
	Myositis	0			3	
3	Prednisone, NSAID, HCQ	0	1	2	3	(c) Mean
	Immunosuppressor	0			3	
4	Proteinuria	0	1	2	3	(d) Mean
	Anti-DNA	0	1	2		
	C3, C4	0	1	2		

Point value of LAI-P = $(a + b + c + d)/4$
HCQ hydroxychloroquine, *LAI-P* lupus activity index in pregnancy

How to recognize a lupus flare in a pregnancy? It is difficult because it can mimic symptoms of normal pregnancy. Multiple predictors of flare have been listed, e.g., disease activity at conception, lupus nephritis, discontinuation of medicines, especially hydroxychloroquine (Table 12.3).

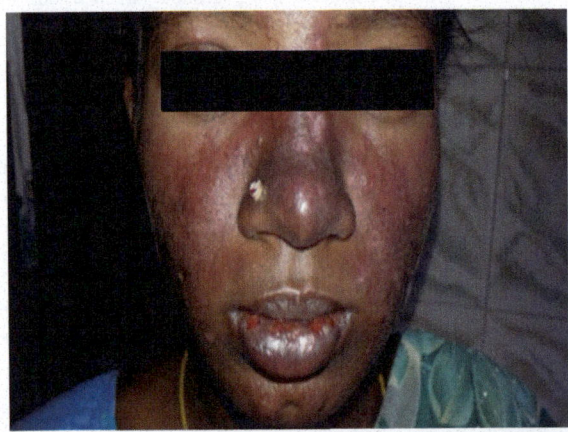

Decline in serum complement levels during pregnancy is associated with poor pregnancy outcomes. SLE disease activity indices have not included pregnancy changes (Tables 12.4 and 12.5).

12 Management of Lupus Flare During Pregnancy

Table 12.3 Recognition of a flare in lupus pregnancy

Organ	Normal	Cause	Lupus	Cause
Cutaneous (a) Facial flush	Centrofacial over cheeks, forehead, upper lip, nose, chin, malar, mandibular		Edematous, erythematous fine scaling, no atrophy	
Palmar erythema	Yes	Estrogen-related vadodilatation	Yes	Vasculitis
Musculoskeletal	Fatigue Back pain Bland knee effusion		Fatigue Lethargy Inflammatory arthritis	
Respiratory system	Dyspnea	Central effects—progesterone	Pleurisy	
Hematological	Mild anemia	Hemodilution	Hemolytic anemia, positive Coomb's test ↑Reticulocyte count ↑LDH	

Table 12.4 Investigations differentiating normal pregnancy and lupus

	Normal		Lupus
First trimester	↑WBC		
30 weeks	Plateau	Neutrophilia	Lymphopenia <1000/mm
	↓Platelet	1–1.5/cm mm (mild)	↓Platelet (to exclude PET/EC)
ESR	↑Mild		↑Inflammatory makers
Proteinuria	Physiologic <300 mg/day		Active urine sediments, proteinuria >300 mg/day
GFR	↑>50%		
BUN	↓		>13 mg%
Serum creatinine	↓		>0.8 mg%
Complement	↑	↑Hepatic synthesis of estrogen	Normal or ↓C3, C4, CH50↓ by 25% or >
Anti-dsDNA	Negative		Positive Second trimester of pregnancy ↑Pregnancy loss

Table 12.5 Differences between normal pregnancy and lupus flare

Feature		Findings indicative of a lupus flare	Findings of normal pregnancy that can mimic a flare
Clinical		Active rash of lupus Inflammatory arthritis Lymphadenopathy	Fatigue Arthralgias Bland effusions of knees
		Fever >38 °C (not related to infection or drug)	Myalgias Malar and palmar erythema Postpartum hair loss
		Pleuritis	Carpal tunnel syndrome Edema of hands, legs, and face Mild resting dyspnea
		Pericarditis	
ESR		Increased	18–46 mm/h <20 weeks gestation 30–70 mm/h ≥20 weeks gestation
Anemia		Hemoglobin <10.5 g/dL	Hemoglobin >11 g/dL during first 20 weeks gestation Hemoglobin >10.5 g/dL after 20 weeks gestation
Thrombocytopenia		Platelet count <95,000/μL	Mild in approximately 8%
Urinalysis		Hematuria or cellular casts	Rare hematuria from vaginal contamination
Proteinuria		≥300 mg/day	<300 mg/day
dsDNA antibodies		Rising titers	Negative or stable titers
Complement		≥25% drop	Usually increased

ESR erythrocyte sedimentation rate

12.1 Comparison of Lupus Pregnancy and Normal Pregnancy

There are various similarities and differences in the hormonal and immune responses between a pregnant lupus patient and woman with normal pregnancy as illustrated (Table 12.6) [8].

Normal pregnancy is associated with hemodilution. There is progesterone-induced smooth muscle relaxation and compression of the ureters by the gravid uterus, the end result being pyelonephritis and symptomatic urolithiasis. The other manifestations mimicking lupus include arthralgia, myalgia, facial and palmar rash, edema of face, hands and legs, hearing loss, shortness of breath, and carpal tunnel syndrome.

Table 12.6 Comparison of immunological and hormonal response between lupus pregnancy and normal pregnancy

S. no.	Parameters	Pregnancy Normal	Pregnancy Lupus	Outcomes
1	TH17-IL17	↑	↑	Preeclampsia, fetal loss
2	Estradiol + progesterone (second and third trimesters)	↑	↓	Impairs placental function and fetal loss
3	IL-10	First trimester—↓ Third trimester—↑	↑ in all trimesters	B-cell stimulation
4	Treg cells	↑	↓	Disease activity
5	Chemokines CXCL-8, IL-8 CXCL-9, MIG CXCL-10, IP-10	↓	↑	↑Flares and complications
6	Ficolin 3	↓	↑	Hemolysis
7	IFN-α	↓	↑	Preeclampsia
8	C4d	↓	↑	↓Placental weight
9	Prolactin	↓	↑	
10	IL-6	↓/N	↑	
11	sTNFαR	↓	↑	

12.2 Checklist for Counselling and Pregnancy Planning for Patients with SLE [8]

1. Risk assessment
   (a) Age
   (b) Previous pregnancies
   (c) Disease activity assessment
   (d) Irreversible damage
2. Autoantibodies
   (a) Antiphospholipid antibodies
   (b) Anti Ro/La
3. Current treatment adjustments
4. Pregnancy-contraindicated if
   (a) SLE Disease Activity Index (SLEDAI >8)
   (b) High irreversible damage
5. Drugs which are contraindicated to be replaced by safe ones-wait for remission for at least 2–3 months
6. Treat active disease
7. Prophylaxis
   (a) *Low-dose Aspirin*: First trimester onwards till delivery to reduce preeclampsia especially in patients with lupus nephritis.

(b) *Prophylaxis*: Preeclampsia and thrombosis in patients with positive antiphospholipid antibodies.
(c) *Pregnancy*: Planned only when the disease is in remission both clinically and by investigations for at least 6 months.
(d) *Thyroid Function*: Should be assessed as hypothyroidism in SLE is associated with poor outcomes.

12.3 Situations Where Pregnancy Is Not Advisable [8]

1. Severe pulmonary hypertension (systemic pressure >50 mmHg).
2. Severe restrictive lung disease (forced vital capacity <1 L).
3. Advanced renal insufficiency (serum creatinine >2.8 mg%).
4. 24 hour urine protein >0.5 g.
5. Advanced heart failure.
6. Previous severe preeclampsia or hemolysis, elevated liver enzymes, low platelet count (HELLP) despite treatment.

12.4 Differences Between Preeclampsia and Lupus Nephritis in Pregnancy

It is important to differentiate preeclampsia from lupus nephritis in pregnancy as depicted in Table 12.7.

12.5 Poor Prognostic Markers [8]

1. Active disease 6 months prior to pregnancy
2. Maternal hypertension
3. Previous fetal loss
4. Active renal lupus
5. Serum creatinine >2.8 mg%
6. SLE onset during pregnancy
7. Presence of APS
8. High anti-dsDNA titers
9. Low complements
10. Proteinuria
11. Thrombocytopenia
12. Comorbid States
    (a) Diabetes mellitus
    (b) Hypertension
    (c) Pulmonary hypertension
    (d) Older age at conception
    (e) Renal failure

Table 12.7 Differences between preeclampsia and lupus nephritis in pregnancy

S. no.	Parameters	Normal	Pre-eclampsia	Lupus nephritis
1	Hypertension	–	After 20 weeks	Anytime
2	Hemolysis	–	Severe	Present
3	Platelets	↓	Normal or ↓	Normal or ↓
4	GFR	↑		
5	Creatinine clearance	↑ by 30%		
6	Serum creatinine	<0.9 (↓)	Normal or ↑	Normal or ↑
7	LFT	Normal expect ↑ ALP	↑	↑
8	Uric acid	↓	↑>5.5 mg%	Normal
9	Anti-dsDNA	Absent	Absent	↑
10	24 hours urine (a) Calcium (b) Protein		<195 mg% –	>195 mg% Doubling of previous value or >3 g/day
11	Urine sediments		Inactive	Active-cellular RBC casts, dysmorphic RBC's and cylinders
12	Other organs		Occasionally- CNS HELLP	Active Non renal +
13	Steroid response		No	Yes
14	Serum sFLT-1		↑	–
15	Placental growth factor		+	–

(f) Preeclampsia (30%), eclampsia, HELLP
(g) Thormbophilia
(h) Sepsis, pneumonia, anemia
(i) Ante-partum and postpartum hemorrhage
(j) Deep vein thrombosis (0.4%) and stroke (0.32%)
(k) Pulmonary thromboembolism

12.6 Definitions

It is worthwhile remembering certain definitions to understand the issues related with lupus pregnancy.

12.6.1 Maternal Flare

Any clinical event attributable to disease activity that required a change in therapy.

12.6.2 Preexisting Lupus Nephritis

Confirmed by renal biopsy, documented proteinuria and on high-dose steroid before pregnancy, on greater than 15 mg prednisolone within 4 months of conception.

12.6.3 Renal Flare

New onset proteinuria greater than 0.5 g/day, urinary cellular casts or by renal biopsy after delivery (from conception to 1 month postpartum).

12.6.4 Acute Kidney Injury

1.5-fold increase in serum creatinine compared to baseline and serum creatinine more than 0.9 mg%

12.6.5 Preeclampsia (Toxemia)

A pregnancy complication occurring in the mother after 20 weeks of pregnancy, which manifests with new onset of high blood pressure (BP) >140/90 mmHg and proteinuria >0.3 g/day, without hypertension and <0.3 g/day at baseline.

12.6.6 Organ Flare [8]

Multi-organ flares are common in pregnant lupus patients especially when there is active disease. About 50% experience a flare during pregnancy. However, renal flares are very difficult to differentiate from preeclampsia, HELLP, and pregnancy-induced hypertension (PIH). LUPUS flares range from 7% to 33%. In active disease, at conception it increases to 60%. Postpartum flares also occur. Many studies have revealed the increased incidence of mucocutaneous, musculoskeletal, and most significantly renal and hematological flares. Active SLE with decreased platelet count in first trimester produces 44% fetal losses. Hypertension and preeclampsia occur in 35% of patients with lupus nephritis. HELLP syndrome occurs in 30–50% of lupus pregnancies as early as 15–20 weeks of gestation. Disease in remission 6–12 months before pregnancy produces less flares.

12.6.7 Lupus Nephritis

A renal flare is associated with proteinuria, hypertension, hematuria, low complement, and anti-dsDNA antibodies. Duration of a renal flare is an independent predictor of chronic kidney disease; preexisting lupus nephritis is associated with more renal flares. In nephrotic syndrome, heparin (either low molecular weight or unfractionated) can be given to prevent thromboembolism [9].

Superimposed preeclampsia is associated with worsening hypertension and 100% increase in proteinuria in patients with baseline hypertension and proteinuria greater than 0.3 g/day, respectively. 50% decrease in proteinuria by 6 months is associated with four times likelihood of achieving complete remission. Successful pregnancies are seen in 65–92% of lupus nephritis patients [10]. Tacrolimus is safe in pregnancy with renal involvement. The approach to manage pregnancy in lupus nephritis is given in Table 12.8 (algorithm).

12.6.8 Class IV Nephritis

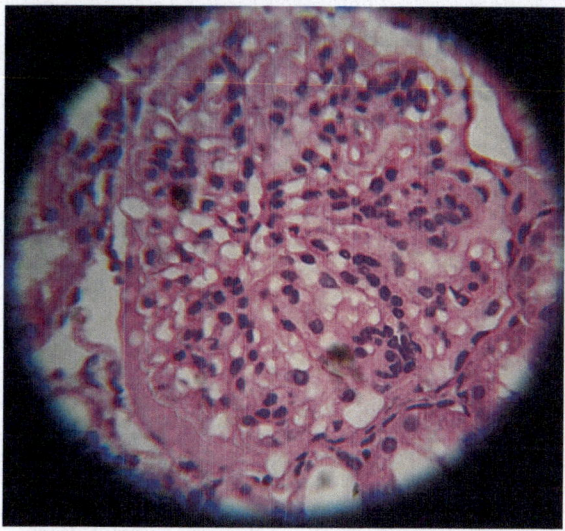

12.7 Renal Transplantation

Successful pregnancies are possible in renal transplant recipients. But there is an increased frequency of preeclampsia, low birth weight, and premature births. Pregnancy outcomes are better in patients on hydroxychloroquine, low-dose aspirin in the first trimester (primary prophylaxis for preeclampsia), clinically inactive SLE, serum creatinine <1.5 mg%, nonsignificant proteinuria <500 mg/day, and well-controlled hypertension.

Table 12.8 Algorithm for management of lupus nephritis in pregnancy

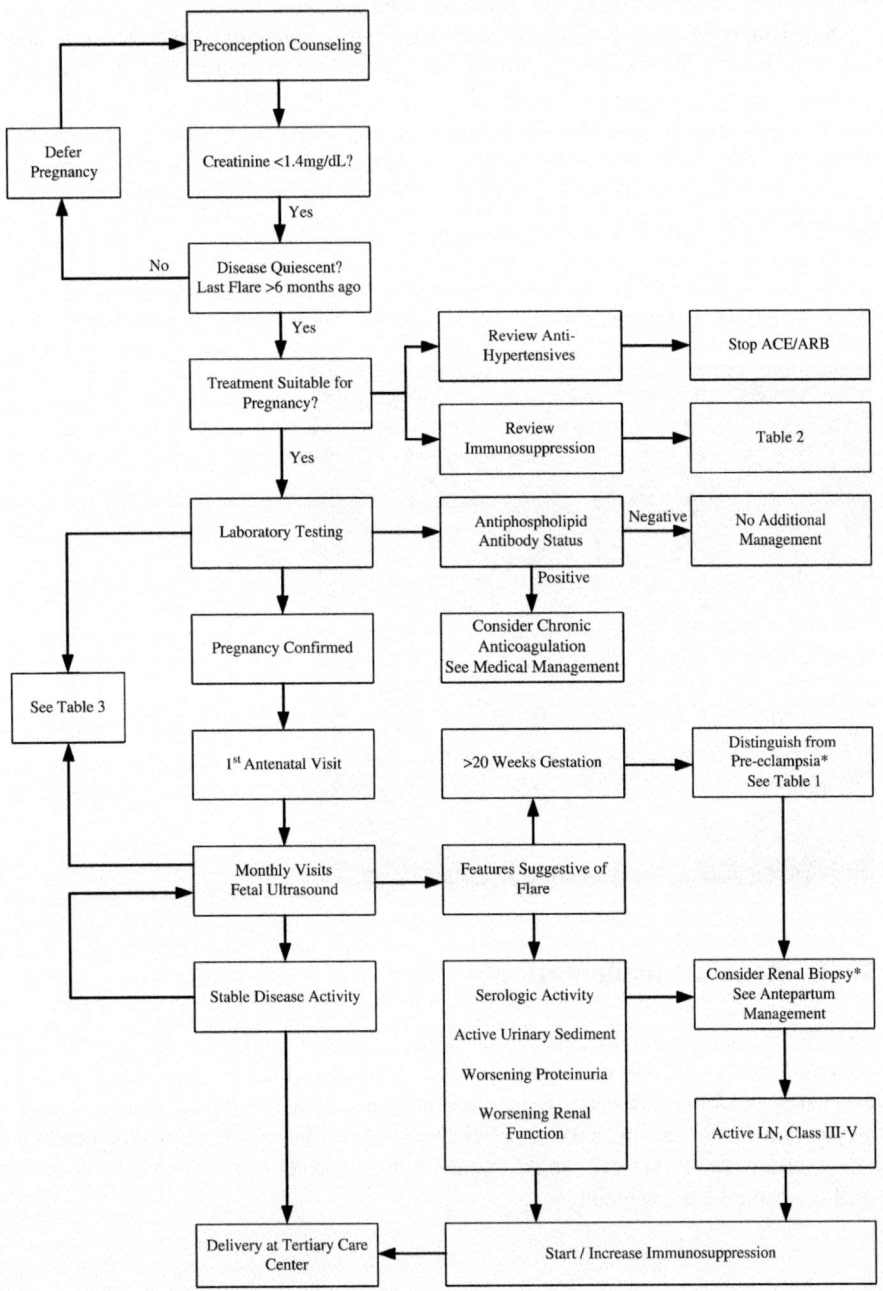

12.8 Other Organ Flares

Multiple studies have shown that whatever flare occurred in pregnancy had been present in the 6 months prior to conception. These were nephritis, serositis followed by hematological, cutaneous, and musculoskeletal flares.

12.9 Lupus Pregnancy and HELLP

The Tennessee Classification System diagnostic criteria for HELLP are hemolysis with increased lactate dehydrogenase (>600 U/L), aspartate aminotransferase (>70 U/L), and platelets <100,000/μL. The prothrombin time remains normal unless there is evidence of disseminated intravascular coagulation or severe liver injury [7].

Treatment of HELLP syndrome based on level IV evidence is rapid delivery after the 34th week of gestation.

12.10 Hematological Flares

Thrombocytopenia in lupus is a well-known phenomenon. Gestational thrombocytopenia is the most common type (75%) of cases, followed by preeclampsia/HELLP syndrome in 15–22% and autoimmune thrombocytopenia. The other important cause of low platelet count in pregnancy is thrombotic thrombocytopenic purpura (TTP) as target treatment can prevent complication like cerebral hemorrhage and organ failure, which can be a true challenge. In TTP the ADAMTS 13 is deficient and in hemolytic uremic syndrome (HUS), the deficiency is severe.

In acquired TTP, the treatment based on level III evidence is plasma exchange within 4–8 h. This reduces the maternal mortality in 90%.

In treatment of autoimmune thrombocytopenia invasive delivery methods should be avoided, the neonatal cord blood platelet should be checked in the immediate postpartum period and the following week. If it is below 50,000 a transcranial ultrasound is done. If it is below 20,000 with or without bleeding—IVIG or steroids are given with or without platelet transfusion to the neonate. Treatment of the mother requires IVIG and prednisolone to increase the count to 20,000–30,000 during pregnancy on just before or after delivery [11].

12.11 Acute Fatty Liver of Pregnancy

Acute fatty liver of pregnancy is a microvesicular fatty infiltration of hepatocytes that develop during the second half of pregnancy. It is a rare complication and resembles Reye's syndrome in its presentation with vomiting, hypoglycemia, lactic acidosis, hyperammonemia, elevated hepatic transaminases, conjugated hyperbilirubinemia, and evidence of disseminated intravascular coagulation. Hypertension, proteinuria, and thrombocytopenia are present in some cases, raising concern for preeclampsia and/or the HELLP syndrome. However, the finding of hypoglycemia points strongly to acute fatty liver as the correct diagnosis.

Treatment of acute fatty liver of pregnancy consists of fluids, glucose administration, correction of coagulopathy and immediate delivery. The value of plasma exchange is doubtful [7].

12.12 Peripheral Smear-Schistocytes (Tables 12.9 and 12.10)

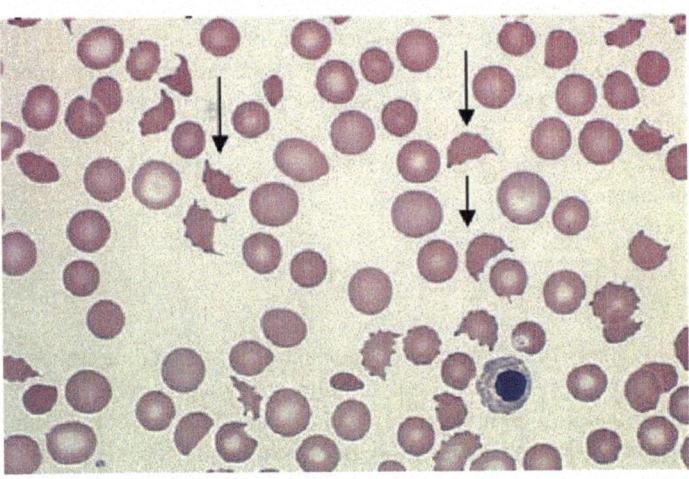

12.13 Antiphospholipid Syndrome

The presence of antiphospholipid antibody syndrome adds on to the thrombotic and obstetric complications and damage. Although formal studies are not available during pregnancy, triple positive patients receive aspirin and LMWH during pregnancy. Warfarin is contraindicated due to risk of warfarin embryopathy syndrome, especially in the first trimester. Reassuring data have put forth direct factor Xa inhibitor Fondaparinux which does not cross the placenta. Hydroxychloroquine is indicated. Role of statins is still under discussion.

12.14 Infections

High disease activity may predispose to infection and vice versa. Management of infections should be proactive. Vaccinations are a must, i.e., Pnemococcal (PCV13, PPSV23) and Influenza during stable disease. Role of Herpes Zoster vaccine in lupus is yet to be defined. Validated scores such as the quick SOFA are used now (systolic BP <100, RR >22/min, altered mental and Glasgow Coma Scale <15). The presence of ≥2 points near the onset of infection indicates poor outcome and a higher mortality rate.

Table 12.9 The differential diagnosis of microangiopathia and thrombocytopenia in pregnancy

Parameter	Preeclampsia	HELLP syndrome	TTP	aHUS	AFLP	APS	SLE
Hypertension	+++	+++	+	++	+	+/−	++
Proteinuria	+++	+++	+/−	+++	+/−	+/−	+++
Upper abdominal pain	+/−	+++	+/−	+/−	++	+/−	+/−
Neurologic deficits	+	+	++	+/−	+	+	+
Thrombocytopenia	+	+++	+++	+++	+	+	+
Hemolysis	+/−	+++	+++	+++	+	+/−	+
Renal dysfunction	+/−	+	+	+++	++	+/−	++
Elevated transaminases	+	+++	+/−	+/−	+++	+/−	+
Disseminated intravascular coagulation	+/−	+	+/−	+/−	+++	+/−	+/−
Peak incidence	Third trimester	Third trimester, postpartum	Second/third trimester	Postpartum	Third trimester		

Table 12.10 Differentiation of preeclampsia, HELLP syndrome, and active lupus nephritis

	Preeclampsia	HELLP syndrome	Active lupus nephritis
Timing in pregnancy	After 20 weeks of gestation	After 20 weeks of gestation	All gestational ages
Complement (C3, C4)	Normal	Normal	Typically decreased
Thrombocytopenia	Absent	Present	Present
Neutropenia	Absent	Absent	Present (benign in Membranous LN)
Active urine sediment	Absent	Absent	
Other organ involvement	Absent	Absent	Present
Anti-double-stranded DNA antibodies	Absent	Absent	Present
Anti-C1q antibodies	Normal	Normal	May be high
Abnormal liver function tests	Absent	Present	Absent
Serum uric acid	Increased	Increased	Normal (may be elevated with reduced GFR)
Hypertension (BP- 140/90 mmHg)	Present	Absent in 10–15%	Variable
Elevation in creatinine (1.2 mg/dL)	Typically absent	May occur in up to 10%	Commonly present

HELLP hemolysis, elevated liver enzymes, low platelet count

12.15 Mimics

Mimics of lupus flares include apart from the pregnancy changes, drug-induced dermatomyositis, psoriasis, Sjogren's syndrome with its complication, fibromyalgia, vasculitis, Kikuchi's disease, etc.

Drugs that are safe in pregnancy and lactation are given in Tables 12.11 and 12.12.

12.16 Glucocorticoids

The lowest possible dose should be given for the fetus with congenital heart block—either dexamethasone or betamethasone (4–8 mg/day) is given till the end of pregnancy. Side effects like cleft lip, palate, or both are associated with the use of glucocorticoids early in the pregnancy. High doses should be avoided in the first trimester. Preterm deliveries, fetal growth restriction, and behavioral childhood problems are encountered with higher doses. In the mother, hypertension, edema, gestational diabetes, and osteoporosis are side effects. Stress dose steroids should be given during labor in the peripartum period for patients already on steroids (24–48 h of hydrocortisone).

Table 12.11 Drugs for lupus in pregnancy and lactation [8]

S. no.	Stages		Names	FDA	Safe in lactation
1.	Antenatal	Without APS	HCQ 200–400 mg	C	Yes
		With APS	HCQ Aspirin-Low dose		
			Heparin, dalteparin		Yes
2.	(a) Flares		Prednisolone 10 mg/day		Yes
			Prednisolone <20 mg/day	C	Yes
			Avoid NSAIDS after 28 weeks Acetaminophen	C	Yes
	(b) Severe flares		Pulse steroid	C	Yes
3.	Breastfeeding		Oral corticosteroids (wait for 4 h after taking pill)	C	
4.	Severe flares immunosuppression				
	(a) Azathioprine		Safe 2 mg/kg/day	D	No
	(b) Cyclosporine		Lowest effective dose	C	No
	(c) Tacrolimus		Last resort		
	(d) IVIG			C	Yes
	(e) Cyclophosphamide			D	No

12.17 Recent Advances

The recent update on the classification criteria for SLE by both ACR and EULAR has reiterated that almost all patients are ANA positive. This has given additional weightage as entry criteria. The international consensus on remission combines the absence of inflammation with prednisolone dose not exceeding 5 mg/day. It also states that visual impairment is rare with hydroxychloroquine. Safety of belimumab and anifrolimumab has to be looked into.

12.18 Key Messages

Lupus pregnancy by itself still remains a challenge. Hence it is not surprising that dealing with flares in lupus pregnancy is like catching a tiger by its tail, considering the fact that both mother and fetus have to be treated with equal importance for normal survival. Grey areas like congenital heart block, other effects on the neonates and development of targeted therapies still remain as challenges. However, the future is not as bleak as it looks.

Table 12.12 Anti-inflammatory and immunosuppressive drugs in pregnancy

Drug name	Comments	FDA class	Breastfeeding
Corticosteroids	Risks of use often outweighed by risk of underlying disease. Risks for orofacial clefts (3 of 1000 births) and premature birth	C	Usually potential compatible
Hydroxychloroquine	Considered safe in pregnancy at 200–400 mg/day. Discontinuation during pregnancy associated with increased risk of lupus flare. May use for maintenance or mild flares.	Not assigned	Usually compatible
NSAID	Avoidance after 28 weeks of gestation because of the effects of related prostaglandin inhibition on the fetal cardiovascular system (closure of ductus arteriosus)	C	Usually NSAID-compatible
Cyclosporine	Can be maintained in pregnancy at lowest effective dose. No significant increase in rate of congenital malformations	C	Not recommended
Tacrolimus	Can be maintained in pregnancy at lowest effective dose. Potential risks of neonatal hyperkalemia and renal dysfunction	C	Not recommended
Rituximab	Limited safety data. May alter fetal and neonatal B cell	C	Not recommended
IVIG (g globulin)	Data are lacking but may be helpful for lupus nephritis flare refractory to medical therapy	C	Compatible
Azathioprine	May use for flare during pregnancy. Consider as alternative to mycophenolate. Avoid doses 1.5–2 mg/kg/day to risk of suppressed neonatal hematopoiesis	D	Not recommended
Mycophenolate mofetil	Contraindicated during pregnancy due to teratogenicity	D	Not recommended
Cyclophosphamide	Useful when maternal disease is life threatening. High risk of fetal loss, but less pronounced in more recent studies	D	Not recommended
Methotrexate	High risk of miscarriage and congenital abnormality. Treatment should be withdrawn 3 months before pregnancy	X	Not recommended

References

1. Ruperto N, Hanrahan LM, Alacorn GS et al (2011) International consensus for a definition of disease flare in lupus. Lupus 20(5):453–462
2. Fortin P, Ferland D, Clarke A (1997) Activity and damage predicts later flares in lupus. Arthritis Rheum 40:S207

3. Fortin P, Ferland D, Moore A (1998) Rates and predictors of lupus flares. Arthrits Rheum 41:S218
4. Touma Z, Gladman D, Ibanez D et al (2011) Development and initial validation of the systemic lupus erythematosus disease activity index 2000 responder index 50. J Rheumatol 38(2):275–284
5. Pastore DEA, Costa D, Parpinelli MA, Surita FG (2018) A critical review on obstetric follow-up of women affected by systemic lupus erythematosus. Rev Bras Ginecol Obstet 40:209–224. https://doi.org/10.1055/s-0038-1625951
6. Ruiz-Irastorza G, Khamashta MA, Gordon C et al (2004) Measuring systemic lupus erythematosus activity during pregnancy: validation of the lupus activity index in pregnancy scale. Arthritis Rheum 51(1):78–82
7. Stojan G, Baer AN (2012) Flares of systemic lupus erythematosus during pregnancy and the puerperium: prevention, diagnosis and management. Expert Rev Clin Immunol 8(5):439–453
8. Rajeswari S (2018) Pregnancy in systemic lupus erythematosus. In: Chaturvedi V (ed) Manual of rheumatology, vol 39. CBS Publishers & Distributors Pvt Ltd, pp 363–365
9. Stanhope TJ et al (2012) Obstetric nephrology: lupus and lupus nephritis in pregnancy. Clin J Am Soc Nephrol 7:2089–2099
10. Rajeswari S (2018) Pregnancy in systemic lupus erythematosus. In: Chaturvedi V (ed) Manual of rheumatology, vol 39. CBS Publishers & Distributors Pvt Ltd, pp 365–366
11. Myers B (2012) Diagnosis and management of maternal thrombocytopenia in pregnancy. Br J Haematol 158:3–15

Lupus Nephritis and Pregnancy

13

Manish Rathi

Abstract

Fertility in lupus patients is considered to be preserved as compared to general healthy population. While pregnancy outcomes have significantly improved in patients with SLE/LN, pregnancy in these patients is still at high risk of complications. Pregnancy may cause both short-term (flares) and long-term effects (progression to end-stage renal disease) on the course of LN. In addition, lupus increases the chances of maternal and fetal complications during pregnancy. Thus a pregnancy should be carefully planned in a lupus patient. The management of such patients is a multidisciplinary approach.

Keywords

Pregnancy · Lupus nephritis · Systemic lupus erythematosus

Case Vignette A 28-year-old female, married for 3 years, presented to the renal clinic with generalized swelling of the body, skin rash, and occasional low-grade fever of 3-month duration. On evaluation, her blood pressure was 150/90 mmHg; she had malar rash, anemia with normal platelets, and total leukocyte counts; ESR was 60. Her ANA was 3+ speckled pattern, anti-dsDNA antibodies were positive, and complement 3 (C3) and 4 (C4) were low. Urinalysis showed 3+ proteinuria, RBCs were 10-15/HPF, and her 24-h urine protein was 3.2 g/day. Serum albumin was 3.1 g/dL, creatinine was 0.8 mg/dL, and liver function tests and coagulation profile were normal. She fulfilled the clinical and laboratory criteria for systemic lupus erythematosus. Renal biopsy revealed class IV LN with activity index of 12/24 and chronicity index of 0/12. She was started on induction therapy with 1 mg/kg oral prednisolone along with 2 g/day of mycophenolate mofetil (MMF) in

---

M. Rathi (✉)
Department of Nephrology, Post Graduate Institute of Medical Education and Research, Chandigarh, India

divided doses. Adjunctive therapy included hydroxychloroquine (5 mg/kg/day), angiotensin receptor blocker (telmisartan 40 mg/day), calcium-vitamin D supplements, and statin (atorvastatin 10 mg/day). At the end of 6 months, her proteinuria reduced to 0.1 g/day, serum creatinine was 0.8 mg/dL, and serum albumin was 4.1 g/dL. Serology for anti-dsDNA was negative and C3 and C4 levels were normal. She was on 5 mg of prednisolone and 1 g/day of MMF with continuation of the adjunctive therapy, on which she was in complete remission for a period of 1 year. She wished to plan her family and was keen on knowing the outcomes and risks of pregnancy.

13.1 Is Fertility Affected by Lupus Nephritis?

Systemic lupus erythematosus (SLE), hence lupus nephritis (LN), predominantly affects females of reproductive-age group. Fertility in lupus patients is considered to be preserved as compared to general healthy population. However, exceptions to this observation are patients being treated with alkylating agents, patients with antiphospholipid antibodies, and those with advanced renal dysfunction [1]. The presence of LN in a patient with SLE imposes a risk of reduction in fertility by two ways: (a) more frequent requirement of treatment with alkylating agent (cyclophosphamide) for severe disease and (b) renal dysfunction, leading to altered hormonal milieu in the form of raised prolactin and reduced gonadotropin-releasing hormone from the hypothalamus. The mean number of pregnancies was found to be lower in lupus patients with LN as compared to those without LN in an observational study from Finland [2]. Women with LN are mostly of the reproductive-age group and improvement in remission induction with relatively safer immunosuppressive agents in these patients has allowed successful outcome of pregnancy in these patients [3].

13.2 Effect of Pregnancy on Lupus Nephritis

While pregnancy outcomes have significantly improved in patients with SLE/LN, pregnancy in these patients is still at high risk of complications. Pregnancy is accompanied by marked hormonal changes and altered immune function to accommodate an allogenic fetus (fetal tolerance), shifting towards a Th2 antibody-mediated immune response from Th1 cell-mediated response. Pregnancy may cause both short-term (flares) and long-term effects (progression to end-stage renal disease) on the course of LN. The risk of SLE flare increases in these settings, as SLE activity is known to correlate with increased estrogen levels and Th2-mediated immune response [4]. The reported rates of LN flare in pregnancy have been conflicting. A systematic review and meta-analysis involving 1842 women with SLE and variable renal function reported lupus flare (of any sort) in 26% of them [5]. LN flare rates of 30–46% have been reported in pregnant women with LN, both during pregnancy and postpartum period [6, 7]. While the incidence of flares during pregnancy increases slightly, the severity of these flares is usually not high and most respond to medications. In addition to LN flare, a pregnant patient with LN also carries risk of progression of renal disease. However, progression to end-stage renal disease is rarely reported, even in those with active LN [8].

Risk factors for LN flare during pregnancy [6–10]:

1. Active disease during 6 months prior to conception
2. Recent LN flare
3. Partial remission
4. Discontinuation of hydroxychloroquine
5. Hypocomplementemia at conception
6. High anti-dsDNA at conception

13.3 Effect of Lupus Nephritis on Pregnancy

13.3.1 Maternal Outcome

In a systematic review on 1842 patients with SLE, both active disease at conception and history of prior LN were associated with maternal hypertension and only prior LN was associated with increased risk of preeclampsia [5]. Preeclampsia has been observed in 8–25% patients with SLE/LN with well-controlled disease at baseline and intensive antepartum vigilance [10, 11]. Preeclampsia occurs earlier in women with SLE and LN compared to women with SLE without LN. While class III and/or IV LN were found to be more associated with hypertension and preeclampsia than class II and/or V LN in a study [12], class of LN and rate of maternal complication or unsuccessful pregnancy were not shown to be associated in a systematic review of nine studies [5]. Nonetheless, with the shortcomings of the systematic review and more aggressive disease course seen in proliferative forms of LN in nonpregnant state, it is important to carefully monitor these patients during pregnancy. The classification of LN, International Society of Nephrology/Renal Pathology Society (ISN/RPS) 2003 with revision in 2018 [13, 14], is based on glomerular injury and shown in Table 13.1 and Fig. 13.1. Preterm delivery was observed in 28–58% of LN patients [10, 11]; proteinuria, active LN, history of renal flares, and arterial hypertension at conception were associated with preterm delivery [10]. Maternal death (mostly due to sepsis followed by disease activity) is reported rarely.

13.3.2 Fetal Outcome

The outcome of pregnancies in 385 SLE patients (including 120 LN patients) with quiescent disease activity was good, with 81% having uncomplicated pregnancies and fetal death being rare. Presence of lupus anticoagulant, Caucasian race, well-controlled hypertension, platelet count above 100×10^9 cells/L, and a physician's global assessment score of ≤ 1 were associated with low fetal/neonatal death (4%) as opposed to high fetal/neonatal death (22%) in those without these factors [11]. Fetal/neonatal loss rates of 8.4–13% and 35% were observed in patients with

Table 13.1 International Society of Nephrology/Renal Pathology Society 2003 classification of lupus nephritis (LN)

Class	Light microscopy	IF/EM
Class I—Minimal mesangial LN	Normal glomeruli	Immune deposits in mesangium
Class II—Mesangial proliferative LN	Pure mesangial hypercellularity of any degree or mesangial matrix expansion	Immune deposits in mesangium along with a few subendothelial or subepithelial deposits
Class III—Focal LN	Segmental or global proliferative lesions in <50% of glomeruli	Subendothelial immune deposits with or without mesangial involvement
III (A)	Focal proliferative lupus nephritis	
III (A/C)	Focal proliferative and sclerosing lupus nephritis	
III (C)	Focal sclerosing lupus nephritis	
Class IV—Diffuse LN	Segmental or global proliferative lesions in >50% of glomeruli	Subendothelial immune deposits with or without mesangial involvement
IV-S (A)	Diffuse segmental proliferative lupus nephritis	
IV-G (A)	Diffuse global proliferative lupus nephritis	
IV-S (A/C)	Diffuse segmental proliferative and sclerosing lupus nephritis	
IV-G (A/C)	Diffuse global proliferative and sclerosing lupus nephritis	
IV-S (C)	Diffuse segmental sclerosing lupus nephritis	
IV-G (C)	Diffuse global sclerosing lupus nephritis	
Class V—Membranous LN	Global or segmental thickening of glomerular basement membrane in >50% of glomeruli	Subepithelial immune deposits with or without mesangial involvement
Class VI—Advanced sclerotic LN	≥90% of glomeruli are globally sclerosed without residual activity	

controlled LN and active LN at conception, respectively; this was predicted by hypocomplementemia at baseline, non-usage of low-dose aspirin, maternal hypertension at baseline, and antiphospholipid antibodies [7, 10, 15]. With renal impairment, outcome is even poorer, with 60% fetal loss in those with serum creatinine >1.5 mg/dL. Low birth weight was reported in 27–46% of pregnancies in patients with active LN [7, 16]. Neonatal lupus syndromes have been associated with the presence of maternal antibodies in the fetus; the most important and permanent is congenital heart block occurring in 15–30% of fetus in the presence of maternal anti-Ro antibodies, maternal hypothyroidism, and fetal genetic polymorphisms [17].

Risk factors for overall adverse maternal and fetal outcome in LN patients [7, 10, 15–19]:

1. *Active LN*
2. *Prior LN*
3. *Partial remission*
4. *Hypertension*
5. *Level of renal dysfunction*
6. *Antiphospholipid antibodies*

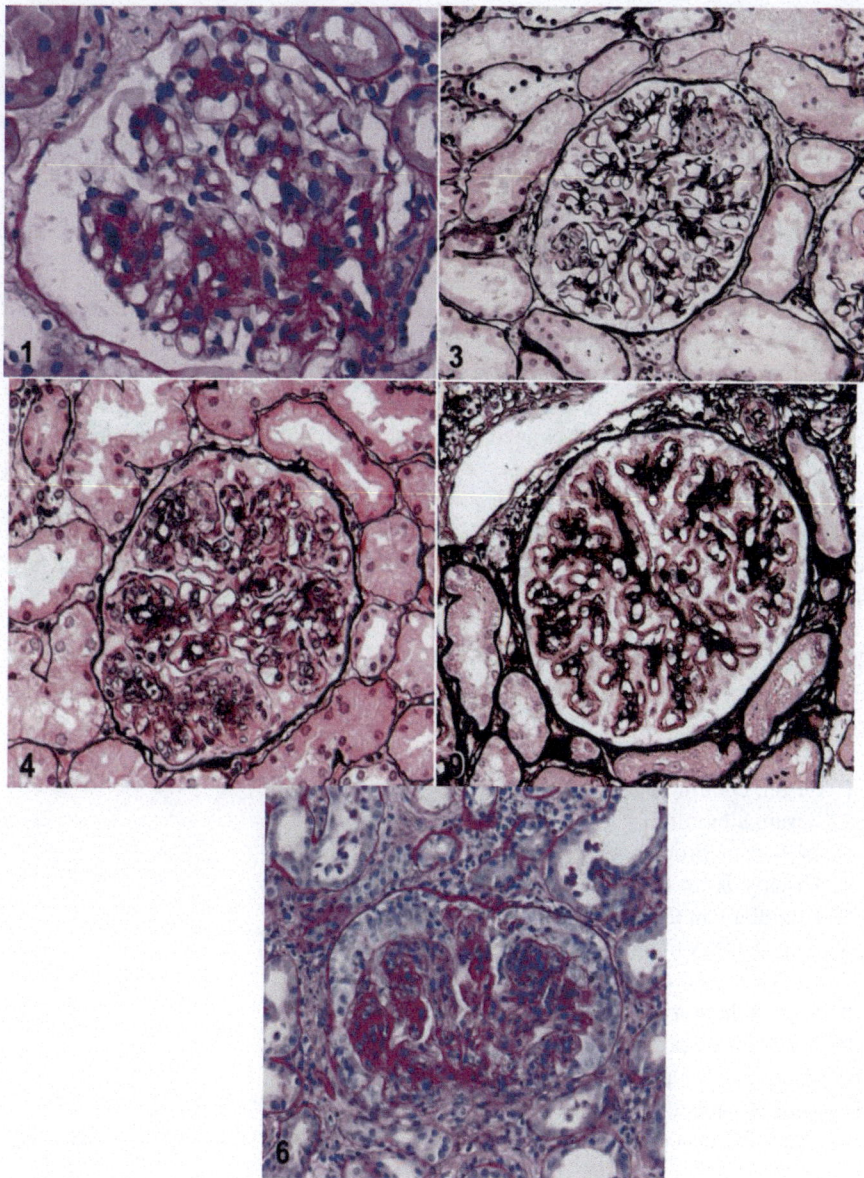

Fig. 13.1 Light microscopy: various classes of lupus nephritis based on ISN/RPS (2003) classification system

7. *Thrombocytopenia*
8. *Hypocomplementemia*

The incidence of all maternal and fetal complications increases with degree of proteinuria and renal dysfunction and chances of successful pregnancy are negligible if the serum creatinine is >2.1 mg/dL [19].

13.3.3 Prepregnancy Checklist

The most important principle of managing pregnancy in a patient with LN is planning, in consultation with the family, the obstetrician, and the nephrologist who is treating the patient. This starts with effective contraceptive counselling in patients with active disease and preconception counselling in those with well-controlled disease on minimal immunosuppressants for at least 6 months.

13.3.3.1 Preconception Counselling
Once the decision regarding pregnancy has been taken a proper preconception counselling is essential. During this period, the nephrologist has to check about the type and degree of renal involvement and whether the patient is suited for pregnancy. The risks and outcomes (as summarized) associated with pregnancy in the presence of well-controlled LN need to be discussed with the patient and family.

13.3.3.2 Clinical Assessment
Detailed clinical history and physical examination, including blood pressure (BP), should be done to assess end-organ damage. There should not be clinically active disease for 6 months prior to conception.

13.3.3.3 Laboratory Assessment
Complete remission of LN should be documented for at least 6 months prior to conception.

1. Serum creatinine
2. Serum albumin
3. 24-h urine protein and creatinine
4. Urinalysis for RBCs, WBCs, casts
5. Complement C3 and C4
6. Anti-dsDNA titers
7. Complete blood count
8. Liver function tests
9. Coagulation profile
10. Antiphospholipid antibodies
11. Anti-Ro and anti-La antibodies
12. ECG+2D-echocardiogram (for patients with suspected pulmonary hypertension)

13.3.3.4 Medication Review
Cyclophosphamide, mycophenolate mofetil, methotrexate, and rituximab are contraindicated in pregnancy and these should be stopped at least 3 months before the conception. It is the manufacturer's recommendation to conceive after at least 1 year of rituximab usage. Azathioprine (maximum 2 mg/kg/day), hydroxychloroquine (5 mg/kg/day), prednisolone (<20 mg/day), and calcineurin inhibitors (cyclosporine and tacrolimus) are usually safe for fetus. Prednisolone is degraded to inactive forms by the placental enzyme 11-beta-hydroxysteroid dehydrogenase 2, protecting the fetus from high levels of the drug. Similarly, antihypertensive drugs like

angiotensin-converting enzyme inhibitors and angiotensin receptor blockers should be stopped; consider stopping prior to conception with monitoring of proteinuria and BP in cases with mild proteinuria; if not, stop as soon as pregnancy is confirmed. Alternative antihypertensives such as amlodipine, nifedipine, labetalol, and methyldopa can be used safely. Statins are contraindicated during pregnancy. If a patient with prior LN in complete remission is not on any immunosuppressive agents or on low-dose steroids, prophylactically starting them or increasing the dose of steroids before or at conception is not advised, as it is not shown to prevent flares.

Case Vignette (Continued) As our index case conformed with the above checklist, prepregnancy counselling was done. Antiphospholipid antibodies and anti-Ro/anti-La antibodies were negative. She was swapped to azathioprine (2 mg/kg/day) from MMF and prednisolone (5 mg/day) along with hydroxychloroquine was continued. Angiotensin receptor blocker (telmisartan) and statin (atorvastatin) were stopped. For BP control, amlodipine (10 mg/day) was added with which BP was well controlled and there was no increase in proteinuria. Folic acid and calcium supplements were started. She was monitored for 3 months after which she was advised to plan her pregnancy. After a period of 5 months, she was confirmed to be pregnant.

13.3.4 Antepartum Management

Regular and close antenatal follow-up by a multidisciplinary team consisting of an obstetrician, a rheumatologist, and a nephrologist is the state-of-the-art principle of managing LN during pregnancy. Clinical review by the team should be done at least monthly, which can be increased depending on the clinical activity or flare. At each visit, a urinalysis should be performed and the serum creatinine should be checked, while the blood counts, complement levels, anti-dsDNA levels, and liver function tests can be checked at three-monthly interval. Fetal ultrasonography is advisable from weeks 7 to 13 for pregnancy dating and monthly from week 16 for fetal anomaly screen and growth monitoring. In mothers with anti-Ro or anti-La antibodies, fetal echocardiography is recommended weekly from weeks 16 to 26 and biweekly thereafter [20]. Low-dose aspirin should be started in all women with LN as soon as pregnancy is confirmed. If the patient is already on warfarin for previous thrombosis or antiphospholipid syndrome (APS), she should be started on anticoagulation in the form of either unfractionated heparin or low-molecular-weight heparin as soon as pregnancy is confirmed or preferably before 6 weeks of gestation.

13.3.5 Differentiating LN Flare from Preeclampsia

Flare of LN can be nephrotic/proteinuric, nephritic, or nephrotic-nephritic type and can occur at any stage of pregnancy or puerperium [19]. A proteinuric flare is sometimes difficult to differentiate from preeclampsia, especially if it occurs after 20th week of gestation. Moreover, the two conditions may be superimposed. Some of the pointers which may favor disease activity are presence of low or falling complement levels, elevated/increasing anti-dsDNA antibodies, presence of active sediments in urine, and other symptoms of flare like arthralgia and skin rash. Hypertension and thrombocytopenia can be seen in both. Elevation of serum uric acid and deranged liver function tests are unusual in LN flare and typically point towards preeclampsia [17, 20]. In doubtful cases, specially early gestations, and/or in cases with rapidly progressive renal failure, a renal biopsy would be useful to confirm the diagnosis and manage. Beyond 28–32 weeks of gestation (after confirming viability), delivery may be the most appropriate management if a patient has worsening hypertension with proteinuria and/or renal dysfunction. This will help in both preeclampsia and LN flare management [20].

13.3.6 Management of Lupus Nephritis Flare in Pregnancy

Management of renal flare is limited by the teratogenicity of most of the efficient immunosuppressant drugs. The possible options are increase in dose of oral steroids, intravenous methylprednisolone pulse steroid, addition/hike in dose of azathioprine, and/or calcineurin inhibitors. The best suitable option should be judged based on the severity of the flare. Intravenous immunoglobulin may be tried in refractory cases. Although cyclophosphamide is contraindicated in pregnancy, its use is justified in cases of rapidly progressive renal failure, neurological involvement, or any other life-threatening flare. Once the fetus becomes viable, delivery is the best step in the management of flare. Patients with proteinuria >3 g/day with serum albumin <3 g/dL should be prescribed with thromboprophylaxis with unfractionated or low-molecular-weight heparin during pregnancy [20]. In case of requirement of dialysis during pregnancy, the intensity and frequency should be at least 20 h/week and 6–7 times/week, respectively, to target blood urea of <20 mmol/L.

13.3.7 Intrapartum Management

The labor in most cases is spontaneous and caesarean section is reserved for obstetrical indications only. If a patient was on a dose of >7.5 mg prednisolone for >2 weeks during antenatal period, parenteral steroids are mandated to cover the stress of labor and delivery, regardless of mode of delivery [19]. Anticoagulants should be stopped 6 h before delivery and then can be restarted.

13.3.8 Postpartum Management

Postpartum follow-up (monthly) is important as flares (after immune reconstitution) and thromboembolism can occur after delivery and until 6 months later. Breastfeeding should be promoted and all drugs which are safe during pregnancy can be given during breastfeeding too [17, 20].

Case Vignette (Continued) Our index patient with prior LN (which is well controlled) and hypertension controlled on single antihypertensive drug had come for her first antenatal visit. There were no additional risk factors such as thrombocytopenia, hypocomplementemia, high anti-dsDNA titers, or antiphospholipid antibodies. Low-dose aspirin was started along with continuation of the drugs mentioned above. A multidisciplinary team approach for follow-up every month (with investigations) was planned. She continued her follow-up regularly and fetal growth was adequate at all visits. At 37 weeks of gestation, she went into spontaneous labor and delivered a healthy baby weighing 3 kg through vaginal route. Postpartum visits were uncomplicated; she was continued on azathioprine and low-dose prednisolone as maintenance therapy with hydroxychloroquine as adjunctive. She had breastfed exclusively for 6 months on the above drugs.

13.4 Conclusion

Though an increased maternal and neonatal morbidity as well as mortality are reported in pregnant LN patients, the outcomes can be optimized by careful selection of patients who are contemplating pregnancy, a planned pregnancy, and a careful management by a multidisciplinary team.

References

1. Chighizola CB, Raimondo MG, Meroni PL (2017) Does APS impact women's fertility? Curr Rheumatol Rep 19:33
2. Ekblom-Kullberg S, Kautiainen H, Alha P, Helve T, Leirisalo-Repo M, Julkunen H (2009) Reproductive health in women with systemic lupus erythematosus compared to population controls. Scand J Rheumatol 38(5):375–380
3. Stanhope TJ, White WM, Moder KG, Smyth A, Garovic VD (2012) Obstetric nephrology: lupus and lupus nephritis in pregnancy. Clin J Am Soc Nephrol 7:2089–2099
4. Zen M, Ghirardello A, Iaccarino L et al (2010) Hormones, immune response, and pregnancy in healthy women and SLE patients. Swiss Med Wkly 140:187–201
5. Smyth A, Oliveira GH, Lahr BD, Bailey KR, Norby SM, Garovic VD (2010) A systematic review and meta-analysis of pregnancy outcomes in patients with systemic lupus erythematosus and lupus nephritis. Clin J Am Soc Nephrol 5:2060–2068
6. Saavedra MA, Cruz-Reyes C, Vera-Lastra O et al (2012) Impact of previous lupus nephritis on maternal and fetal outcomes during pregnancy. Clin Rheumatol 31(5):813–819
7. Imbasciati E, Tincani A, Gregorini G et al (2009) Pregnancy in women with pre-existing lupus nephritis: predictors of fetal and maternal outcomes. Nephrol Dial Transplant 24:519–525
8. Clowse ME (2007) Lupus activity in pregnancy. Rheum Dis Clin N Am 33:237–252
9. Rahman FZ, Rahman J, Al-Suleiman SA, Rahman MS (2005) Pregnancy outcome in lupus nephropathy. Arch Gynecol Obstet 271:222–226
10. Moroni G, Doria A, Giglio E et al (2016) Fetal outcome and recommendations of pregnancies in lupus nephritis in the 21st century. A prospective multicentre study. J Autoimmun 74:6–12
11. Buyon JP, Kim MY, Guerra MM et al (2015) Predictors of pregnancy outcomes in patients with lupus: a cohort study. Ann Intern Med 163:153–163

12. Carmona F, Font J, Moga I et al (2005) Class III-IV proliferative lupus nephritis and pregnancy: a study of 42 cases. Am J Reprod Immunol 53:182
13. Weening JJ, D'Agati VD, Schwartz MM et al (2004) The classification of glomerulonephritis in systemic lupus erythematosus revisited. J Am Soc Nephrol 15(2):241–250
14. Bajema IM, Wilhelmus S, Alpers CE et al (2018) Revision of the International Society of Nephrology/Renal Pathology Society classification for lupus nephritis: clarification of definitions, and modified National Institutes of Health activity and chronicity indices. Kidney Int 93(4):789–796
15. Soubassi L, Haidopoulos D, Sindos M et al (2004) Pregnancy outcome in women with pre-existing lupus nephritis. J Obstet Gynaecol 24(6):630–634
16. Wagner SJ, Craici I, Reed D et al (2009) Maternal and foetal outcomes in pregnant patients with active lupus nephritis. Lupus 18(4):342–347
17. Lateef A, Petri M (2013) Managing lupus patients during pregnancy. Best Pract Res Clin Rheumatol 27(3):435–447
18. Gladman DD, Tandon A, Ibanez D, Urowitz MB (2010) The effect of lupus nephritis on pregnancy outcome and fetal and maternal complications. J Rheumatol 37(4):754–758
19. Germain S, Nelson-Piercy C (2006) Lupus nephritis and renal disease in pregnancy. Lupus 15:148–155
20. Bramham K, Soh MC, Nelson-Piercy C (2012) Pregnancy and renal outcomes in lupus nephritis: an update and guide to management. Lupus 21:1271–1283

Pregnancy in Systemic Vasculitis

14

Puneet Mashru and Chetan Mukhtyar

Abstract

Conception, pregnancy and childbirth are a biological necessity, a unique privilege and birthright and yet something that mothers suffering with vasculitis cannot take for granted. Takayasu arteritis and Behcet's disease mainly, but also ANCA associated vasculitis and IgA vasculitis are of relevance in this population. A diagnosis of systemic vasculitis has meant a lower chance of stable relationships, lower fertility, lower conception rates and worse foetal outcomes. Systemic vasculitis or it's treatment may affect fertility by direct involvement of the reproductive organs, teratogenicity, induced infertility, or by producing a state inducing an inability of the maternal body to carry a foetus to term. Unfortunately, there is sometimes the need for medical termination. Pregnancy outcomes are poorer in women with a diagnosis of vasculitis, but this may be truer for women with Takayasu arteritis than Behcet's disease. In spite of the many challenges in looking after expectant mothers with systemic vasculitis, we suggest some basic principles in this chapter to improve maternal and foetal outcomes. This is largely an evidence-free zone and this stream of medicine involving motherhood, babies and life-threatening rare diseases will remain emotive and therefore difficult, calling for the best that clinicians can offer.

Keywords

Systemic vasculitis · Pregnancy · Maternal outcomes · Foetal outcomes · Multi-disciplinary team working

---

P. Mashru
Sir H N Reliance Foundation Hospital, Mumbai, India

C. Mukhtyar (✉)
Norfolk and Norwich University Hospital, Norwich, UK

University of East Anglia, Norwich, UK
e-mail: Chetan.mukhtyar@nnuh.nhs.uk

14.1 Introduction

The systemic vasculitides are multisystem disorders characterised by inflammation of vessel wall that may lead to stenosis or aneurysm resulting in either ischaemic or haemorrhagic clinical manifestations. The clinical presentation depends upon the size of vessel involved. Small vessel diseases are most likely to cause organ-specific manifestations, and large vessel diseases are most likely to cause constitutional and ischaemic manifestations. For a full description of the classification of the vasculitides we would direct the reader to the 2012 Chapel Hill Consensus Conference nomenclature [1]. The clinical course can be variable in individuals but every single one of the entities is capable of inflicting severe organ damage very rapidly. The use of small-molecule conventional oral immunosuppressive drugs like cyclophosphamide and large-molecule parenteral biologic immunosuppressive drugs has significantly improved survival in these conditions [2]. Remission is achievable in most patients with systemic vasculitis [3]; but the diseases (and the treatments) still manage to inflict irreversible damage [4] which adversely affects the quality of life [5].

Primary systemic vasculitis has a bimodal distribution of incidence. In this chapter we will mainly focus on Takayasu arteritis (TAK) and Behcet's disease (BD) which are more likely to affect young women of childbearing age, as compared to other vasculitides. IgA vasculitis and anti-neutrophil cytoplasm antibody-associated vasculitis (AAV) are the other vasculitides of interest in this population [6]. Secondary vasculitis as part of systemic lupus erythematosus is also a consideration in this patient group.

Pregnancy can be considered as a birthright as well as a privilege for women. Traditionally, the diagnosis of any autoimmune rheumatic disease, not just systemic vasculitis, meant lower chance of stable relationships, lower fertility, lower conception rates and worse foetal outcomes because of the disease as well as the toxic chemotherapy used to treat the conditions [7, 8]. Even now, these remain a major issue, but adequate planning and treatment can help maximise the potential for a successful foetomaternal outcome.

14.2 Immunological Changes in Pregnancy

During pregnancy, the female body undergoes several physiological changes—increasing cardiac output, higher blood volume, tachycardia and decreased peripheral vascular resistance resulting in lower blood pressure are some examples. There are several immunological changes that also normally occur in pregnancy [9]. These changes are necessary for foetal survival, without which each pregnancy would end up with spontaneous abortion. After all, pregnancy is a state where the female body is learning to tolerate a 50% foreign tissue. There appears to be a fall in total T-cell numbers without a change in the numbers of helper/inducer T cells or suppressor/cytotoxic T cells. There may even be an increase in T regulatory cells improving tolerance to 'non-self' antigens. There has been a demonstration of increased potential of lymphocytes to respond to mitogenic activity in normal pregnancy, but this increased potential does not actually lead to a natural increase in activity suggesting the presence of tolerance mechanisms [9].

So, how does the presence of allogeneic tissue in the uterus affect autoimmune diseases generally, and vasculitis specifically? The honest answer is that we do not know for certain. But there are some clues to the physiological mechanisms at play from studies in other autoimmune diseases. In a study of pregnant women with rheumatoid arthritis, women with greater HLA class II incompatibility with the foetus showed a greater tolerance to the disease, resulting in a better disease course after delivery [10]. This suggests that maternal immunology undergoes changes which may be commensurate to the amount of 'non-self' antigen exposure via foetal tissue. How might this happen? There seems to be a basic shift in TH1/TH2 cytokine balance in pregnant women which may happen to a greater extent in women with autoimmune rheumatic diseases. Placental and maternal hormonal changes in pregnancy lead to a Th2 shift in the prevalent cytokine profile and at the same time there may be an active downregulation of Th1 cytokines aiding in the amelioration of disease [11, 12]. While remaining pregnant is not a viable therapeutic option, the recognition of these changes has certainly helped in understanding the immunology of rheumatic diseases and may even help with the development of therapeutic targets.

14.3 Effects of Systemic Vasculitis on Fertility

To understand the effect on fertility, we must first define infertility. By convention, infertility is defined as a failure to conceive after 1 year of regular, contraceptive-free intercourse. It is thought that this is incident in about 10% of normal couples. Fertility is further defined by the ability to carry a foetus to term. Loss of 2–3 consecutive pregnancies is defined as recurrent pregnancy loss and a further 1% of couples suffer with this complication. Autoimmune rheumatic diseases are rare causes of infertility and recurrent pregnancy loss.

Systemic vasculitis may affect fertility in different ways.

14.3.1 Direct Involvement of Reproductive Organs

Systemic vasculitis can directly affect the ovary and testes. At presentation, these can mimic cancers leading to surgical intervention and resultant subfertility or infertility [13, 14]. Even in patients where the disease is recognised, there may be enough damage to the parenchyma causing long-term subfertility or infertility. Testicular inflammation because of vasculitis can be reversed in most cases and very rarely would lead to testicular necrosis and infertility [15].

14.3.2 Drug Toxicity via Teratogenicity

Cyclophosphamide is activated by cytochrome P-450 enzymes to produce its active metabolite phosphoramide mustard. Phosphoramide mustard disrupts DNA linkages in cell leading to apoptosis. At the most basic level, this is responsible for its chemotherapeutic and immunomodulatory effects. However, this is also highly teratogenic. Cyclophosphamide embryopathy commonly leads to neurological and skeletal deformities—craniofacial malformations, cleft palate, hydrocephaly, micrognathia, hearing defects, craniosynostosis, limb defects and digital defects, and vertebral fusions have all been described related to prenatal maternal cyclophosphamide exposure [16].

14.3.3 Drug Toxicity via Induced Infertility

Prior treatment of vasculitis with cyclophosphamide in women results in a diminished ovarian reserve as demonstrated by a fall in anti-Müllerian hormone (AMH) levels [17]. AMH is a hormone produced by the granulosa cells of growing ovarian follicles that helps in maturation of oocytes. Falls in AMH effectively mean the loss of ovarian reserve. Since an older woman would have fewer viable oocytes compared to a younger woman, the effect of cyclophosphamide may be greater on an older ovary compared to a younger ovary. It may take a smaller cumulative dose of cyclophosphamide to render older women infertile [18]. Cyclophosphamide, leflunomide and methotrexate are all thought to impair spermatogenesis—but this may be reversible [19]. The authors do not routinely offer cryopreservation of ova or sperm, but this remains a topic of discussion and should be offered if the expectant parents should want it with the full knowledge of the pitfalls and local success rates of these procedures.

14.3.4 Infertility via Inability to Carry Foetus to Term

A sick body is unable to bear the strains of carrying a foetus to term. In patients with a relapse of vasculitis during pregnancy, there is a risk of spontaneous abortion even with the use of only corticosteroid-heavy treatment [20]. Even in the absence of an overt relapse, there is a small but definite risk of miscarriage [21]. In one study of 26 pregnancies in 10 women with Takayasu arteritis, 5 pregnancies (19%) had a spontaneous loss of pregnancy [22]. This is comparable to the results of a mixed cohort of pregnant women with vasculitis. Sangle et al. found that 13/51 (25%) pregnancies resulted in a spontaneous abortion compared to 27/156 (17%) control pregnancies [23]. Anecdotally, outcomes are worse in Takayasu arteritis than in ANCA-associated vasculitis. Croft et al. studied 15 pregnancies in 13 women across 5 centres in the UK resulting in 13 single births, 1 twin birth and 1 medical termination for an unplanned pregnancy [24]. At least in part this may be related to the presence of antiphospholipid antibodies in patients with Takayasu arteritis. Jordan et al. found that 10/22 patients with Takayasu arteritis had persistent antiphospholipid antibodies and when present it led to worse pregnancy outcomes [25].

14.3.5 Need for Medical Termination Due to Danger to Maternal/Foetal Health

Oral contraception is associated with a higher risk of venous thromboembolism and this is exacerbated by the presence of vasculitis. Not uncommonly, there is a greater reliance on other forms of contraception in couples where the female partner is suffering from vasculitis. This leads to an increased risk of accidental pregnancy and thus a greater risk of exposure to teratogenic drugs and thus at least a theoretically increased risk for the need for medical termination of pregnancy due to foetal exposure to teratogenic drugs. Cardiac failure, pulmonary hypertension and eclampsia are all recognised complications for women with heart and/or renal involvement. The maternal body may not be able to bear the physiological increase in blood volume and cardiac output leading to the need for medical termination.

14.4 Prenatal and Antenatal Care

We suggest the following principles for planning and caring for pregnant women with vasculitis:

1. Women of childbearing age with vasculitis should be looked after at centres where multidisciplinary care is available. This should include clinicians with an interest in vasculitis, obstetricians with experience of looking after women with complex medical problems and nursing or midwifery input from a practitioner with experience of caring for pregnancies with comorbidities [24].
2. Pregnancy should only be planned when the disease is in remission. However, women with severe damage—congestive cardiac failure, end-stage renal disease, poor respiratory reserve, refractory hypertension, pulmonary hypertension, etc.—should be informed of the risk to their life and adverse foetal outcomes at the planning stage.
3. All teratogenic drugs should be stopped about 3 months prior to planned conception. Detailed guidance on drug avoidance is available from the British Society for Rheumatology [26]. Azathioprine, hydroxychloroquine, prednisolone and intravenous immunoglobulin are safe in pregnancy.
4. Preconception assessment should include general health assessment, vaccination, smoking and alcohol intake status and looking for risk factors like diabetes, arterial hypertension, obesity and thyroid disease.
5. Post-conception care must include more than usual monitoring for mother and foetus. Vigilance should be exercised in the mother for disease relapse, pre-

eclampsia and gestational diabetes, and in the foetus for intrauterine growth and congenital malformations.
6. When possible, labour must be planned electively. During labour, careful attention should be paid to blood pressure control. There should have been prior discussion and planning about the need for instrumentation and caesarean section with a documented plan for surgical conversion.

14.5 Pregnancy Outcomes

In general, the presence of vasculitis is a bad influence on pregnancy outcomes. Women with vasculitis have more pregnancy-related complications. A British cohort compared outcomes of 51 pregnancies in 29 women suffering from systemic vasculitis to 156 pregnancies in 62 age, body mass index and ethnicity-matched healthy controls [23]. Of 51 pregnancies, the mothers with vasculitis suffered 13 miscarriages, 3 had pre-eclampsia and 2 had intrauterine death. This was significantly worse to the outcomes of the 156 control pregnancies where 20 mothers had 27 miscarriages, 1 had pre-eclampsia and 1 had antepartum haemorrhage. Mothers with vasculitis delivered at a median gestational age of 36 weeks compared with 40 weeks for control ($P < 0.03$). The babies of the affected mothers were 0.5 kg lower in birth weight (3.0 kg vs. 3.5 kg). Similarly, poor outcomes were demonstrated in a prospective Italian cohort of 65 pregnancies in 50 mothers with systemic vasculitides—higher risk of preterm deliveries and higher risk of intervention in the form of caesarean sections were seen.

Having said that the presence of vasculitis produces adverse outcomes, this is not universally true and does depend on the nature of the vasculitis, all other things remaining equal. If we consider the two important vasculitides affecting women of childbearing age group—Takayasu arteritis and Behcet's disease—we get slightly different results. There is Indian data available for pregnancy outcomes in Takayasu arteritis. In a case-control study, Mandal et al. described 16 patients with TA who had 29 pregnancies and compared outcomes to 60 controls [27]. Maternal complications were significantly more compared to the control group. Twenty pregnancies were delivered by C-section (71%). Maternal complications included preterm labour (17% vs. 3%; $P < 0.001$), post-partum haemorrhage (17% vs. 2%; $P < 0.001$), pregnancy-induced hypertension (100% vs. 2%; $P < 0.001$) and pre-eclampsia (93% vs. 0%; $P < 0.001$). There were 26 live births with a risk of increased intrauterine growth restriction (IUGR) (52% vs. 2%; $P < 0.001$) and more neonates required intensive care (59% vs. 5%; $P < 0.001$). One maternal death was reported due to cerebrovascular accident. In a larger French cohort of 96 mothers who had 240 pregnancies, maternal outcomes were observed depending on whether the diagnosis preceded pregnancy or was diagnosed concurrently to pregnancy. 98 pregnancies in 52 women were compared with mothers who were diagnosed before pregnancy (142 pregnancies in 52 women) [28]. It was noted that in women with concomitant diagnosis of TA there was a 13-fold increased risk of obstetric complications with

40% frequency of obstetric complications including intrauterine foetal growth restriction, foetal death, pre-eclampsia/eclampsia and premature delivery.

If mothers with Takayasu arteritis seem to do so badly, the mothers with Behcet's disease do not seem to be affected in a systematic review of literature of 11 case series and 21 case reports [29]. In fact, the condition may even improve during pregnancy, perhaps for the reasons described earlier in the chapter. In a French study of 76 pregnancies in women with Behcet's disease, it was seen that the mean (standard deviation) annual relapse rate was 0.49 (0.72) during pregnancy compared to 1.46 (2.42) during nonobstetric period [30]. This difference in outcomes from Takayasu arteritis may be related to the fact that Takayasu arteritis is generally associated with a greater burden of damage, especially cardiovascular. This may be why mothers with Behcet's disease who have a history of deep venous thrombosis have a higher risk of obstetric complications (odds ratio 7.25, 95% confidence interval 1.21–43.46, $P = 0.029$). The use of colchicine is likely to be protective in preventing relapse of venous thromboembolism and improving disease activity during pregnancy.

14.6 Effects of Pregnancy on Systemic Vasculitis and Pharmacotherapy

Pregnancy does not seem to adversely affect the disease course of systemic vasculitis. There is evidence to suggest that Behcet's disease improves in pregnancy [30]. This is in spite of reduction of immunosuppression. As discussed earlier in the chapter, this may be because of a true amelioration of disease mechanisms. However, pregnancy brings unique challenges pertaining to differential diagnosis between relapse and complications of pregnancy. Is the hypertension and proteinuria related to vasculitis or pre-eclampsia? That can be challenging. Thus, it is important to have a multidisciplinary approach for the care of these patients with a vasculitis expert and an obstetrician experienced in managing complex cases. Managing relapses during pregnancy poses a challenge, as most conventional immunosuppressive agents cannot be used. Increased doses of corticosteroids are often used in these situations but that is not enough in most cases and other agents are required [31]. The British Society of Rheumatology 2016 guidelines have described in detail regarding the drugs that can be used in pregnancy and lactation [26]. They are briefly discussed below:

- Corticosteroids: Prednisolone and methylprednisolone are compatible in all trimesters of pregnancy and breastfeeding. Use of corticosteroids may increase the risk of IUGR. Mothers with hypertension, kidney disease and fluid retention should be monitored carefully. Babies of mothers on large doses of prednisolone should be monitored for adrenal suppression.
- Methotrexate, leflunomide and mycophenolate mofetil are contraindicated during pregnancy and breastfeeding.
- Cyclophosphamide is also contraindicated in pregnancy and breastfeeding due to toxicity to foetus. There may not be a choice to its use when a relapse is organ or

life threatening and if rituximab is not indicated or available. There is some anecdotal use in pregnancy [32].
- Rituximab has been used successfully in pregnancy [33]. Accidental exposure in first trimester is unlikely to be harmful but if used in second and third trimesters can lead to B-cell depletion in the neonate and thus appropriate vaccination precautions would be needed.
- TNFα inhibitors are safe drugs in pregnancy [34]. Certolizumab pegol is safest because the size of the molecule prevents it from crossing the placenta, but it is not currently available in India. Infliximab after 16 weeks of pregnancy and adalimumab and etanercept in the third trimester should be avoided but if these are necessary it will affect vaccination schedules for the baby. TNFα inhibitors are compatible with breastfeeding.
- Intravenous immunoglobulin is safe in pregnancy. It can be used in relapsing and grumbling disease where clinically appropriate [35]. It cannot replace the use of rituximab and cyclophosphamide in life-threatening situations like alveolar haemorrhage and rapidly progressive glomerular nephritis.
- Azathioprine is safe in pregnancy and breastfeeding and potentially could be switched too at the stage of conception planning.
- Plasma exchange can sometimes be a safe effective way to tide over a crisis in vasculitides which are mediated by humoral immunity and where there are high titres of antibodies.

14.7 Conclusions

Conception, pregnancy and childbirth are a biological necessity, a unique privilege and birthright and yet something that mothers suffering from vasculitis cannot take for granted without the help of multidisciplinary input. In spite of being something that is responsible for the existence of a species, it is an incompletely understood immunological entity. There is a true amelioration of pro-inflammatory processes without which every pregnancy might end in spontaneous abortion. This amelioration results in a short-lived ceasefire of hostilities between the vasculitis and the maternal physiology. However, outcomes may remain poor in mothers who have already suffered damage, especially irreversible cardiovascular damage.

There is a great need for multidisciplinary clinics which can provide a point of entry for expectant mothers with vasculitis. Early input in the form of conception planning, choice of medication, antenatal monitoring, modification of risk factors and dedicated multidisciplinary input can improve outcomes. Unfortunately, some expectant mothers with major pulmonary, cardiovascular or renal involvement may have to be counselled against pregnancy for the well-being of not only them, but also the planned child. Relapses in pregnancy can be difficult to diagnose. When they occur, corticosteroids will form the mainstay of treatment, but drugs like azathioprine, anti-TNFα, intravenous immunoglobulins and if absolutely necessary even cyclophosphamide or rituximab can be used.

We are never going to get high-quality data for pregnancy outcomes in mothers with vasculitis. The disease is rare and the ethical considerations for designing studies in this group of patients are many. But that should not stop us from considering the production of registries that are mandated. In a large country like India with several research-active institutes, this data can be easily produced with a spirit of collaboration and research. But no matter how much research is done in this area, this stream of medicine involving motherhood, babies and life-threatening rare diseases will remain emotive and therefore difficult, calling for the best that clinicians can offer.

References

1. Jennette JC, Falk RJ, Bacon PA, Basu N, Cid MC, Ferrario F et al (2013) 2012 Revised International Chapel Hill Consensus Conference Nomenclature of Vasculitides. Arthritis Rheum 65(1):1–11
2. Guillevin L, Mukhtyar C, Pagnoux C, Yates M (2018) Conventional and biological immunosuppressants in vasculitis. Best Pract Res Clin Rheumatol 32(1):94–111
3. Mukhtyar C, Hellmich B, Jayne D, Flossmann O, Luqmani R (2006) Remission in antineutrophil cytoplasmic antibody-associated systemic vasculitis. Clin Exp Rheumatol 24(6):S93
4. Mukhtyar CB, Flossmann O, Luqmani RA (2006) Clinical and biological assessment in systemic necrotizing vasculitides. Clin Exp Rheumatol 24(2 Suppl 41):S92–S99
5. Walsh M, Mukhtyar C, Mahr A, Herlyn K, Luqmani R, Merkel PA et al (2011) Health-related quality of life in patients with newly diagnosed antineutrophil cytoplasmic antibody-associated vasculitis. Arthritis Care Res (Hoboken) 63(7):1055–1061
6. Pathak H, Mukhtyar C (2016) Pregnancy and systemic vasculitis. Indian J Rheumatol 11(6):145
7. McDuffie FC (1985) Morbidity impact of rheumatoid arthritis on society. Am J Med 78(1A):1–5
8. Pagnoux C, Mahendira D, Laskin CA (2013) Fertility and pregnancy in vasculitis. Best Pract Res Clin Rheumatol 27(1):79–94
9. MacLean MA, Wilson R, Thomson JA, Krishnamurthy S, Walker JJ (1992) Immunological changes in normal pregnancy. Eur J Obstet Gynecol Reprod Biol 43(3):167–172
10. van der Horst-Bruinsma IE, de Vries RR, de Buck PD, van Schendel PW, Breedveld FC, Schreuder GM et al (1998) Influence of HLA-class II incompatibility between mother and fetus on the development and course of rheumatoid arthritis of the mother. Ann Rheum Dis 57(5):286–290
11. Østensen M, Förger F, Nelson JL, Schuhmacher A, Hebisch G, Villiger PM (2005) Pregnancy in patients with rheumatic disease: anti-inflammatory cytokines increase in pregnancy and decrease post-partum. Ann Rheum Dis 64(6):839–844
12. Wegmann TG, Lin H, Guilbert L, Mosmann TR (1993) Bidirectional cytokine interactions in the maternal-fetal relationship: is successful pregnancy a TH2 phenomenon? Immunol Today 14(7):353–356
13. Kariv R, Sidi Y, Gur H (2000) Systemic vasculitis presenting as a tumorlike lesion. Four case reports and an analysis of 79 reported cases. Medicine (Baltimore) 79(6):349–359
14. Suo L, Perez LC, Finch CJ (2019) Testicular granulomatous vasculitis mimicking testicular torsion in an anti-neutrophil cytoplasmic antibody-associated vasculitis patient. SAGE Open Med Case Rep 7. https://doi.org/10.1177/2050313X18823451
15. Barber TD, Al-Omar O, Poulik J, McLorie GA (2006) Testicular infarction in a 12-year-old boy with Wegener's granulomatosis. Urology 67(4):846.e9–846.10
16. Rengasamy P (2017) Congenital malformations attributed to prenatal exposure to cyclophosphamide. Anti-Cancer Agents Med Chem 17(9):1211–1227

17. Clowse ME, Copland SC, Hsieh TC, Chow SC, Hoffman GS, Merkel PA et al (2011) Ovarian reserve diminished by oral cyclophosphamide therapy for granulomatosis with polyangiitis (Wegener's). Arthritis Care Res (Hoboken) 63(12):1777–1781
18. Slater CA, Liang MH, McCune JW, Christman GM, Laufer MR (1999) Preserving ovarian function in patients receiving cyclophosphamide. Lupus 8(1):3–10
19. Ding J, Shang X, Zhang Z, Jing H, Shao J, Fei Q et al (2017) FDA-approved medications that impair human spermatogenesis. Oncotarget 8(6):10714–10725
20. Kumar A, Mohan A, Gupta R, Singal VK, Garg OP (1998) Relapse of Wegener's granulomatosis in the first trimester of pregnancy: a case report. Br J Rheumatol 37(3):331–333
21. Pagnoux C, Le Guern V, Goffinet F, Diot E, Limal N, Pannier E et al (2011) Pregnancies in systemic necrotizing vasculitides: report on 12 women and their 20 pregnancies. Rheumatology (Oxford) 50(5):953–961
22. Hidaka N, Yamanaka Y, Fujita Y, Fukushima K, Wake N (2012) Clinical manifestations of pregnancy in patients with Takayasu arteritis: experience from a single tertiary center. Arch Gynecol Obstet 285(2):377–385
23. Sangle SR, Vounotrypidis P, Briley A, Nel L, Lutalo PM, Sanchez-Fernandez S et al (2015) Pregnancy outcome in patients with systemic vasculitis: a single-centre matched case-control study. Rheumatology (Oxford) 54(9):1582–1586
24. Croft AP, Smith SW, Carr S, Youssouf S, Salama AD, Burns A et al (2015) Successful outcome of pregnancy in patients with anti-neutrophil cytoplasm antibody-associated small vessel vasculitis. Kidney Int 87(4):807–811
25. Jordan NP, Bezanahary H, D'Cruz DP (2015) Increased risk of vascular complications in Takayasu's arteritis patients with positive lupus anticoagulant. Scand J Rheumatol 44(3):211–214
26. Flint J, Panchal S, Hurrell A, van de Venne M, Gayed M, Schreiber K et al (2016) BSR and BHPR guideline on prescribing drugs in pregnancy and breastfeeding—part I: standard and biologic disease modifying anti-rheumatic drugs and corticosteroids. Rheumatology (Oxford) 55(9):1693–1697
27. Mandal D, Mandal S, Dattaray C, Banerjee D, Ghosh P, Ghosh A et al (2012) Takayasu arteritis in pregnancy: an analysis from eastern India. Arch Gynecol Obstet 285(3):567–571
28. Comarmond C, Mirault T, Biard L, Nizard J, Lambert M, Wechsler B et al (2015) Takayasu arteritis and pregnancy. Arthritis Rheumatol 67(12):3262–3269
29. Ben-Chetrit E (2014) Behcet's syndrome and pregnancy: course of the disease and pregnancy outcome. Clin Exp Rheumatol 32(4 Suppl 84):S93–S98
30. Noel N, Wechsler B, Nizard J, Costedoat-Chalumeau N, Boutin d LT, Dommergues M et al (2013) Behcet's disease and pregnancy. Arthritis Rheum 65(9):2450–2456
31. Yates M, Watts RA, Bajema IM, Cid MC, Crestani B, Hauser T et al (2016) EULAR/ERA-EDTA recommendations for the management of ANCA-associated vasculitis. Ann Rheum Dis 75(9):1583–1594
32. Dayoan ES, Dimen LL, Boylen CT (1998) Successful treatment of Wegener's granulomatosis during pregnancy: a case report and review of the medical literature. Chest 113(3):836–838
33. Sangle SR, Lutalo PM, Davies RJ, Khamashta MA, D'Cruz DP (2013) B-cell depletion therapy and pregnancy outcome in severe, refractory systemic autoimmune diseases. J Autoimmun 43:55–59
34. Diav-Citrin O, Otcheretianski-Volodarsky A, Shechtman S, Ornoy A (2014) Pregnancy outcome following gestational exposure to TNF-alpha-inhibitors: a prospective, comparative, observational study. Reprod Toxicol 43:78–84
35. Jayne DR, Chapel H, Adu D, Misbah S, O'Donoghue D, Scott D et al (2000) Intravenous immunoglobulin for ANCA-associated systemic vasculitis with persistent disease activity. QJM 93(7):433–439

Managing APLA During Pregnancy

15

Arghya Chattopadhyay and Varun Dhir

Abstract

Anti-phospholipid syndrome (APS) is a systemic autoimmune disease resulting in vascular thrombosis and pregnancy morbidity affecting both mother and foetus. In obstetric APS, the aim of management is ensuring adequate anticoagulation and maternal and foetal well-being through regular monitoring. Perinatal counseling is important to reassure the couple that a good outcome is possible through proper monitoring and regular follow up with both the rheumatology and obstetric teams. In the case of vascular APS, the switch to heparin needs to be done as soon as pregnancy is detected, whereas, in obstetric APS, heparin needs to be started at this time. The dose of heparin is different in the case of vascular APS patients getting pregnant compared to only obstetric APS. Low-dose aspirin is generally added to both regimens. In the post-partum period, heparin is continued till 6 weeks and then discontinued in obstetric APS. In contrast, in vascular APS, reinitiation of vitamin K oral antagonist should be done as this is safe in lactation.

Keywords

Pregnancy · Anti-phospholipid · Anticoagulation · APLA · Anticardiolipin

15.1 Introduction

Anti-phospholipid syndrome (APS) is a systemic autoimmune disease resulting in vascular thrombosis and pregnancy morbidity affecting both mother and foetus. There are broadly two phenotypes or clinical subsets in this entity with different

---

A. Chattopadhyay · V. Dhir (✉)
Rheumatology Unit, Department of Internal Medicine, Post Graduate Institute of Medical Education and Research, Chandigarh, India

© Springer Nature Singapore Pte Ltd. 2020
S. K. Sharma (ed.), *Women's Health in Autoimmune Diseases*,
https://doi.org/10.1007/978-981-15-0114-2_15

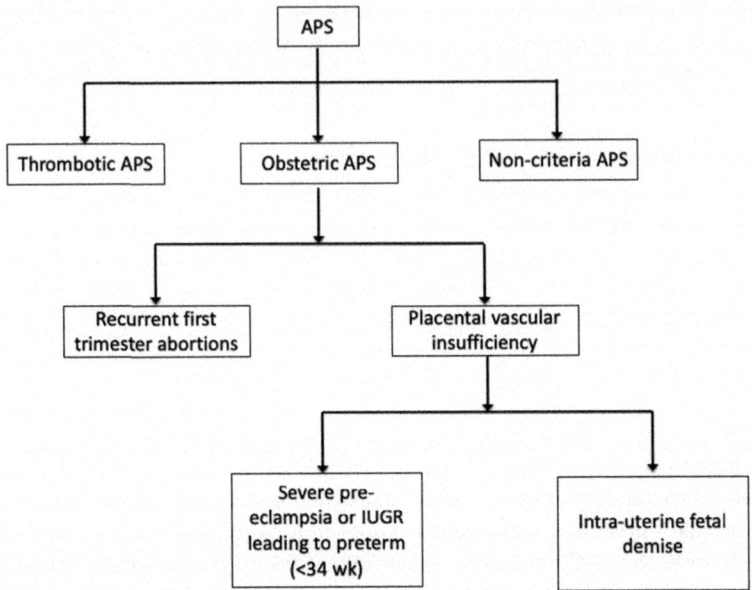

Fig. 15.1 Classification of antiphospholipid syndrome

clinical courses and outcomes—obstetric APS and thrombotic APS [1, 2]. These are defined using classification criteria—the latest being the Sydney APS classification criteria of 2006 [3]. In addition, a third group, namely patients with non-criteria manifestations and positive APLA, is often added to the above two groups (Fig. 15.1).

Like other autoimmune diseases, APS also requires two elements for its diagnosis—autoantibodies (antiphospholipid antibodies or APLA) and clinical features (thrombotic or obstetric events). An additional requirement (in addition to other autoimmune diseases) is the demonstration of persistence of autoantibodies—by a repeat test at least 12 weeks later. It is important to reiterate that mere presence of autoantibodies (even if persistent) is not sufficient to classify a patient as having APS.

The detection of APLA is not uncommon in healthy volunteers; in one study, among healthy blood donors, 10% were found to be positive for anticardiolipin antibodies (aCL) and 1% for lupus anticoagulant (LA). However, only 1% remain persistently positive for the same after 1 year. On the other hand 20–30% of lupus patients, 6% women with pregnancy complications, 10% with venous thrombosis, 11% with a myocardial infraction, and 17% with young stroke (<50 years) are positive for APLA (Fig. 15.2) [4].

There is a female preponderance for this disease (5:1) and it usually affects middle-aged people (average age in the Europhospholipid cohort was 34 years). These factors carry a huge connotation as this is the group likely to have a pregnancy. Thus, the management of this disease in pregnancy is crucial to a successful outcome and minimisation of risk to the mother and the foetus.

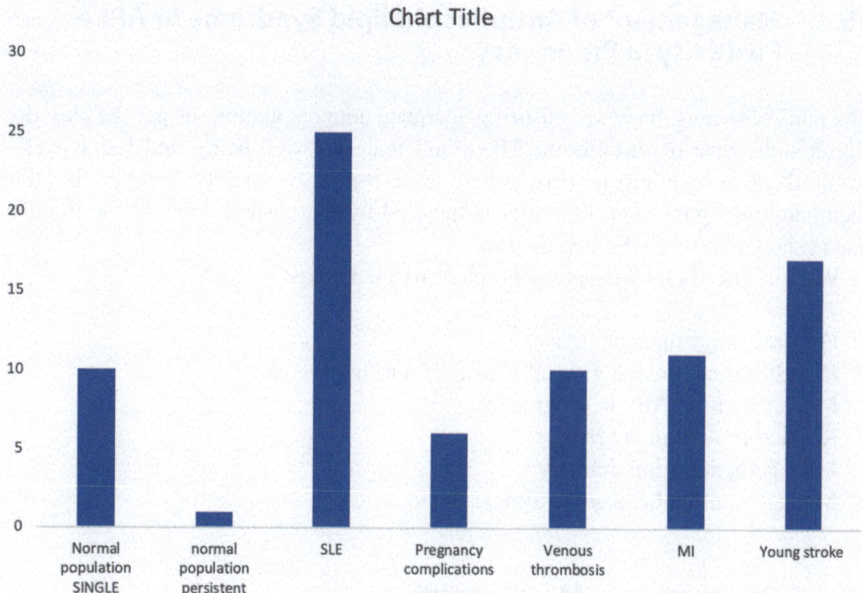

Fig. 15.2 Prevalence of APLA in various situations

15.2 When Should APLA Testing Be Done for a Lady in or Before Pregnancy?

General screening for APLA antibody is discouraged. According to Scientific and Standardization Subcommittee of the International Society of Thrombosis and Haemostasis (SSC-ISHT) guideline, APS antibody testing should be carried out in a subject with unprovoked venous or arterial thrombosis, thrombosis at an unusual site and pregnancy complications [5]. Pregnancy complications are defined by criteria manifestations, which include one or more unexplained foetal death at or >10 weeks' gestation; one or more premature birth at or <34 weeks of gestations due to severe pre-eclampsia, eclampsia, severe placental insufficiency; or three or more unexplained consecutive spontaneous abortions at or <10 weeks of gestations. Women have extra-criterial obstetrical clinical manifestations like late pre-eclampsia (>34 weeks), late premature birth, placental abruption, three non-consecutive miscarriages, two unexplained miscarriages and two or more unexplained in vitro fertilisation failures [6] that may also be considered for testing according to the physician's discretion. All women who have diagnosed with a case of lupus should undergo APLA testing at the time of planning for pregnancy, due to its prognostic value. Specifically, these patients would be more prone for pre-eclampsia and IUGR, and thus closer foetal and maternal monitoring during pregnancy.

15.3 Management of Antiphospholipid Syndrome or APLA Positivity in Pregnancy

The aims of management are ensuring adequate anticoagulation (as per the classification—obstetric or thrombotic APS), and maternal well-being and foetal well-being through monitoring (Fig. 15.3). The former is mainly handled by the rheumatologist/physician, the latter is handled by the obstetrician and the middle one is shared between the two doctors.

We will discuss the management under five headings:

1. Pre-pregnancy management
2. Risk stratification and general measures during pregnancy
3. Management of APS in pregnancy
4. Refractory APS in pregnancy
5. Management during delivery
6. Management in the post-partum period

15.3.1 Pre-pregnancy Management

This consists of having a conversation with the patient and her spouse. It is important to let them know that even with anticoagulation the chance of having a successful pregnancy is 70–80%. It is also important to let them know the risks of anticoagulation, in terms of bleeding events that can occur at 1–3% per year. If the lady is already on vitamin K antagonists (warfarin, acenocoumarol), she needs to be informed that she needs to switch to heparin as soon as the pregnancy is detected. She needs to go for a planned pregnancy and keep a strict vigil, in terms of her menstrual cycles and

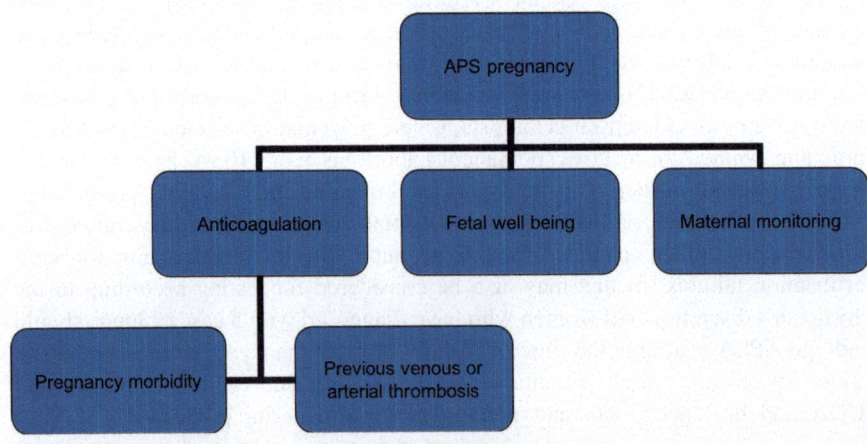

Fig. 15.3 Broad aims of management of an APS pregnancy

should get a urine pregnancy test in case she gets pregnant. This will enable minimal exposure of the embryo to vitamin K antagonists which are teratogenic.

This is also a good time to let them know the measures they can start taking right away. They can start low-dose aspirin if they are trying for a baby. Also, the lady needs to get her regular check-up done and meet an obstetrician for a planned pregnancy and correction of any other factors that may impair a successful pregnancy (anaemia, thyroid status, hypertension, diabetes, etc.).

15.3.2 Risk Stratification and General Measures

Women with diagnosed 'obstetric APS' should undergo pre-pregnancy counselling for risk assessment, and evaluation for the presence of 'APS non-criteria manifestations' [7], other associated connective tissue disorders, any major organ involvement, other comorbidities, lifestyle risk factors like smoking and alcohol, and medications that can affect foetal growth and development. Risk factors like multiple previous pregnancy loss, thrombotic APS, concomitant lupus, hypocomplementemia at the time of conception, LA positivity and triple positivity are associated with adverse pregnancy outcome. The global APS score (GAPSS) [8] is a composite score that may be used to predict the risk of thrombosis (first/recurrent) and pregnancy morbidity.

A close follow-up preferably with a monthly visit and additional third-trimester ultrasonographic surveillance (monthly from third trimester onwards) is recommended for the early detection of growth retardation and planning for delivery [7]. Blood pressure and 24-h urinary protein should be monitored regularly in patients with renal involvement.

All patients should be on folic acid, preferably 3 months before the conception, along with calcium and vitamin D supplementation. During puerperium, early mobilisation should be encouraged along with compressive stockings if any history of thrombosis is present.

15.3.3 Management of APS in Pregnancy [1, 9, 10] (Table 15.1)

This can be divided into four categories, as follows:

(a) *Fulfilling criteria for obstetric APS*

The current standard of care is prophylactic dose of unfractionated heparin (UFH) or low-molecular-weight heparin (LMWH) along with low-dose aspirin (LDA) (75–100 mg/day). LDA may be started before pregnancy and LMWH/UFH at the time of confirmation of pregnancy. A platelet count should be done before starting any kind of therapy—in mild thrombocytopenia ($>50 \times 10^9$) with no other risk factors for bleeding anti-thrombotic therapy can be continued (after risk-benefit assessment), but if the platelets are lower than 50×10^9, usually any kind of anti-platelet therapy or heparin is avoided. Baseline coagulation tests should be done to assess any prior abnormality (which may have a bleeding risk).

Table 15.1 Treatment for various scenarios of APS in pregnancy

	Pre-pregnancy	Pregnancy	Time of delivery	Post-partum
Obstetric APS	Add low-dose aspirin	Start heparin prophylactic dose *plus* low-dose aspirin	Shift to unfractionated heparin from 36 to 37 weeks, stop aspirin[a]	Restart heparin 12 h after delivery, till 6–12 weeks post-partum; breastfeeds
Thrombotic APS	Continue on warfarin, vigilant for pregnancy	Shift to heparin therapeutic dose *plus* low-dose aspirin	Shift to unfractionated heparin from 36 to 37 weeks, stop aspirin[a]	Restart warfarin (overlap with heparin), can breastfeed
SLE with APS	Continue on hydroxychloroquine; rest as per above	Same	Same	Same
Not fulfilling criteria but APLA positive	Reassurance, may consider low-dose aspirin in high-risk profile	Consider low-dose aspirin	Stop aspirin 1–2 weeks before	–

[a]May not stop aspirin as per a recent American college of obstetricians and gynecologists committe opinion

Table 15.2 Usual doses of anticoagulation used before or during pregnancy

Agent used	Dosing
Heparin prophylactic dose	UFH[a] = 5000 units SC BD Enoxaparin[b] 1 mg/kg SC OD or 0.5 mg SC BD
Heparin full dose (therapeutic dose)	UFH = 500 U/kg/day in two doses SC BD → titrate to keep APTT 1.5–2× (60–90 s); usually start at 10,000 SC BD or 12,500 SC BD Enoxaparin 1 mg/kg SC BD
Low-dose aspirin	75–100 mg/day
Warfarin[c]	Start at 5 mg OD, repeat INR after 2–3 days and 7 days, keep INR 2–3

[a]Unfractionated heparin usually comes in strengths of 5000 or 10,000 U/mL (preferred) or 1000 U/mL; store in refrigerator
[b]Pre-filled syringes, usually come in 0.4 mL (40 mg) or 0.6 mL (60 mg) dose
[c]Teratogenic in first trimester

LMWH has certain advantages over UFH; namely single daily dose, less chance of heparin-induced thrombocytopenia and reduced risk of osteoporosis. However, UFH is markedly cheaper (ten times lower cost), and needs to be given twice a day, without any monitoring (Table 15.2). If LMWH is used, it must be shifted to UFH 1 week prior to delivery, and aspirin must be stopped. UFH is generally stopped for 12 h before and after delivery.

(b) *Fulfilling criteria for thrombotic APS*

Patients with 'thrombotic APS' usually get pregnant while on secondary thromboprophylaxis with oral vitamin K antagonist (example: warfarin, acenocoumarol). It is important to counsel the patients regarding a planned pregnancy to get a urine pregnancy test done at the earliest to avoid prolonged exposure to VKA to the foetus. Generally, in most cases, switching before pregnancy is not feasible as this increases cost and puts the lady at a higher risk of bleeding for an uncertain duration of time before she conceives.

It is important to discontinue vitamin K antagonist (VKA) (example: warfarin, acenocoumarol) once the pregnancy is confirmed and shift to a therapeutic dose of LMWH or UFH to avoid foetal warfarin syndrome. Its main teratogenic effects are during the period of organogenesis (6th–12th weeks of gestations). The preferred agent is low-molecular-weight heparin (for reasons above), which must be given as per the weight of the patient (enoxaparin 1 mg/kg/day BD or dalteparin) with low-dose aspirin 75–100 mg/day (Table 15.2). A platelet count should be done before starting any kind of therapy—in mild thrombocytopenia (>50 × 10^9) with no other risk factors for bleeding anti-thrombotic therapy can be continued (after risk-benefit assessment), but if the platelets are lower than 50 × 10^9, usually any kind of anti-platelet therapy or heparin is avoided. However, no monitoring is recommended with LMWH.

However, as this treatment has to be given for 9 months, there is a substantial cost involved in LMWH (daily cost approximately INR 500–1000, monthly cost approximately INR 15–30,000). As compared to this, UFH is at least ten times less expensive. The usual therapeutic dose of UFH is 500 units/kg/day, approximately 30,000 units for a 60 kg woman. However, generally it can be started at 20–25,000 units/day and then titrated upwards. This should be given by subcutaneous route in two divided doses. In this case, the aPTT needs to be monitored to keep it at 60–90 s (control 40 s or 1.5–2× control). Furthermore, considering the high dose, heparin with a higher concentration (5000–10,000 units/mL) and not lower concentration (1000 units/mL) needs to be used to keep the subcutaneous injection to be feasible.

In case LMWH is used, it must be shifted to UFH a few days before delivery, and UFH must be withheld 12 h before and after delivery, especially if any spinal anaesthesia is to be given. Another option when financial and logistic issues preclude the use of heparin is to reinstitute oral vitamin K antagonist (VKA) (example: warfarin, acenocoumarol) from 13th week to 36th week. However, this requires regular monitoring of INR to reach a therapeutic dose, which may be different from the dose used before pregnancy.

(c) *APS associated with lupus*

Treatment of APS in a patient with lupus warrants the addition (or continuation) of hydroxychloroquine (5–6 mg/kg/day) to the management as per above.

(d) *Anti-phospholipid antibody (APLA) carrier/not fulfilling criteria for obstetric APS*

Treatment of APLA carrier or those who are not fulfilling the criteria depends on baseline risk stratification. Women with a high-risk profile can be managed with addition of LDA.

15.3.4 Refractory Obstetric APS

Despite treatment, there is a failure to a successful pregnancy in 20–30% cases. There is no specific guideline for the treatment of refractory obstetric APS. There is no standard evidence-based therapy. The first option should be a strictly controlled anticoagulation (at a higher intensity than used in previous pregnancies).

Experimental off-label drugs may be considered in rare cases, not responding to standard anticoagulation, and other factors have been ruled out—however, their benefit-risks must be considered carefully. Corticosteroids have been used, with a caveat that their use has been associated with poor pregnancy outcomes in randomised controlled studies. IVIG (400 mg/kg/day for 5 consecutive days or 1 g/kg/day for 2 consecutive days) or plasmapheresis (3–5 consecutive days) has also been tried. Hydroxychloroquine (5–6 mg/kg/day), pravastatin (20 mg/day) and certolizumab pegol have shown benefits in initial trials.

15.3.5 Antithrombotic Therapy During Delivery

Management of anti-platelets and anticoagulation is an essential component of peripartum management. The time (period of gestation) when low-dose aspirin should be stopped is controversial and depends on anaesthesiologist experience and hospital protocol. LMWH should be switched to UFH at 36–37 weeks, which should be stopped 12 h before the elective induction of labour, spinal anaesthesia or caesarean section. Heparin can be restarted as soon as possible after delivery, in consultation with the obstetrician, generally around 12 h.

15.3.6 Management During the Post-partum Period

(a) *Management of mother*: During the post-partum period the same treatment should be continued as during pregnancy for another 4–6 weeks. Those patients with thrombotic APS (previous thrombosis) may either continue therapeutic dose of LMWH or be shifted to VKA, which is equally safe during breastfeeding.
(b) *Management of foetus*: Children born to the APS mother can have IgG isotype antibody positivity due to transplacental transfer. aCL usually disappears by 12 months, but beta-2 GPI may be persistently positive without any clinical significance. Though children born to the APS mother have normal physical growth and intelligence they may require special attention regarding neurological development and extra learning support.

15.4 Some Case Scenarios Normally Encountered

Scenario 1
Pregnant for first time with SLE and positive APLA

Mrs. N, 25-year-old lady who got married 1 year ago, is planning on getting pregnant. She has a past history of systemic lupus erythematosus since the past 3 years, mainly involving the skin and joints in the form of malar rash, photosensitivity and arthritis. She is doing well on low-dose prednisolone and hydroxychloroquine since the past 2 years. She is concerned that her APLA workup revealed a persistently high anticardiolipin IgG (30 and 45 GPL, respectively, 12 weeks apart). She has never had any vascular event. What is the appropriate treatment?

The appropriate treatment in this case is reassurance. The patient must be reassured that antiphospholipid antibodies are present in up to 40% of patients with systemic lupus erythematosus but only in 5–10% do these patients develop antiphospholipid syndrome. In addition, the presence of these antibodies is associated with a higher risk of pre-eclampsia, IUGR and immaturity on a population basis; however, in a single patient (and in a majority of cases), they do not lead to any problems. There is no strong evidence for any therapy. However, low-dose aspirin may be added after getting her baseline platelet count done. If a decision is taken to start this, it would need to be stopped in case of any bleeding and in third trimester. However, the American college of obstetricians and gynecologists in a committe opinion opined that low dose aspirin does not need to be discontinued as it does not lead to excessive bleeding during delivery.

Scenario 2
Pregnant for second time with previous one abortion at 7 weeks and positive APLA

Mrs. P, a 27-year-old lady who got married 3 years ago, is pregnant for the second time. In her first pregnancy she had a spontaneous abortion at 7 weeks and is anxious about her current pregnancy. She was tested elsewhere and had a positive anti-B2 GP1 antibody (40 units). She has never been ill before. What will you advise her?

The appropriate treatment will be reassurance. First-trimester abortions are very common (30% of all pregnancies) and occur due to a variety of causes. At this stage it is the best for her to not worry about her 'positive antibodies' and focus on being positive. A repeat testing for APLA is also not warranted as if positive (persistent positive) still no therapy is warranted. Obviously, if positive again, it will add to the mental agony of the patient!

Scenario 3
Pregnant with many previous abortions and APLA positive

Mrs. A, a 30-year-old lady, has a significant history of multiple first-trimester abortions. She is referred for a rheumatology opinion—and on testing for APLA—is found to be triple positive—LAC, beta-2 GPI and ACL. On repeat testing 12 weeks later, LAC and ACL are persistently positive. What is her management?

This lady fulfils the obstetric criteria for obstetric APS. As she is trying to conceive, she can be started on low-dose aspirin at 75–100 mg/day (after a platelet count). She should be started on heparin as soon as her pregnancy gets confirmed. This may be in the form of low-molecular-weight heparin once a day (1 mg/kg of enoxaparin) or unfractionated heparin (much cheaper) at 5000 U subcutaneously twice a day. She is advised that this treatment needs to be continued throughout pregnancy and till 6–12 weeks post-partum. There is no need for any testing, apart from a baseline platelet count and repeat after 6 weeks on starting heparin. Her obstetrician and rheumatologist need to discuss and decide the best time to switch to UFH (if on LMWH)—generally 1 week before delivery or 36 weeks, and stopping aspirin around the same time. UFH needs to be started post-delivery and she can breastfeed on it.

Scenario 4
Vascular APS getting pregnant

Ms. Z, a 25-year-old lady with deep venous thrombosis 1 year ago, who was found to be anticardiolipin antibody positive twice, is planning to get pregnant. She is on warfarin. Her obstetrician has sent to the rheumatologist to advise on further management. What is the plan we draw up?

This lady will require full-dose anticoagulation during pregnancy. As warfarin is teratogenic, it must be stopped at the time she is detected pregnant and shifted to full-dose heparin. She is counselled that she should have a planned pregnancy and be vigilant about her menstrual cycle, so that she can detect any delay in menstruation and get a urine pregnancy test done at the earliest to avoid prolonged foetal exposure to warfarin.

One she gets pregnant, she is advised to shift to low-molecular-weight heparin (1 mg/kg twice a day of enoxaparin) or unfractionated heparin (10–15,000 units twice a day, inexpensive, more painful due to higher volume, testing required). If she goes for the latter she needs to keep her APTT between 60 and 90 s (usual control 40 s). This will entail testing the same repeatedly and adjusting the dose appropriately. Generally the APTT should be done 6 h after the subcutaneous injection.

15.5 Miscellaneous Issues

Some issues not discussed in this chapter will get a brief mention here. Newer anticoagulants like direct thrombin inhibitors and direct-Xa inhibitors namely dabigatran, rivaroxaban, etc. have been introduced recently and have a major advantage of not requiring to be titrated as per prothrombin time and INR (compared to vitamin K antagonists like warfarin). However, their role in APLA is not yet clear, specifically in obstetric APS. Many of them could be teratogenic. Another issue is catastrophic APS. Catastrophic APS is an accelerated form of this disease which occurs in 1% and is often precipitated by an infection or sudden cessation of anticoagulation in known APS patients. It presents with multi-organ dysfunction and should be considered as a differential with septicaemia, TTP, HELLP, etc. It is characterised by mild thrombocytopenia and microangiopathic haemolytic anaemia and microvascular thrombosis in multiple organs (by definition in at least three in a single week). Its treatment involves both anticoagulation and immunosuppressive, namely pulse steroids.

15.6 Conclusions

Antiphospholipid syndrome is an intriguing disorder, ranging from thrombotic manifestations to obstetric manifestations. Testing in those not fulfilling clinical criteria for APS is not recommended as it does not change therapy if positive, but adds to the mental agony of a patient. It is important to realise that although the treatment of both obstetric and thrombotic APLA will include low-dose aspirin, the dose of heparin used will be markedly different—prophylactic dose in the former to full dose in the latter.

Although low-molecular-weight heparin is the most convenient (and probably safest) option, it is markedly expensive and thus UFH (at least ten times cheaper) is often used in developing countries for financial reasons. UFH is very convenient when used at prophylactic doses; however, it requires monitoring at therapeutic doses. It is important to make adjustments in the type of heparin and aspirin 1 week prior to planned delivery. At delivery, UFH is generally stopped 12 h before and resumed 12 h later. It should be continued for 6–12 weeks post-partum in obstetric APS and changed to warfarin in thrombotic APS.

References

1. Gerardi MC, Fernandes MA, Tincani A, Andreoli L (2018) Obstetric anti-phospholipid syndrome: state of the art. Curr Rheumatol Rep 20(10):59
2. Meroni PL, Borghi MO, Grossi C, Chighizola CB, Durigutto P, Tedesco F (2018) Obstetric and vascular antiphospholipid syndrome: same antibodies but different diseases? Nat Rev Rheumatol 14(7):433–440
3. Miyakis S, Lockshin MD, Atsumi T, Branch DW, Brey RL, Cervera R et al (2006) International consensus statement on an update of the classification criteria for definite antiphospholipid syndrome (APS). J Thromb Haemost 4(2):295–306
4. Garcia D, Doruk E (2018) Diagnosis and management of the antiphospholipid syndrome. N Engl J Med 378(21):2010–2021
5. Devreese KM, Pierangeli SS, de Laat B, Tripodi A, Atsumi T, Ortel TL, For the Subcommittee on Lupus Anticoagulant/Phospholipid/Dependent Antibodies (2014) Testing for antiphospholipid antibodies with solid phase assays: guidance from the SSC of the ISTH. J Thromb Haemost 12:792–795
6. Uthman I, Noureldine MHA, Ruiz-Irastorza G et al (2019) Management of antiphospholipid syndrome. Ann Rheum Dis 78:155–161
7. Andreoli L, Bertsias GK, Agmon-Levin N, Brown S, Cervera R, Costedoat-Chalumeau N et al (2017) EULAR recommendations for women's health and the management of family planning, assisted reproduction, pregnancy and menopause in patients with systemic lupus erythematosus and/or antiphospholipid syndrome. Ann Rheum Dis 76(3):476–485

8. Sciascia S, Sanna G, Murru V, Roccatello D, Munther A (2013) GAPSS: the global antiphospholipid syndrome score. Rheumatology (Oxford) 52(8):1397–1403
9. Schreiber K, Sciascia S, de Groot PG, Devreese K, Jacobsen S, Ruiz-Irastorza G et al (2018) Antiphospholipid syndrome. Nat Rev Dis Primers 4:17103
10. Antovic A, Sennström M, Bremme K, Svenungsson E (2018) Obstetric antiphospholipid syndrome. Lupus Sci Med 5:e000197

Managing Pregnancy in Systemic Sclerosis

16

Shefali K. Sharma

Abstract

In the past it was encouraged that systemic sclerosis patients didn't get pregnant due to higher risk of poor maternal and fetal outcomes. However, now if we plan pregnancy when the disease is quiescent, under close monitoring and appropriate therapy we are likely to get successful pregnancy. It is encouraged to plan pregnancy when the disease is quiescent. The physical Investigations that need to be done prior to getting pregnant are:

Blood pressure measurement
Kidney function tests
Autoantibody tests
Echocardiography (heart scan)
Lung function tests

Generally scleroderma does not worsen during pregnancy, but the most dreaded complication is scleroderma renal crisis. Even though ACE inhibitors are associated with increased risk of congenital malformations, they are recommended during pregnancy in scleroderma. So for all patients who become pregnant close monitoring for cardiopulmonary complications and renal crisis should be done. It is best to adopt a multidisciplinary approach for such patients.

Keywords

Systemic sclerosis · Pregnancy

In the past it was encouraged that scleroderma patients do not become pregnant due to higher risk of poor maternal and foetal outcomes. However, now if we plan

S. K. Sharma (✉)
Department of Internal Medicine, PGIMER, Chandigarh, India

© Springer Nature Singapore Pte Ltd. 2020
S. K. Sharma (ed.), *Women's Health in Autoimmune Diseases*,
https://doi.org/10.1007/978-981-15-0114-2_16

pregnancy when the disease is quiescent, under close monitoring and appropriate therapy we are likely to get a successful pregnancy. The most dreaded maternal complication of scleroderma is renal crisis. Even though ACE inhibitors are associated with increased risk of congenital malformations, they are recommended during pregnancy in scleroderma. So for all patients who become pregnant close monitoring for cardiopulmonary complications and renal crisis should be done. It is best to adopt a multidisciplinary approach for such patients.

This chapter discusses about fertility in systemic sclerosis (SSc), pregnancy outcomes, maternal complications during pregnancy and management issues during pregnancy.

16.1 Fertility in Systemic Sclerosis

This may be difficult to determine as many issues may be involved like the ability to get pregnant, and also the desire to get pregnant in spite of a crippling disease. Luckily for us most patients have completed family when they come to us in late 20s or 30s.

There are no cases of infertility in limited systemic sclerosis. The cases of infertility in diffuse are related to the fibrosis of the genital tract, making conception difficult. Recent studies have not identified decreased overall fertility in SSc [1–3].

Steen et al. concluded that SSc patients have reasonably good pregnancy outcomes compared with other rheumatic diseases. Infertility is not frequently encountered. For good obstetric outcomes for the mother and child pregnancy should be planned well, i.e., when the disease is in remission [4, 5].

16.2 Pregnancy Outcomes

The pregnancy outcomes of patients with SSc are variable. The studies by Black and Slate showed that miscarriages were increased in patients of SSc [6, 7]. However, as the patients belonged to low-income group it could be argued that they had inherent risks for miscarriages. Some studies showed that miscarriages were increased even before the onset of clinical SSc [8].

Study by Steen et al. documented the frequency of miscarriage to be 9% in patients of SSc and it was 7.5% in pregnancies of healthy controls. This study also observed that the frequency of miscarriage was more after the disease than before (15% vs. 8%). But the risk of miscarriage in SSc patients was not significant.

Should a patient who has suffered from scleroderma renal crisis plan a pregnancy? In this scenario the pregnancy will be a high-risk one. Then probably pregnancy carries a significant risk. If the blood pressure is not controlled by non-ACE inhibitors then an ACE inhibitor will have to be added. Both ACE inhibitor and non-ACE inhibitor medication will have to be combined, and the patient will have to be closely monitored for oligohydramnios or other signs of foetal abnormalities.

16.3 Prematurity

SSc had increased incidence of premature infants as compared to controls. Steen et al. did a retrospective case-control study of pregnancies in patients who had SSc before; small full-term infants, i.e. below 5.5 lb, occurred significantly more frequently in patients who had SSc (10%), in comparison to rheumatoid arthritis (4%), and normal controls (2%).

Certain case reports have documented increased infant mortality in SSc patients. Most of them were associated with acute exacerbation of scleroderma. Neonatal deaths have been reported but they are not statistically significant.

Recent studies from Spain, India and Brazil have confirmed that although there are increased risks of miscarriage, prematurity and very rarely infant death, the chances are not so much as to discourage women to become pregnant.

16.4 Effects of Pregnancy on Systemic Sclerosis

The main reason for worry in a pregnant patient of SSc is scleroderma renal crisis. The blood pressure elevation in scleroderma pregnancies must be treated promptly and aggressively with ACE inhibitors. As we know that ACE inhibitors are contraindicated in pregnancy, particularly during the third trimester, and as it has been associated with infant kidney dysfunction, it is essential to control hypertension and the associated renal crisis in pregnant SSc patients [9], which is potentially life-saving.

If a SSc patient has had scleroderma renal crisis it is not a contraindication to plan pregnancy provided that the disease is stable for a considerable period of time prior to planning a pregnancy. In this scenario ACE inhibitors may be used to control blood pressure if other medications are not effective [10].

In a scleroderma pregnancy with hypertension and proteinuria, diagnosis of scleroderma renal crisis can be confused with pre-eclampsia of pregnancy.

Pregnancy may not be advisable in patients with severe visceral involvement; the presence of severe cardiomyopathy (ejection fraction <30%), pulmonary hypertension, severe restrictive lung disease (forced vital capacity <50%) and renal insufficiency are associated with an adverse outcome of pregnancy [10].

Musculoskeletal complaints like carpal tunnel syndrome, leg cramps, arthralgias and back pain are common in SSc pregnancies.

As we are aware gastro-oesophageal reflux worsening is a common problem in healthy pregnancy more so in SSc pregnancies, particularly during third trimester as the uterus enlarges. SSc patients suffer from Mallory–Weiss syndrome during early or late pregnancy [11, 12]. This can be associated with life-threatening bleeding and recurrent vomiting that needs prompt treatment and hospitalization.

Some patients may experience increase in dyspnoea and pulmonary hypertension.

16.5 Management of Pregnancy

Pregnancy in SSc may be uneventful, with good maternal and foetal outcomes. SSc is a multisystem disease and complications do occur; however, careful antenatal evaluations, discussion of potential problems and participation in monitoring programme are mandatory to optimize outcomes.

1. Because women with diffuse SSc are at greater risk for developing serious cardiopulmonary and renal problems early in the disease, they should be encouraged to delay pregnancy until the disease stabilizes.
2. At the onset of pregnancy SSc patient should be evaluated to determine the type of disease, extent and type of systemic involvement and duration of symptoms. Patients with diffuse SSc or who have anti-topoisomerase or RNA polymerase III antibodies are at greater risk of a more aggressive disease.
3. When there are serious concerns like severe cardiomyopathy (ejection fraction <30%), moderate-to-severe pulmonary arterial hypertension, severe restrictive lung disease (forced vital capacity <50% of predicted), renal insufficiency and malabsorption, the decision to continue pregnancy will be based on specific abnormalities, not because of SSc being the cause.
4. Stop the drugs that are contraindicated during pregnancy like methotrexate and D-penicillamine. Avoid corticosteroids. Minimize use of proton pump inhibitors, calcium channel blockers and antihistamines.
5. Hydroxychloroquine is safe during pregnancy. Low-dose prednisone did not show an increased risk for oral cleft [13] or any association with renal crisis [14]. Antihistaminic and proton pump inhibitors may be used for the treatment of oesophageal reflux, nausea and vomiting. Intravenous immunoglobulin therapy may be given during pregnancy. But cyclophosphamide is contraindicated during pregnancy.
6. More frequent monitoring of foetal size and uterine activity is necessary.
7. Frequent blood pressure monitoring is recommended and aggressive therapy with antihypertensives when required. If elevated blood pressure is due to scleroderma renal crisis then ACE inhibitors should be started immediately. Before the use of ACE inhibitors the prognosis of scleroderma renal crisis was bad. Their immediate use saves both mother and child. The benefit to mother outweighs the risk of toxicity to foetus. Patients who have been treated with ACE inhibitors during the third trimester of pregnancy stand at an increased risk for serious kidney problems in the baby.
8. ACE inhibitors can result in foetal abnormalities including anhydramnios, renal atresia, pulmonary hypoplasia and foetal death. This is more so when used in the latter half of pregnancy. This is called fetopathy [15, 16]. The exact incidence is not known. In case a patient of SSc has renal crisis during pregnancy ACE inhibitors are mandatory.
9. Close observation and treatment of premature labour are required to avoid beta-adrenergic agonists.
10. Procure a venous access.

11. Epidural anaesthesia is preferred.
12. Special warming of delivery room and intravenous fluids should be done and patients should be kept warm.
13. Epidural anaesthesia is preferred.
14. Care should be given to the episiotomy and caesarean section incisions.

The worst clinical scenario will be a progression of skin or rapid deterioration of internal organs. If such a situation occurs in first trimester then elective termination of pregnancy can be considered. However, if it occurs in the third trimester then preterm birth with aggressive treatment should be instituted.

16.6 Management of Delivery

Pregnant SSc patients are an anaesthetic challenge. Thick skin causes difficulty in venous access. Vaginal constriction, taut abdominal skin and contractures interfere with taking blood pressure and positioning during delivery.

General anaesthesia should be avoided as patients have microstomia. Regional anaesthesia like epidural block is preferred as it not only provides anaesthesia but vasodilation as well.

16.7 Conclusion

Pregnancy is not a contraindication in systemic sclerosis. The increased risk for premature and small infants may be minimized with good obstetric and neonatal care. Risk of scleroderma renal crisis is unique to these pregnancies. Careful planning, close monitoring and aggressive management with optimal immunosuppression allow these women to have normal babies.

References

1. Goirdano M et al (1985) Pregnancy and systemic sclerosis. Arthritis Rheum 28:237–238
2. Silman A, Black C (1988) Increased incidence of spontaneous abortion and infertility in women with scleroderma before disease onset. A controlled study. Ann Rheum Dis 47:441–444
3. Wanchu A, Misra R (1996) Pregnancy outcomes in systemic sclerosis. JAPI 44(9):637–640
4. Steen VD, Medsger TA Jr (1999) Fertility and pregnancy outcomes in women with systemic sclerosis. Arthritis Rheum 42(4):763–768
5. Steen VD (1999) Pregnancy in women with systemic sclerosis. Obstet Gynecol 94(1):15–20
6. Black CM, Stevens WM (1989) Scleroderma. Rheum Dis Clin N Am 15(2):193–212
7. Slate WG, Graham AR (1968) Scleroderma and pregnancy. Am J Obstet Gynecol 101(3):335–341
8. Siamopoulou-Mavridou A, Manoussakis MN, Mavridis AK et al (1988) Outcome of pregnancy in patients with autoimmune rheumatic disease before the disease onset. Ann Rheum Dis 47(12):982–987
9. Karlen JR, Cook WA (1974) Renal scleroderma and pregnancy. Obstet Gynecol 44(3):349–354

10. Traub YM, Shapiro AP, Rodnan GP et al (1983) Hypertension and renal failure in progressive systemic sclerosis. Review of a 25-year experience with 68 cases. Medicine (Baltimore) 62(6):335–352
11. Steen VD, Conte C, Day N et al (1989) Pregnancy in women with systemic sclerosis. Arthritis Rheum 32(2):151–157
12. Kahl LE, Blair C, Ramsey Goldman R et al (1990) Pregnancy outcomes in women with primary Raynaud's phenomenon. Arthritis Rheum 38(8):1249–1255
13. Altieri P, Cameron JS (1988) Scleroderma renal crisis in a pregnant women with late partial recovery of renal function. Nephrol Dial Transplant 3(5):677–680
14. Baethge BA, Wolf RE (1989) Successful pregnancy with scleroderma renal disease and pulmonary hypertension in a patient using angiotensin converting enzyme inhibitors. Ann Rheum Dis 48(9):776–778
15. Mehta N, Modi N (1989) ACE inhibitors in pregnancy. Lancet 2(8654):96–97
16. Pryde PG, Barr M Jr (2001) Low dose, short acting, angiotensin converting enzyme inhibitors as rescue therapy in pregnancy. Obstet Gynecol 97(5):799–800

Management and Monitoring of Anti-Ro/La positive Mother

17

G. S. R. S. N. K. Naidu and M. B. Adarsh

Abstract

Neonatal lupus erythematosus is a clinical syndrome that occurs in the babies of mothers who are positive for anti-Ro and anti-La autoantibodies and characterized by cardiac and cutaneous manifestations. The risk of developing neonatal lupus during first pregnancy is about 2% but the risk of recurrence in mothers with past history of neonatal lupus is higher, up to 18–20%. Cardiac involvement in the form of complete heart block is the most dreaded and is usually irreversible and is associated with increased morbidity and mortality. The cardiac manifestations can develop as early as 16 weeks of gestation; hence, in utero cardiac screening is recommended for at-risk fetuses starting from 16 weeks. Hydroxychloroquine has been shown to prevent the development of cardiac manifestations but the role of other treatments like fluorinated steroids, intravenous immunoglobulin, and plasma exchange is still doubtful. Pediatric cardiologist should be involved in the management as infants with complete heart block will need pacemaker implantation immediately after birth.

Keywords

Neonatal lupus erythematosus · Anti-Ro antibody · Anti-La antibody · Congenital heart block

17.1 Introduction

Anti-Ro/SS-A and anti-La/SS-B antibodies are autoantibodies against ribonucleoproteins that are commonly associated with autoimmune diseases like Sjogren's syndrome and systemic lupus erythematosus (SLE). The Ro antigen is constituted of two different proteins, Ro52 and Ro60 kDa [1]. Neonatal lupus erythematosus is

G. S. R. S. N. K. Naidu (✉) · M. B. Adarsh
Post Graduate Institute of Medical Education and Research, Chandigarh, India

a clinical syndrome that occurs in the fetus or infant of mothers who are positive for serum anti-Ro and/or anti-La autoantibodies. It is characterized by the presence of cutaneous, cardiac, hematologic, and hepatobiliary manifestations.

17.2 Pathogenesis

Immunoglobulin G (IgG) crosses the placenta from mother to fetus beginning from 12–13 weeks of gestation and linearly increases to reach maximum concentrations in fetal circulation in the third trimester [2]. IgG anti-Ro and La autoantibodies cross the placenta and cause damage to developing tissues by inducing inflammation and fibrosis. These autoantibodies form immune complexes with fetal antigens exposed on apoptotic cells or by molecular mimicry with L-type calcium channels leading to damage [3]. Even though more than 98% of infants with neonatal lupus have maternal transfer of anti-Ro and anti-La antibodies, only 1–2% of mothers with these antibodies have infants developing manifestations of neonatal lupus [4]. The risk increases in subsequent pregnancies with up to 18–20% risk of recurrence. The risk of congenital heart block (CHB) is about 2% in mothers with anti-Ro autoantibody positivity and it increases to 3.1% if the mother is positive for both anti-Ro and anti-La autoantibodies [5].

17.3 Clinical Features of Neonatal Lupus

The clinical features of neonatal lupus can be divided into reversible and nonreversible manifestations (Table 17.1).

Cardiac involvement, noted in about 25%, is the most distinctive and dreaded manifestation and is usually irreversible. The classic cardiac involvement in neonatal lupus is first-, second-, or third-degree congenital atrioventricular (AV) block in a structurally normal heart. It commonly manifests during 18–24 weeks of gestation but can sometimes manifest as early as 16 weeks of gestation. Complete heart block once established is usually irreversible, develops due to fibrosis and calcification of AV nodal area, and presents in utero with bradycardia (40–80 beats/min). Other less common cardiac manifestations include valvular abnormalities, sinus bradycardia, QT prolongation, cardiomyopathy, congestive heart failure, endocardial fibroelastosis, and hydrops fetalis. Mortality rates up to 19% were documented with autoimmune complete heart block with majority occurring in utero [6]. Hydrops fetalis, myocarditis, low ventricular rate (<50/min), and earlier gestational age at diagnosis are associated with high mortality.

Cutaneous involvement is noted in about 40% of infants with neonatal lupus and usually develops few days or weeks after birth. The lesions resemble the lesions of acute to subacute cutaneous lupus seen in patients with SLE. The lesions are erythematous, nonscarring, macular, annular, or elliptical and commonly affect the head and scalp followed by trunk, extremities, or rarely whole body. These lesions usually resolve over few months and rarely persist for more than a year.

Table 17.1 Clinical manifestations of neonatal lupus erythematosus

Irreversible manifestation	Reversible manifestations
Cardiac involvement • AV block (first, second, third degree) • Sinus bradycardia • QT prolongation • Cardiomyopathy • Congestive heart failure • Valvular abnormality • Ventricular or atrial septal defect	*Cutaneous involvement* • Subacute cutaneous lupus • Photosensitivity • Telangiectasias • Atrophy
	Hematologic involvement • Anemia • Neutropenia • Thrombocytopenia • Aplastic anemia
	Hepatobiliary involvement • Elevated aminotransferases • Cholestasis • Hepatomegaly • Splenomegaly
	Neurological involvement • Macrocephaly • Hydrocephalus

Hematological and hepatobiliary manifestations are noted in about 35% of infants and are usually mild and self-limiting. They rarely present as isolated manifestations and are always associated with cardiac or cutaneous manifestations. Neurological involvement is very rare, manifests as macrocephaly with or without hydrocephalus, and is usually reversible.

17.4 Obstetric and Perinatal Outcomes of Ro/La-Positive Mothers

The obstetric outcomes, including mode of delivery, incidence of prematurity, growth retardation, intrauterine death, perinatal mortality, and infections, of asymptomatic anti-Ro/anti-La-positive mothers were found to be similar to those of the general population except for the incidence of neonatal lupus. But the perinatal outcomes were poor if the mother had SLE, due to higher incidence of prematurity and growth retardation [7–9].

Few studies have shown increased incidence of SLE among children of anti-Ro-positive mothers and the incidence correlated with the titers of anti-Ro autoantibodies [10, 11]. However, the incidence of SLE was not found to be higher among children who had neonatal lupus, but they were found to have higher incidence of juvenile immune arthritis and Hashimoto's thyroiditis [12]. At 10 years of follow-up, SLE developed in 18.6% and Sjogren's syndrome developed in 27.9% of asymptomatic mothers who had a baby with neonatal lupus [13]. The risk of developing a systemic autoimmune disease on follow-up was twice in mothers who are positive for both anti-Ro and anti-La autoantibodies compared to mothers with only anti-Ro positivity.

17.5 Management

Congenital heart block is a potentially life-threatening manifestation of neonatal lupus and can manifest in utero, as early as 16 weeks of gestation. Hence, the management of neonatal lupus includes prenatal counselling, fetal screening, maternal evaluation, and treatment of heart disease.

17.5.1 Counselling

Among mothers with anti-Ro and anti-La autoantibody positivity, the risk of having a child with neonatal lupus is approximately 2%. However, the risk is higher, up to 18–20%, among women who had a previous pregnancy complicated by cardiac manifestations of neonatal lupus. Hence, the expecting parents should be counselled regarding the risk of neonatal lupus and the need for fetal screening for early detection and subsequent management of cardiac abnormalities.

17.5.2 Fetal Screening

Fetal screening for cardiac abnormalities should be done in all mothers with anti-Ro and anti-La autoantibody positivity and especially in those with previous history of child with neonatal lupus. Fetal echocardiography is a noninvasive screening method for structural heart disease and assessment of heart rhythm and function. Up to 80% of cases develop cardiac abnormalities between 16 and 26 weeks of gestation; hence weekly screening is advised between 16 and 26 weeks and less frequently after 26 weeks of gestation. Neonates without cardiac abnormalities at birth should be monitored till 1 month of age, as up to 2% of them can develop heart blocks during this period. Asymptomatic infants with transient second-degree AV block should be evaluated at 3 months of age while infants with first-degree AV block should be evaluated at 1 year of age with electrocardiogram and echocardiography.

17.5.3 Maternal Evaluation

All mothers of neonates having congenital heart block should be screened for anti-Ro and anti-La autoantibodies. In a systematic review of 1416 affected mothers, 86% were positive for anti-Ro antibodies while only 55% were positive for anti-La antibodies [5]. Anti-Ro52 antibodies are more frequent than anti-Ro60 antibodies and are suspected to play an important role in the development of CHB in the fetus. Mothers who are negative for anti-Ro and anti-La antibodies should be tested specifically for anti-Ro52 and anti-Ro60 (by both recombinant antigen and native antigen). Mothers who are positive for these antibodies should be screened for underlying systemic autoimmune diseases like SLE and primary Sjogren's syndrome. The commonest autoimmune disease noted in these mothers is SLE (up to 30%) followed by primary Sjogren's syndrome (up to 20%). Twenty-five percent of mothers remain asymptomatic while 25% have undifferentiated connective tissue disorder.

17.5.4 Prevention of Cardiac Disease

Various drugs have been used to prevent high-degree AV blocks in utero but none of them were proven to be beneficial. Fluorinated steroids like dexamethasone and betamethasone, which can reach the fetal circulation, were thought to reduce inflammation and fibrosis in cardiac tissue and help in preventing high-degree heart blocks. However, the efficacy of fluorinated steroids in preventing the progression of cardiac disease or death is not conclusively proven [14]. There is a high risk of fetal complications like intrauterine growth retardation and oligohydramnios apart from maternal complications like infections, osteoporosis, and diabetes with use of fluorinated steroids. Hence, presently, fluorinated steroids are not recommended for preventing cardiac manifestations or death of fetuses at risk of developing cardiac neonatal lupus.

Intravenous immunoglobulin (IVIg) is a potential therapeutic option in preventing cardiac manifestations of neonatal lupus as IVIg can increase the catabolism and decrease placental transfer of anti-Ro and anti-La antibodies. Even though case reports have shown that IVIg may prevent the development of cardiac neonatal lupus, two prospective studies with 20 patients each failed to demonstrate the efficacy of IVIg in preventing cardiac manifestations in at-risk fetuses [15, 16]. However, we need to keep in mind that the dose of IVIg used in both the studies was 400 mg/kg given at an interval of 3 weeks. Whether using a higher dose of IVIg will be beneficial needs to be studied.

Plasma exchange can help in lowering the levels of anti-Ro and anti-La antibodies and aid in preventing cardiac damage in at-risk fetuses. However, the data on plasma exchange is limited to few case reports with varied results and compounded by the concomitant use of steroids and IVIg in some case reports [14].

Hydroxychloroquine (HCQ) has shown a lot of promise in reducing the recurrence of cardiac neonatal lupus in few case-control studies [17, 18]. In a small randomized placebo-controlled trail, use of HCQ was shown to be protective against the development of congenital abnormalities [19]. Based on the present available data, HCQ should be advised to all mothers with anti-Ro and anti-La antibodies, especially to those mothers who had a previous child with cardiac neonatal lupus.

17.5.5 Management of Heart Blocks

Complete heart block is irreversible and associated with increased morbidity and mortality. Pediatric cardiologist needs to assess the infant soon after birth and plan for pacemaker implantation at the earliest. Pacemaker is indicated in infants with congenital third-degree AV block with ventricular rate less than 55/min or less than 70/min with structural heart disease or a wide QRS escape rhythm, complex ventricular ectopy, or ventricular dysfunction [20].

References

1. Franceschini F, Cavazzana I (2005) Anti-Ro/SSA and La/SSB antibodies. Autoimmunity 38:55–63
2. Palmeira P, Quinello C, Silveira-Lessa AL et al (2012) IgG placental transfer in healthy and pathological pregnancies. Clin Dev Immunol 2012:985646
3. Izmirly P, Saxena A, Buyon JP (2017) Progress in the pathogenesis and treatment of cardiac manifestations of neonatal lupus. Curr Opin Rheumatol 29:467–472
4. Hon KL, Leung AKC (2012) Neonatal lupus erythematosus. Autoimmune Dis 2012:301274
5. Gordon P, Khamashta MA, Rosenthal E et al (2004) Anti-52 kDa Ro, anti-60 kDa Ro, and anti-La antibody profiles in neonatal lupus. J Rheumatol 31:2480–2487
6. Brito-Zeron P, Izmirly PM, Ramos-Casals M et al (2015) The clinical spectrum of autoimmune congenital heart block. Nat Rev Rheumatol 11:301–312
7. Brucato A, Cimaz R, Caporali R et al (2011) Pregnancy outcomes in patients with autoimmune diseases and anti-Ro/SSA antibodies. Clin Rev Allergy Immunol 40:27–41
8. Martínez-Sánchez N, Perez-Pinto S, Robles-Marhuenda A et al (2017) Obstetric and perinatal outcome in anti-Ro/SSA-positive pregnant women: a prospective cohort study. Immunol Res 65:487–494
9. Costedoat-Chalumeau N, Amoura Z, Lupoglazoff JM et al (2004) Outcome of pregnancies in patients with anti-SSA/Ro antibodies a study of 165 pregnancies, with special focus on electrocardiographic variations in the children and comparison with a control group. Arthritis Rheum 50:3187–3194
10. Jaeggi E, Laskin C, Hamilton R et al (2010) The importance of the level of maternal anti-Ro/SSA antibodies as a prognostic marker of the development of cardiac neonatal lupus erythematosus: a prospective study of 186 antibody-exposed fetuses and infants. J Am Coll Cardiol 55:2778–2784
11. Lehman TJA, Reichlin M, Santner TJ et al (1989) Maternal antibodies to Ro (SS-A) are associated with both early onset of disease and male sex among children with systemic lupus erythematosus. Arthritis Rheum 32:1414–1420
12. Martin V, Lee LA, Askanase AD et al (2002) Long-term follow-up of children with neonatal lupus and their unaffected siblings. Arthritis Rheum 46:2377–2383
13. Rivera TL, Izmirly PM, Birnbaum BK et al (2009) Disease progression in mothers of children enrolled in the Research Registry for Neonatal Lupus. Ann Rheum Dis 68:828–835
14. Saxena A, Izmirly PM, Mendez B et al (2014) Prevention and treatment in utero of autoimmune associated congenital heart block. Cardiol Rev 22:263–267
15. Friedman DM, Llanos C, Izmirly PM et al (2010) Evaluation of fetuses in a study of intravenous immunoglobulin as preventive therapy for congenital heart block: results of a multicenter, prospective, open-label clinical trial. Arthritis Rheum 62:1138–1146
16. Pisoni CN, Brucato A, Ruffatti A et al (2010) Failure of intravenous immunoglobulin to prevent congenital heart block: findings of a multicenter, prospective, observational study. Arthritis Rheum 62:1147–1152
17. Izmirly PM, Kim MY, Llanos C et al (2010) Evaluation of the risk of anti-SSA/Ro-SSB/La antibody-associated cardiac manifestations of neonatal lupus in fetuses of mothers with systemic lupus erythematosus exposed to hydroxychloroquine. Ann Rheum Dis 69:1827–1830
18. Izmirly PM, Costedoat-Chalumeau N, Pisoni CN et al (2012) Maternal use of hydroxychloroquine is associated with a reduced risk of recurrent anti-SSA/Ro-antibody-associated cardiac manifestations of neonatal lupus. Circulation 126:76–82
19. Levy RA, Vilela VS, Cataldo MJ et al (2001) Hydroxychloroquine in lupus pregnancy: a double-blind placebo-controlled study. Lupus 10:401–404
20. Epstein AE, DiMarco JP, Ellenbogen KA et al (2013) 2012 ACCF/AHA/HRS focused update incorporated into the ACCF/AHA/HRS 2008 guidelines for device-based therapy of cardiac rhythm abnormalities: a report of the American College of Cardiology Foundation/American Heart Association task force on practice guidelines and the Heart Rhythm Society. J Am Coll Cardiol 61:e6–e75

Management of Sjögren's Syndrome During Pregnancy

18

Pulukool Sandhya

Abstract

There is a scarcity of data on the management of primary Sjögren's syndrome (pSS) in pregnancy. As there is a higher risk of complications in pregnant women with pSS, including the possibility of neonatal lupus, these women should be managed by a multidisciplinary team. At the preconceptional stage itself, there is a need to ensure that the disease activity is well controlled and the patient is not on any teratogenic drugs. It is also important to verify that there is no severe organ involvement that could adversely impact maternal and fetal health. Disease activity needs to be monitored throughout pregnancy. Baseline antibody profile (anti-Ro52, anti-Ro60, and anti-La) should be performed in all women planning pregnancy and if they are seropositive, appropriate counseling about possible risks of neonatal lupus should be done without imparting undue anxiety. Weekly fetal echocardiography is done from 16th to 28th weeks of gestation and less frequently till term hoping that impending complete heart block can be detected and treated, though evidence to support this protocol is weak. Fluorinated steroids are associated with adverse effects and have not been found to have survival advantage or decrease requirement for pacing. Routine use of fluorinated steroids should be avoided and may be considered only in certain scenarios such as recent-onset incomplete heart block and in case of myocardial involvement/hydrops. Hydroxychloroquine protects against occurrence of cardiac and cutaneous lupus and hence is a potential preventive therapy.

Keywords

Sjögren's syndrome · Pregnancy · Anti-Ro 52 · Anti-Ro 60 · Anti-La · Congenital heart block · Hydroxychloroquine · Dexamethasone

P. Sandhya (✉)
Department of Rheumatology, St Stephens Hospital, New Delhi, India

© Springer Nature Singapore Pte Ltd. 2020
S. K. Sharma (ed.), *Women's Health in Autoimmune Diseases*,
https://doi.org/10.1007/978-981-15-0114-2_18

18.1 Introduction

Primary Sjögren's syndrome (pSS) is an autoimmune disease characterized by lymphocytic infiltration of the exocrine glands. The disease is well known for sicca symptoms though sicca symptoms may not always be conspicuous [1, 2]. It is increasingly being recognized that systemic manifestations can be presenting features of the disease [1]. Like other autoimmune diseases, pSS occurs predominantly in women. Though in Western countries the age at onset is perimenopausal, in India the onset of the disease is at least a decade earlier [2] and in those with predominant systemic features, the disease can manifest in their 30s [3].

Pregnancy is an important issue in women with chronic autoimmune diseases that requires shared decision-making between the treating rheumatologist, obstetrician, and the patient. Hormonal and immunological changes during pregnancy can modulate the expression of autoimmune disease; concurrently, the underlying autoimmune disease can also affect maternal and fetal outcomes. Both mother and fetus, therefore, need to be monitored regularly throughout pregnancy. Knowledge of potential complications related to the disease enables early detection and institution of appropriate management which is vital to an optimal outcome.

18.2 Considerations Before Pregnancy

Women with pSS should undergo a thorough clinical evaluation, risk assessment, laboratory evaluation as required, and detailed counseling in the preconceptional period as given in Table 18.1 and detailed below. She should be evaluated for disease activity and any systemic involvement that could have an adverse effect on maternal and fetal health during the course of pregnancy. The EULAR Sjögren's syndrome disease activity index (ESSDAI) is a recently introduced disease activity scoring that incorporates the following domains—cutaneous, respiratory, renal, articular, muscular, peripheral nervous system, central nervous system, glandular, constitutional, lymphadenopathic, hematological, and biological [4]. Though there is no specific data on pSS, it is logical to assume based on literature from other autoimmune diseases that the disease activity in pSS needs to be well controlled for at least 6 months, prior to pregnancy. Teratogenic drugs such as methotrexate, cyclophosphamide, and mycophenolate should be discontinued in the preconceptional period itself and switched to drugs that are compatible with pregnancy and further, it should be ensured that disease is well controlled post-switching also [5].

Women with pSS should also be evaluated for organ involvement that could be a contraindication to pregnancy. For instance, pulmonary arterial hypertension (PAH) could occur in up to 20% of pSS [6]. Lung and renal involvement were seen in 11% and 5% of patients with pSS, respectively [7]. As in lupus, pregnancy should be avoided in case of severe ILD, heart failure, PAH, and chronic kidney disease. Comorbidities such as hypertension, thyroid disorders, and blood sugars should be adequately controlled.

Table 18.1 : Key points to consider before pregnancy

What to check	How to check	Action
1. Systemic disease activity	– Clinical – ESSDAI	ESSDAI >5 [9]—Consider deferring pregnancy till disease activity is controlled
2. Organ involvement and comorbidities	– Clinical – CBC, LFT, KFT, ESR, sugars, thyroid function test, urinalysis—tests for organ-specific involvement as required, e.g., arterial blood gas, pulmonary function test, and echocardiography Evaluate for hypercoagulable conditions	Pregnancy contraindicated • CKD • Severe PAH • Severe ILD • Heart failure Defer pregnancy till blood pressure, sugars, and thyroid function abnormalities are corrected Heparin/aspirin as indicated
3. Drugs	Check for teratogenic drugs	Discontinue teratogenic drugs-methotrexate, cyclophosphamide, mycophenolate Leflunomide-cholestyramine washout required
4. Prior pregnancy outcome	Details of fetal mortality or morbidity—Recurrent spontaneous abortions, IUD, prematurity, neonatal lupus, IUGR, SGA Maternal mortality—eclampsia, preeclampsia, HELLP, syndrome, abruptio placenta, oligohydramnios, thrombosis	Evaluate and manage for APS antibodies and immunological profile—see point number 5 Severe HELLP or eclampsia—contraindication to pregnancy Evaluation by gynecologist
5. Antibodies	– Anti-Ro52, anti-Ro60, anti-La – Lupus anticoagulant – Anticardiolipin antibodies of IgG and/or IgM subtype – Anti-b2 glycoprotein-I antibodies of IgG and/or IgM subtype	Commence/continue HCQ APS features—heparin/aspirin as indicated

ESSDAI EULAR Sjögren's syndrome disease activity index; *CBC* Complete blood count; *LFT* Liver function test; *KFT* Kidney function test; *TFT* Thyroid function test; *CKD* Chronic kidney disease; *PAH* Pulmonary arterial hypertension; *ILD* Interstitial lung disease; *MTX* Methotrexate; *MMF* Mycophenolate; *CYC* Cyclophosphamide; *LEF* Leflunomide; *IUD* Intrauterine death; *IUGR* Intrauterine growth restriction; *SGA* Small for gestational age; *HELLP* Hemolysis, elevated liver enzymes, low platelet count; *aPL* Antiphospholipid; *aCL* Anti-cardiolipin; *anti-B2GP1* Anti-b2 glycoprotein-I; *APS* Antiphospholipid syndrome

All women with pSS contemplating pregnancy should have been tested for anti-Ro52 and anti-Ro60 and anti-SSB (anti-La). Women testing positive for these antibodies need to be counseled in detail regarding the risk of neonatal lupus. The high rate for recurrence in case of a previously affected child needs to be explained and counseled. A word of caution though; it should be understood that this is a rare complication and parents should not be subjected to undue anxiety. As hydroxychloroquine (HCQ) has been found to reduce the risk of neonatal lupus (cardiac and cutaneous), it is advisable that HCQ is started in the preconceptional period and continued throughout pregnancy [8, 9].

Details of previous pregnancy and adverse fetal and maternal outcome should be analyzed in detail. Adverse pregnancy outcome and fetal mortality and morbidity may be due to neonatal lupus in the setting of pSS. Though antiphospholipid antibody syndrome (APS) is less frequent in pSS, the antiphospholipid antibodies should be ordered if features of thrombosis and/or characteristic pregnancy morbidity are present [10]. If there are features of APS, she should be managed accordingly.

18.3 Consideration During Pregnancy

To ensure optimum outcome, mother and fetus should be monitored regularly and managed by a multidisciplinary team. Overview of management is depicted in Fig. 18.1. Unlike lupus which is known to flare during pregnancy, the effect of pregnancy on pSS disease activity is not known. Needless to say, disease activity needs to be monitored during pregnancy but there is no guideline regarding the timing or frequency of monitoring. Consultation with a rheumatologist should be scheduled

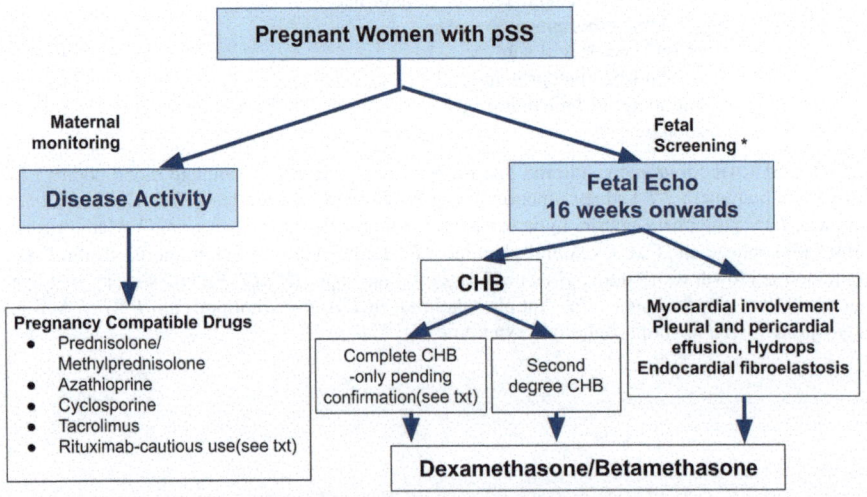

Fig. 18.1 Overview of management in pregnancy. *Only weak evidence

at least once in every trimester and more frequently in case of a disease flare. There are no validated disease scores for use in pregnancy. The laboratory domains of ESSDAI include hematological-(hemoglobin, leukocyte count, and platelet count) and biological (globulin levels and complements) variables [4]. Physiologic changes in pregnancy are known to alter these parameters. Cutoff values of these parameters would need to be modified accordingly for use in pregnancy [12]. Further, unlike C3, C4, and anti-dsDNA in lupus, there are no lab parameters that can reliably predict disease flare in pSS even in the nonpregnant stage. In such a scenario, close clinical evaluation followed by relevant tests to assess disease in a particular domain should be followed. For instance, in case of renal involvement, blood pressure, renal function, electrolyte, and urine evaluation should be done. Arterial blood gas analysis may be required in select cases such as in patients with renal tubular acidosis.

Pregnancy-compatible drugs need to be continued under close monitoring of a rheumatologist to minimize the occurrence of disease flares. Azathioprine, cyclosporine, tacrolimus, and prednisolone can be used during pregnancy to control disease activity [5]. Use of steroids can lead to diabetes, hypertension, preeclampsia, oligohydramnios, premature rupture of membranes, small-for-gestational-age births, adrenal insufficiency, and neurodevelopmental defects in the offspring. Hence, it is advisable that steroids are used in the lowest dose and the disease is controlled with immunosuppressants. Further, adverse effects of these drugs need to be weighed against the risk posed by untreated maternal disease to the mother and fetus. Limited data shows that rituximab is not teratogenic. Cautious use of rituximab is permitted during pregnancy though there is a risk of neonatal B-cell depletion when used in the later half of pregnancy. Hence, when indicated, it is recommended that rituximab is preferably used 6 months before pregnancy [5]. Pilocarpine is listed as a FDA category C drug. In the absence of adequate data in pregnancy, cautious use is recommended [13]. As hydroxychloroquine (HCQ) is safe in pregnancy and has a protective effect, continuing the drug throughout pregnancy is advisable.

18.3.1 Neonatal Lupus

Neonatal lupus encompasses clinical features resulting from passive transplacental transfer of maternal antibodies anti-SSA (anti-Ro52, anti-Ro60) and anti-SSB (anti-La 48 kDa) causing inflammation and damage to fetal tissue [14]. This complication is related to antibody status rather than maternal diagnosis. Neonatal lupus is seen in offsprings of asymptomatic mothers or mothers with lupus, pSS, or other connective tissue diseases with antibody positivity. In fact many a time, diagnosis of neonatal lupus can unmask an otherwise asymptomatic Sjögren's mother. It is to be noted that the data on neonatal lupus in literature is derived from anti-Ro-positive mothers as a whole and are therefore not specific for pSS.

The most characteristic and life-threatening manifestation of neonatal lupus is cardiac involvement. Maternal antibodies acting in concert with fetal, maternal, and environmental factors can damage the fetal conduction system especially the atrioventricular (AV) node as well as endocardium and myocardium. This results in congenital heart block (CHB), endocardial fibroelastosis, and cardiomyopathy; the latter two predict a worse prognosis [15]. Cardiac involvement generally develops in utero, most often between 16 and 24 weeks, but can also be seen at birth or in the immediate neonatal period. CHB is seen in 2% of anti-Ro-positive pregnancies with a recurrence of 19% in subsequent pregnancies [16]. CHB is usually complete and irreversible and presents with fetal heart rate <100/minute. Advanced CHB with low ventricular rate results in hydrops fetalis and death resulting in mortality of 20% [17]. CHB also has high morbidity and around 70% require pacing [17]. In CHB-affected pregnancies, 81% result in live births. Premature birth was seen in 38% whereas most of the deliveries occurred between 34–37 weeks. In 75% of cases mode of delivery was by caesarean section [17].

In addition to cardiac manifestations, dermatologic, hematologic, and hepatobiliary features have been described in neonatal lupus [14]. In contrast to the cardiac manifestations, the noncardiac manifestations are transient and resolve with the disappearance of the maternal antibodies at around 6 months.

18.3.2 Management of Neonatal Lupus (Cardiac)

There are no evidence-based recommendations for fetal screening, prophylaxis, or treatment of pSS mothers with anti-Ro positivity. Considering the severity of complications, it is of paramount importance that these patients with high-risk pregnancy are managed by a multidisciplinary team consisting of rheumatologists, obstetricians, fetal medicine specialists, and pediatricians. Management essentially consists of monitoring fetal heart and initiating treatment when significant abnormalities are detected and continued monitoring to assess response to treatment.

As the highest period of risk for developing cardiac events is between 16 weeks to 28 weeks, weekly monitoring by fetal echocardiography during this period, followed by less frequent monitoring till term, is the protocol followed at most centers [17]. Fetal echocardiography estimates first-degree AV block by calculating the mechanical PR interval which is the time from onset of left atrial contraction to the onset of left ventricular ejection [18]. In addition to detecting fetal heart rate and rhythm abnormalities, echocardiography also detects ventricular and valvular defects. There is a suggestion that premature atrial contractions, pericardial effusion, atrial echodensities, and tricuspid regurgitation detected on echocardiography could be a forerunner of CHB [16, 18].

The concept of fetal heart monitoring would be meaningful if the following are true—(a) phase of cardiac injury exists that heralds CHB (b) this phase is amenable to treatment (c) this phase can be identified precisely and within the therapeutic window by monitoring. Unfortunately, the current system of monitoring is far from ideal.

A number of questions typically come to the treating clinician's mind: Is PR interval prolongation a forerunner of CHB? Is weekly monitoring by fetal echocardiography appropriate enough? These questions have been partly answered by previous studies. Studies suggest that PR prolongation may not always be deleterious and could be a transient phenomenon. The PRIDE study revealed that CHB development was not always preceded by PR prolongation identified by weekly monitoring [18]. This study suggests that the progression from normal sinus rhythm to CHB is abrupt and unpredictable and there may not be a "warning event". Therefore, weekly monitoring is inadequate to capture the rapidity of events. In this scenario, maternal home-based Doppler monitoring of fetal heart rate twice daily followed by echocardiography is possibly a practical and more sensible alternative. A recent study using this methodology suggests that progression from normal to CHB happens rapidly and the critical window for treatment may be less than 12 hours [19]. Though in the study, the rate of CHB was low and reversibility with treatment was seen in only one out of the three affected cases, the methodology seems to hold promise and needs to be tested in a larger set of high-risk patients before it could be widely recommended.

The other key question in management relates to the existence of therapeutic window and whether there is an effective treatment which could reverse the critical cardiac injury from progressing. This is of importance as no treatment has been found to reverse complete CHB. Fluorinated steroids (dexamethasone and betamethasone) have been the most widely used treatment; because fluorinated compounds can cross the placenta and are bioavailable to the fetus. In incomplete heart block, steroids/ other immunosuppressants are expected to act by blocking inflammation and fibrosis of the conduction system as well as other cardiac tissues. In earlier case reports and series, steroids were reportedly effective in the treatment of myocardial dysfunction, pleural effusions, ascites, and hydrops fetalis but this was not seen in large series [20–22]. The study which reported efficacy and survival benefit for steroids suffers from poor methodology and has to be interpreted cautiously [23]. Further, concerns have been raised about the routine use of steroids for the following reasons. Firstly, dexamethasone has not been able to reverse second-degree CHB or demonstrate any survival benefit in large international series, systematic meta-analysis, and prospective study [22, 24–30]. Secondly, steroids are associated with both maternal and fetal adverse effects. Thirdly, differentiation between complete and incomplete forms of CHB is extremely difficult in utero. Moreover, incomplete CHB is also known to reverse spontaneously without treatment. Additionally, the exact preceding event to CHB at which point a window of opportunity exists has not been clearly defined so far. In a recent review, the suggestion has been to commence steroids for a brief duration in the following scenarios after carefully weighing and explaining risks and benefits to the mother: (a) recent complete heart block till the diagnosis of CHB is confirmed, (b) incomplete heart block, and (c) myocardial dysfunction, pleural and pericardial effusion, and hydrops [31].

Treatment options other than steroids have also been tried with varying success. Intravenous immunoglobulins (IVIG) at a dose of 400 mg/kg could not prevent progression of CHB in a prospective open-label trial [30]. In a small prospective cohort study, a combination of weekly plasmapheresis, fortnightly IVIG, and daily betamethasone was found to have some benefit in halting the progression of second-degree heart block [32]. $\beta 2$-Adrenergic receptor agonist has also been used in treatment with variable results. In utero cardiac pacing is risky and fraught with complications [15]. Prenatal use of hydroxychloroquine has been found to have a protective effect on cardiac and cutaneous manifestations [8, 9] and a prospective

PATCH trial is underway to verify the protective effect on mothers with prior CHB [15].

The future of effective treatment for cardiac neonatal lupus depends on improvement in monitoring devices and identifying risk factors. Wearable sensor devices that enable continuous monitoring and facilitate early detection while providing ease of in-home monitoring and are expected to revolutionize the field [15]. There is a need to identify fetal and maternal risk factors that could classify risk and apply intensive monitoring for those at highest risk while sparing others at low risk of undue anxiety and economic implications of monitoring. Considering rarity of the condition large trials may not be feasible but prospective studies are needed to define optimal risk and effective treatment strategies. Novel therapeutic approaches to reverse CHB and effective pacing strategies could potentially reduce fetal loss and fetal morbidity.

18.4 Other Considerations in Pregnancy and Delivery

Beyond neonatal lupus, data on other pregnancy outcomes in pSS are scarce. As compared to healthy controls, women with pSS had higher mean maternal age, babies with lower birth weight and were more likely to deliver by caesarean section or vacuum extraction [33, 34].

18.5 Considerations on Fertility and pSS

Fertility and parity rates in pSS have been reported to be comparable to those of the general population [35]. In a single-center retrospective study from India, only 4 out of 332 (1.2%) pSS patients had infertility [2]. Two had primary infertility whereas the other two had secondary infertility. In the only study on IVF and pSS, pSS was incidentally detected in 7 out of 42 infertile women with ANA positivity undergoing in vitro fertilization. These patients had unexplained implantation failure during prior embryo transfer. Interestingly, use of steroids in these patients during subsequent IVF resulted in successful implantation [36].

In conclusion, women with pSS have adverse pregnancy outcomes. Hence, they have to be evaluated and counseled in detail prior to planning pregnancy. The prepregnancy checklist should include the following-screen for systemic involvement and disease activity, check for teratogenic drugs, assess prior pregnancy outcome and tests for anti-Ro and anti-La antibodies and also antiphospholipid antibodies. Drugs compatible with pregnancy should be prescribed. As HCQ can reduce the risk of cardiac and cutaneous lupus, continuation of HCQ throughout pregnancy is advisable. The most dangerous complication is CHB. It is currently unclear if CHB can be reliably predicted and treated effectively by weekly fetal echocardiography considering the rapidity of events and narrow therapeutic window period. Fluorinated steroids have adverse effects and may be considered only in case of incomplete CHB at risk of progressing to complete CHB and involvement of myocardium, valvular lesion, or hydrops. Better monitoring techniques coupled with effective treatment strategies are expected to improve outcome.

References

1. Brito-Zerón P, Theander E, Baldini C, Seror R, Retamozo S, Quartuccio L et al (2016) Early diagnosis of primary Sjögren's syndrome: EULAR-SS task force clinical recommendations. Expert Rev Clin Immunol 12(2):137–156
2. Sandhya P, Jeyaseelan L, Scofield RH, Danda D (2015) Clinical characteristics and outcome of primary Sjogren's syndrome: a large Asian Indian cohort. Open Rheumatol J 9:36–45
3. Mohanasundaram K, Mani M, Chinnadurai S, Mahendran B, Balaji C, Bhoorasamy A et al (2016) Study on demography and outcome of extraglandular manifestations of primary Sjögren's syndrome. Indian J Rheumatol 11:202–206
4. Seror R, Ravaud P, Bowman SJ, Baron G, Tzioufas A, Theander E et al (2010) EULAR Sjogren's syndrome disease activity index: development of a consensus systemic disease activity index for primary Sjogren's syndrome. Ann Rheum Dis 69(6):1103–1109
5. Flint J, Panchal S, Hurrell A, van de Venne M, Gayed M, Schreiber K et al (2016) BSR and BHPR guideline on prescribing drugs in pregnancy and breastfeeding—part I: standard and biologic disease modifying anti-rheumatic drugs and corticosteroids. Rheumatology (Oxford) 55(9):1693–1697
6. Vassiliou VA, Moyssakis I, Boki KA, Moutsopoulos HM (2008) Is the heart affected in primary Sjögren's syndrome? An echocardiographic study. Clin Exp Rheumatol 26(1):109–112
7. Mariette X, Criswell LA (2018) Primary Sjögren's syndrome. N Engl J Med 378(10):931–939
8. Izmirly PM, Costedoat-Chalumeau N, Pisoni CN, Khamashta MA, Kim MY, Saxena A, Friedman D, Llanos C, Piette J-C, Buyon JP (2012) Maternal use of hydroxychloroquine is associated with a reduced risk of recurrent anti-ssa/ro-antibody–associated cardiac manifestations of neonatal lupus. Circulation 126(1):76–82
9. Barsalou J, Costedoat-Chalumeau N, Berhanu A, Fors-Nieves C, Shah U, Brown P et al (2018) Effect of in utero hydroxychloroquine exposure on the development of cutaneous neonatal lupus erythematosus. Ann Rheum Dis 77(12):1742–1749
10. Fauchais AL, Lambert M, Launay D, Michon-Pasturel U, Queyrel V, Nguyen N et al (2004) Antiphospholipid antibodies in primary Sjögren's syndrome: prevalence and clinical significance in a series of 74 patients. Lupus 13(4):245–248
11. Seror R, Bootsma H, Saraux A, Bowman SJ, Theander E, Brun JG et al (2016) Defining disease activity states and clinically meaningful improvement in primary Sjögren's syndrome with EULAR primary Sjögren's syndrome disease activity (ESSDAI) and patient-reported indexes (ESSPRI). Ann Rheum Dis 75(2):382–389
12. Abbassi-Ghanavati M, Greer LG, Cunningham FG (2009) Pregnancy and laboratory studies: a reference table for clinicians. Obstet Gynecol 114(6):1326–1331
13. Razeghinejad MR, Nowroozzadeh MH (2010) Anti-glaucoma medication exposure in pregnancy: an observational study and literature review. Clin Exp Optom 93(6):458–465
14. Kumar S (2016) Neonatal lupus: an update. Indian J Rheumatol 11(Suppl S2):139–144
15. Pruetz JD, Miller JC, Loeb GE, Silka MJ, Bar-Cohen Y, Chmait RH (2019) Prenatal diagnosis and management of congenital complete heart block. Birth Defects Res 111(8):380–388
16. Brucato A (2008) Prevention of congenital heart block in children of SSA-positive mothers. Rheumatology 47(Suppl 3):iii35–iii37
17. Brito-Zerón P, Izmirly PM, Ramos-Casals M, Buyon JP, Khamashta MA (2015) The clinical spectrum of autoimmune congenital heart block. Nat Rev Rheumatol 11(5):301–312
18. Friedman DM, Kim MY, Copel JA, Davis C, Phoon CKL, Glickstein JS et al (2008) Utility of cardiac monitoring in fetuses at risk for congenital heart block: the PR Interval and Dexamethasone Evaluation (PRIDE) prospective study. Circulation 117(4):485–493

19. Cuneo BF, Sonesson S-E, Levasseur S, Moon-Grady AJ, Krishnan A, Donofrio MT et al (2018) Home monitoring for fetal heart rhythm during anti-Ro pregnancies. J Am Coll Cardiol 72(16):1940–1951
20. Rosenthal D, Druzin M, Chin C, Dubin A (1998) A new therapeutic approach to the fetus with congenital complete heart block: preemptive, targeted therapy with dexamethasone. Obstet Gynecol 92(4 Pt 2):689–691
21. Saleeb S, Copel J, Friedman D, Buyon JP (1999) Comparison of treatment with fluorinated glucocorticoids to the natural history of autoantibody-associated congenital heart block: retrospective review of the research registry for neonatal lupus. Arthritis Rheum 42(11):2335–2345
22. Eliasson H, Sonesson S-E, Sharland G, Granath F, Simpson JM, Carvalho JS et al (2011) Isolated atrioventricular block in the fetus: a retrospective, multinational, multicenter study of 175 patients. Circulation 124(18):1919–1926
23. Jaeggi ET, Fouron J-C, Silverman ED, Ryan G, Smallhorn J, Hornberger LK (2004) Transplacental fetal treatment improves the outcome of prenatally diagnosed complete atrioventricular block without structural heart disease. Circulation 110(12):1542–1548
24. Izmirly PM, Saxena A, Kim MY, Wang D, Sahl SK, Llanos C et al (2011) Maternal and fetal factors associated with mortality and morbidity in a multi-racial/ethnic registry of anti-SSA/Ro-associated cardiac neonatal lupus. Circulation 124(18):1927–1935
25. Fredi M, Andreoli L, Bacco B, Bertero T, Bortoluzzi A, Breda S et al (2019) First report of the Italian Registry on immune-mediated congenital heart block (Lu.Ne Registry). Front Cardiovasc Med 6:11
26. Levesque K, Morel N, Maltret A, Baron G, Masseau A, Orquevaux P et al (2015) Description of 214 cases of autoimmune congenital heart block: results of the French neonatal lupus syndrome. Autoimmun Rev 14(12):1154–1160
27. Van den Berg NWE, Slieker MG, van Beynum IM, Bilardo CM, de Bruijn D, Clur SA et al (2016) Fluorinated steroids do not improve outcome of isolated atrioventricular block. Int J Cardiol 225:167–171
28. Izmirly PM, Saxena A, Sahl SK, Shah U, Friedman DM, Kim MY et al (2016) Assessment of fluorinated steroids to avert progression and mortality in anti-SSA/Ro-associated cardiac injury limited to the fetal conduction system. Ann Rheum Dis 75(6):1161–1165
29. Ciardulli A, D'Antonio F, Magro-Malosso ER, Saccone G, Manzoli L, Radolec M et al (2019) Maternal steroid therapy for fetuses with immune-mediated complete atrioventricular block: a systematic review and meta-analysis. J Matern Fetal Neonatal Med 32(11):1884–1892
30. Friedman DM, Kim MY, Copel JA, Llanos C, Davis C, Buyon JP (2009) Prospective evaluation of fetuses with autoimmune-associated congenital heart block followed in the PR Interval and Dexamethasone Evaluation (PRIDE) Study. Am J Cardiol 103(8):1102–1106
31. Brucato A, Tincani A, Fredi M, Breda S, Ramoni V, Morel N et al (2017) Should we treat congenital heart block with fluorinated corticosteroids? Autoimmun Rev 16(11):1115–1118
32. Ruffatti A, Cerutti L, Favaro M, Del Ross T, Calligaro A, Hoxha A et al (2016) Plasmapheresis, intravenous immunoglobulins and betamethasone—a combined protocol to treat autoimmune congenital heart block: a prospective cohort study. Clin Exp Rheumatol 34(4):706–713
33. Hussein SZ, Jacobsson LTH, Lindquist PG, Theander E (2011) Pregnancy and fetal outcome in women with primary Sjogren's syndrome compared with women in the general population: a nested case-control study. Rheumatology 50(9):1612–1617
34. De Carolis S, Salvi S, Botta A, Garofalo S, Garufi C, Ferrazzani S et al (2014) The impact of primary Sjogren's syndrome on pregnancy outcome: our series and review of the literature. Autoimmun Rev 13(2):103–107
35. Skopouli FN, Papanikolaou S, Malamou-Mitsi V, Papanikolaou N, Moutsopoulos HM (1994) Obstetric and gynaecological profile in patients with primary Sjögren's syndrome. Ann Rheum Dis 53(9):569–573
36. Ishihara O, Saitoh M, Hayashi N, Kinoshita K, Takeuchi T (2001) Successful treatment of embryo implantation failure in patients with the Sjögren syndrome with low-dose prednisolone. Fertil Steril 75(3):640–641

Maternal Mortality and Morbidity in Autoimmune Diseases

19

Pooja Sikka and Rinnie Brar

Abstract

Women with autoimmune disorders can present with a myriad of symptoms during pregnancy that sometimes causes catastrophic illness. With greater understanding of the interaction between pregnancy and autoimmune disorders as well as interdisciplinary cooperation among physicians, the maternal and infant prognosis can be greatly improved. Pregnancy should be planned after control of active disease and discussion of risks associated with pregnancy. Systemic lupus erythematosus is the most important disorder and can cause severe complications such as nephropathy, encephalopathy, pulmonary hypertension, multiple organ dysfunction and maternal and infant mortality. Women with autoimmune diseases are also at risk of puerperal sepsis. Other important issues include hypertension, preeclampsia, pulmonary hypertension, cardiac dysfunction and hypercoagulable states. Management should be carried out by a multidisciplinary team comprising of obstetricians, rheumatologists, nephrologists, cardiologists, pulmonary physicians and neonatologists. A one-stop clinic for this special pregnant population should be established for these patients.

Keywords

Autoimmune disease · Pregnancy · Systemic lupus erythematosus · Antiphospolipid antibody syndrome

---

P. Sikka (✉) · R. Brar
Department of Obstetrics and Gynaecology, Postgraduate Institute of Medical Education and Research (PGIMER), Chandigarh, India

© Springer Nature Singapore Pte Ltd. 2020
S. K. Sharma (ed.), *Women's Health in Autoimmune Diseases*,
https://doi.org/10.1007/978-981-15-0114-2_19

Due to improved access to healthcare, maternal deaths due to the direct obstetric causes such as haemorrhage, hypertension and sepsis are on a declining trend. However, to reach our target of attaining an optimal level of health for all women, our focus also needs to encompass chronic medical disorders, such as autoimmune diseases, which are responsible for significant maternal morbidity and mortality during pregnancy.

Autoimmune diseases are usually chronic debilitating disorders. However, they may also present acutely and may have flare-ups, which can be severe. Owing to the various dynamic interactions between the immune system and physiological alterations during pregnancy, pregnancy can lead to worsening of autoimmune diseases. Various autoimmune diseases affecting women are systemic lupus erythematosus (SLE), systemic sclerosis, scleroderma, rheumatoid arthritis, Takayasu arteritis, dermatomyositis and antiphospholipid antibody (APLA) syndrome. The risks of maternal complications from autoimmune diseases in pregnancy are not well documented. Since reliable data for rare complications is not available, the extent of risk to a woman with these diseases is difficult to assess. Majority of data available is from lupus pregnancies. A 7% risk of major morbidity associated with autoimmune diseases has been reported during pregnancy. In a review of 13,555 pregnancies in women with SLE, maternal morbidity and mortality rate has been reported to be 325 per 100,000.

Autoimmune diseases affect women more than men and thus their occurrence in pregnancy is common. These diseases often manifest for the first time during pregnancy. In such scenarios, these disorders often pose diagnostic challenges to physicians due to overlap of clinical profile with pregnancy-specific disorders, such as eclampsia, acute fatty liver of pregnancy (AFLP) and HELLP syndrome, and due to multi-systemic involvement by these diseases, such as SLE presenting with renal involvement as acute glomerulonephritis or with central nervous system involvement, catastrophic APLA syndrome presenting with multi-organ failure, scleroderma presenting as interstitial lung disease (ILD) and acute respiratory failure. Diagnosis may also be delayed since imaging studies are avoided because of risks of radiation exposure to the foetus. The delays in diagnosis worsen the disease prognosis.

With a greater understanding of the profile of autoimmune diseases and the impact of and on pregnancy, as well as improved interdisciplinary cooperation among physicians, the maternal and infant prognosis has greatly improved. Historically, if there were previous renal involvement in a case of SLE, even if it were quiescent at present, patients were counselled to avoid pregnancy. Today, patients are counselled to conceive while the disease is inactive and in remission for a significant period of time. However, owing to its varied presentations, the disease can still worsen when pregnancy supervenes. A better understanding of the occurrence of adverse pregnancy outcomes in these women is essential for informing patients of the potential risks during pregnancy.

There are several management strategies, and many novel therapies are under trials, even for complicated autoimmune diseases. However, despite intensive care, some patients still have a poor prognosis, or even die of worsening disease. This is especially true of diseases such as SLE.

19.1 Why Is Morbidity and Mortality the Highest in SLE?

Owing to multi-systemic involvement, SLE can adversely affect the pregnancy and cause severe complications, such as lupus nephritis, lupus encephalopathy, pulmonary hypertension, haemolytic anaemia, cardiac dysfunction, multiple-organ dysfunction and even maternal and infant death. The presence of lupus nephritis, anti-Ro/SSA antibody, anti-La/SSB, hypertension, Raynaud's phenomenon and aggravated lupus are all predictors of poor pregnancy outcomes. The higher risks of mortality are not only because of the disease per se, but also because of the delay in initiating treatment, due to concerns for the foetus.

19.2 Renal Concerns

Apart from the high immunological risk in pregnant SLE women, pregnancies inevitably cause renal problems during the gestational course. Up to 75% of pregnant SLE patients with or without abnormal serum creatinine changes exhibit a spectrum of renal abnormalities. Physiological renal compensation, including glomerular hypertrophy and hyperfiltration, occurs to meet the increased requirements of pregnancy. In healthy women, these physiological changes stabilize naturally without any sequelae after delivery. However, patients with chronic kidney disease probably fail to compensate for increased requirements during pregnancy. Data suggest that insufficient adaption of the kidneys is associated with the risk of chronic kidney failure and progression to end-stage renal disease necessitating dialysis, or even renal transplantation after delivery. Increased risk of disease activity flare-up in these patients contributes to short- and long-term adverse effects on the kidneys, which can potentially lead to accelerated progression to end-stage renal disease.

The significantly higher risk of hypertensive disorders, including gestational hypertension and pre-eclampsia, in pregnant patients with SLE is considered to be highly associated with the flare-up of lupus nephritis and has been suggested to lead to cardiovascular diseases in the future. Similar association with hypertensive disorders of pregnancy has also been noted in pregnant women with systemic sclerosis.

19.3 Risks of Underlying Interstitial Lung Disease (ILD) and Pulmonary Arterial Hypertension (PAH)

Autoimmune diseases, such as rheumatoid arthritis (RA), scleroderma and SLE, often have detrimental effects on the pulmonary functions, and lead to ILD and PAH. ILD is associated with a high rate of mortality especially after 5 years of disease onset. Prognosis of patients with severe pulmonary impairment (FVC <55% and DLCO <40% of predicted normal values) is unfavourable with up to 42% dying within 10 years of disease onset. Pulmonary haemorrhage is a rare but serious and frequently fatal event. Its clinical course is similar to lupus pneumonitis, with rapid progression and deterioration of patient health status.

The European societies for cardiology and respiratory diseases have limited guidelines on managing PAH during pregnancy, but these suggest that pregnancy should be discouraged in women with underlying PAH. Hence, counselling about contraception including medical sterilization is important. In case a woman gets pregnant, high maternal and foetal risks and the option of termination of pregnancy should be discussed. If pregnancy is continued, disease-targeted therapies, effective close collaboration between obstetricians and the PAH team and planned elective delivery are important because of substantially high risk of maternal and foetal morbidity and mortality.

Studies prior to the introduction of prostaglandin therapy estimated a 50% chance of mortality of both mother and baby in pregnant women with PAH. More recent studies estimate the probability of death to be 18–40%, and this is higher in women with rheumatologic disorders, often due to complications from pre-eclampsia and disease flare-ups. Majority of these deaths are attributed to right-heart failure, although they are often multifactorial, involving respiratory failure, kidney failure and obstetric haemorrhage. Without prostanoid treatment, mortality rates are unacceptably high, and with therapy these risks are reduced, although comprehensive data is lacking.

19.4 Maternal Heart Is Also Not Spared

Cardiac impairment is quite frequent in SLE. Mitral regurgitation is one of the most common cardiac manifestations; however, it is usually haemodynamically insignificant. Valvular vegetations of variable size, from small nodules to large verrucous vegetations (Libman-Sacks endocarditis), are the most frequent cause of the valve dysfunction and/or insufficiency. Diastolic impairment is the most frequent finding on echocardiogram; however, systolic dysfunction can also occur. Women with autoimmune disorders are also at risk of developing peripartum cardiomyopathy, which is associated with significant maternal morbidity and mortality.

19.5 Pregnancy, Coagulation and Autoimmune Disorders

Pregnancy is a hypercoagulable state. Certain autoimmune diseases are also associated with prothrombotic tendencies, such as APLA. Life-threatening conditions related to APLA syndrome in pregnancy include mainly vascular thrombosis, leading to pulmonary embolisms, arterial occlusions, cerebrovascular events, myocardial infarctions and microangiopathic haemolysis. Pre-eclampsia, eclampsia and HELLP syndrome are potentially fatal antiphospholipid syndrome-related disorders connected with pregnancy.

19.6 Cerebral Involvement

The risk of cerebral infarction and sudden death is significantly increased in pregnant women with SLE. Cerebral infarction may present either as a classical stroke or as a transitory ischaemic attack. Behavioural and mood disorders, psychomotor restlessness and different levels of consciousness disorders may accompany episodes. There is also a strong association between these events and antiphospholipid antibodies.

19.7 Beware of the Risk of Sepsis

Women with autoimmune diseases are at risk of puerperal sepsis. This is mainly due to immune suppression either due to the disease process or due to the drug therapy. Caesarean delivery has been proven to be the most common risk factor associated with maternal sepsis and pregnancies with autoimmune disorders are at high risk of caesarean deliveries due to intrauterine growth restriction, preterm-induced deliveries and other associated comorbidities like pulmonary hypertension. High clinical suspicion and aggressive treatment with broad-spectrum antibiotics can prevent morbidity to a large extent.

19.8 Therapy of Autoimmune Diseases and Pregnancy

Timely and expertly administered therapy suppresses the disease activity and helps in improving pregnancy outcomes. However, therapy in itself is associated with unwarranted maternal and foetal side effects of the various drugs used. These drugs are primarily steroids and steroid-sparing immunosuppressant drugs. Glucocorticoid use in pregnancy is associated with a higher risk of hypertension and diabetes, and increased risk of puerperal sepsis. Biologic agents such as TNF inhibitors, rituximab and anakinra are not used as frequently in pregnant patients as in non-pregnant patients due to foetal concerns, thus limiting the option of therapeutic agents available for reducing disease activity to a desirable level. Counselling of pregnant patients with regard to safety profile of these agents needs to be thorough so that optimal therapy can be chosen, thereby reducing maternal morbidity associated with untreated and uncontrolled disease.

19.9 Conclusions

Autoimmune disorders during pregnancy are associated with increased maternal and infant morbidity and mortality. Active disease during pregnancy is associated with adverse outcomes. Various life-threatening issues can arise during pregnancy, abortion, medical termination of pregnancy and post-partum period. These can effectively be tackled only by a multidisciplinary team comprising obstetricians trained in medical disorders, rheumatologists, nephrologists, cardiologists, pulmonary physicians and neonatologists. A one-stop clinic for this special pregnant population should be established where their comprehensive health needs can be taken care of.

Suggested Reading

1. Dörner T, Furie R (2019) Novel paradigms in systemic lupus erythematosus. Lancet 393:2344–2358
2. Benagiano G, Benagiano M, Bianchi P et al (2019) Contraception in autoimmune diseases. Best Pract Res Clin Obstet Gynaecol 60:111–123
3. Benagiano M, Bianchi P, D'Elios MM et al (2019) Autoimmune diseases: role of steroid hormones. Best Pract Res Clin Obstet Gynaecol 60:24–34
4. De Carolis S, Moresi S, Rizzo F et al (2019) Autoimmunity in obstetrics and autoimmune diseases in pregnancy. Best Pract Res Clin Obstet Gynaecol 60:66–76
5. Alijotas-Reig J, Esteve-Valverde E, Ferrer-Oliveras R et al (2019) The European Registry on Obstetric Antiphospholipid Syndrome (EUROAPS): a survey of 1000 consecutive cases. Autoimmun Rev 18:406–414
6. Belizna C, Pregnolato F, Abad S et al (2018) HIBISCUS: hydroxychloroquine for the secondary prevention of thrombotic and obstetrical events in primary antiphospholipid syndrome. Autoimmun Rev 17:1153–1168
7. Mekinian A, Alijotas-Reig J, Carrat F et al (2017) Refractory obstetrical antiphospholipid syndrome: features, treatment and outcome in a European multicenter retrospective study. Autoimmun Rev 16:730–734
8. Andreoli L, Bertsias GK, Agmon-Levin N et al (2017) EULAR recommendations for women's health and the management of family planning, assisted reproduction, pregnancy and menopause in patients with systemic lupus erythematosus and/or antiphospholipid syndrome. Ann Rheum Dis 76:476–485
9. Andreoli L, Crisafulli F, Tincani A (2017) Pregnancy and reproductive aspects of systemic lupus erythematosus. Curr Opin Rheumatol 29:473–479
10. Limper M, Scirè CA, Talarico R et al (2018) Antiphospholipid syndrome: state of the art on clinical practice guidelines. RMD Open 4:e000785
11. Spinillo A, Beneventi F, Locatelli E et al (2016) The impact of unrecognized autoimmune rheumatic diseases on the incidence of preeclampsia and fetal growth restriction: a longitudinal cohort study. BMC Pregnancy Childbirth 16:313
12. Kamper-Jørgensen M, Gammill HS, Nelson JL (2018) Preeclampsia and scleroderma: a prospective nationwide analysis. Acta Obstet Gynecol Scand 97:587–590
13. Lidar M, Langevitz P (2012) Pregnancy issues in scleroderma. Autoimmun Rev 11:A515–A519
14. Sobanski V, Launay D, Depret S et al (2016) Special considerations in pregnant systemic sclerosis patients. Expert Rev Clin Immunol 12:1161–1173

Anti-rheumatic Drugs in Pregnancy

20

Ashok Kumar and Anunay Agarwal

Abstract

Rheumatic diseases frequently occur in women in the reproductive age group. Although patients are advised to avoid pregnancy unless the disease has been in remission for at least 6 months, many patients present with pregnancy and active rheumatic disease. Rheumatologists, therefore, need to know which drugs are safe in pregnancy. Some diseases like RA naturally remit during pregnancy while others like SLE pose unpredictable challenges. Steroid can be used in all the three trimesters of pregnancy as well as during lactation. Prednisolone and methylprednisolone are the preferred compounds. Non-selective NSAIDs can be used in pregnancy, with caution especially during the first trimester. These should be avoided in the third trimester due to risk of closure of ductus arteriosus. Among DMARDs for RA, only hydroxychloroquine, sulphasalazine, calcineurin inhibitors and azathioprine are safe during pregnancy. Anti-TNF drugs have been found safe during pregnancy. Safety data do not exist on other biological drugs and small molecules. Low molecular weight heparin is safe throughout pregnancy. Warfarin is best avoided during pregnancy but can be used after 16th week of gestation. Tadalafil and Sildenafil can be used during pregnancy albeit with caution. Bisphosphonates should be stopped at least 6 months prior to planned pregnancies.

Keywords

Pregnancy · Anti-inflammatory drugs · Antirheumatic drugs · Biological drugs · JAK inhibitors

A. Kumar (✉) · A. Agarwal
Department of Rheumatology, Fortis Flt. Lt. Rajan Dhall Hospital, Vasant Kunj, New Delhi, India

20.1 Introduction

Rheumatic diseases are more prevalent in women than in men, and frequently affect women in the childbearing age group [1]. Pregnancies do occur in these patients. Ideally, these should be planned when the disease is in remission. Patients, whose disease has been in remission for at least 6 months, do better [2]. Almost 50% of pregnancies are unplanned. The disease may be severe enough to merit treatment or even escalation of existing therapy during pregnancy and lactation. Hence it is imperative for the treating physician to know which drugs can be safely used in these patients.

With improved quality of life consequent to modern treatment, more and more women with rheumatic diseases feel confident in undertaking pregnancy. Some diseases like RA naturally remit during pregnancy; others like SLE pose unpredictable challenges. Good disease control is mandatory for a successful pregnancy. The onus falls on the treating rheumatologist to choose the most effective therapy with the best safety profile when managing these patients.

Fertility in general is not affected in women with rheumatic diseases although fewer pregnancies are reported in these patients, which most likely is out of personal choice. Contraception should be an integral part of counselling of patients in reproductive-age group, undergoing treatment for rheumatic diseases.

The British Society for Rheumatology published its guidelines in 2016 on the use of anti-rheumatic drugs during pregnancy and lactation [3, 4].

20.2 Anti-inflammatory and Synthetic Disease Modifying Drugs

20.2.1 Steroids

Steroid can be used in all the three trimesters of pregnancy as well as during lactation. Prednisolone and methylprednisolone are the preferred compounds. Only one-eighth to one-tenth of maternal circulating level of prednisolone is attained in the foetal circulation [5]. This is because steroid is converted into 11-keto form, which is relatively inactive. Betamethasone and dexamethasone (fluorinated forms) are less well metabolised by the placenta.

It is noteworthy that increased blood pressure, osteopenia/osteoporosis, susceptibility to infections and insulin resistance can be caused by both the pregnant state and steroid intake. Patients taking bisphosphonate for osteoporosis should discontinue the drug at least 6 months before pregnancy. There have been reports of increase in the incidence of cleft lip and palate after foetal exposure to steroids. Studies have shown variable results and the risk is minimal.

Although one course of dexamethasone or betamethasone can be administered for the protection of the foetus from the risk of death, respiratory distress syndrome and cerebral haemorrhages, multiple courses are not recommended as they have been shown to interfere with the neurological development of the foetus.

Only 5–25% of the maternal prednisolone is secreted in breast milk, so the levels reaching the infant would be very low (even with higher doses like 80 mg/day). Prednisolone can be used in lactating mothers.

20.2.2 NSAIDs

NSAIDs are used intermittently for pain relief in patients with rheumatic diseases. COX-1 and COX-2 are both involved in ovulation and implantation. There have been reports of transient infertility associated with NSAID usage. NSAIDs also exert this action by inhibiting the rupture of luteinised follicle. Although there have been a few reports of decrease in sperm count of men on long-term NSAIDs, paternal exposure to non-selective NSAIDs is permissible.

There have been reports of miscarriages due to the use of NSAIDs during pregnancy. The odds ratio ranged from 1.3 to 7 (NSAIDs used 1–12 weeks before miscarriage) [6]. The odds ratio increased in a study with prolonged use around the time of conception. This is attributed to the interference with implantation and placental circulation. A meta-analysis showed no increase in miscarriages with the use of low-dose aspirin in the first trimester [7]. NSAIDs also have tocolytic properties and have been used to delay premature labour.

There have been reports of midline defects in women using low-dose aspirin during the first trimester. All NSAIDs have a potential to cause premature closure of ductus arteriosus. This was reversible with indomethacin. Both selective and non-selective COX inhibitors have been reported to cause reduced foetal renal perfusion, which was reversible with drug cessation. Oligohydramnios have also been reported which appears to be dose dependent. High-dose aspirin and indomethacin intake close to the delivery have also been reported to cause CNS haemorrhages in the newborns. NSAIDs are mostly secreted in very small quantities in breast milk and are generally considered safe for lactation. However, precautions should be taken, like feeding just before taking the drug.

In summary, non-selective NSAIDs can be used in pregnancy (with caution especially during the first trimester). These should be avoided in the third trimester due to risk of closure of ductus arteriosus. Selective COX-2 inhibitors should be avoided. Low-dose aspirin can be continued in the third trimester. NSAIDs including low-dose aspirin are safe during lactation and with paternal exposure.

20.2.3 Hydroxychloroquine

This antimalarial drug has a proven safety and efficacy in patients with systemic lupus erythematosus or inflammatory arthritis who are planning pregnancy or are pregnant or lactating. HCQ has also been shown to protect foetal cardiac conduction pathways in anti-SS-A-positive pregnant women. HCQ should be continued while planning a pregnancy. A prospective study by Clowse et al. found no statistically significant difference in the rates of miscarriage, stillbirth, pregnancy loss or congenital deformities between the group of women continuing HCQ throughout pregnancy and those who discontinued the drug [8]. Also, they found that the lupus activity was much higher in the latter group (they also needed a higher dose of steroid). No ocular adverse effects have been reported in children born to mothers on long-term HCQ. Although low doses of antimalarials are secreted in breast milk, no adverse effects have been reported in such breastfed babies.

20.2.4 Methotrexate

This folate antagonist is the anchor drug in the management of inflammatory arthritis. Also, it is efficacious in scleroderma, psoriasis and autoimmune inflammatory myositis and other rheumatic conditions. Active metabolites can remain in the body, months after stopping therapy. It is known to be a teratogenic and abortifacient drug. The congenital abnormalities associated with exposure to MTX include central nervous system anomalies, cranial ossification and growth retardation. Exposure to MTX during early pregnancy carries the highest risk of nervous system involvement.

Most data for MTX in pregnancy comes from its use in oncology practice. Even though much higher doses than what are prescribed for rheumatic conditions were used, US FDA classifies MTX as category X drug. Features of adults with the 'foetal methotrexate syndrome' comprise hypertelorism, low-set ears, micrognathia, limb deformities and low IQ [9].

The current recommendation is that all couples should be advised contraception while on MTX. If pregnancy is planned, MTX should be stopped at least 3 months prior. This recommendation is for both women and men. Should a pregnancy occur while on MTX, the drug should be stopped immediately and an assessment of foetal risk should be obtained. Folate supplementation should continue throughout pregnancy (5 mg/day). MTX is also secreted in breast milk and is contraindicated during lactation.

20.2.5 Leflunomide

Leflunomide was developed from a specific anti-inflammatory drug development programme. It is a reversible competitive inhibitor of dihydro-orotate dehydrogenase. Dihydro-orotate dehydrogenase is a rate-limiting enzyme in the synthesis of pyrimidines. Due to extensive enterohepatic circulation it can be detected in the plasma for a few years after discontinuation of the drug.

Exposure to leflunomide during pregnancy in humans has not been reported to cause a higher incidence of birth defects as compared to normal population. However, since it was found to be embryotoxic in animal studies it is categorised in category X. Women of childbearing age to be started on leflunomide should be counselled and advised for contraception. Also, they should test negative for pregnancy before starting therapy.

Cholestyramine washout is mandated to clear the drug. Recommended dose is 8 g thrice a day orally for a total of 11 days or until the plasma levels fall below 0.02 mg/L [10]. The plasma levels should be reconfirmed twice (at least 2 weeks apart). Leflunomide is also contraindicated during lactation. Limited evidence suggests that leflunomide may be compatible with paternal exposure.

20.2.6 Sulphasalazine

Sulphasalazine is a conjugate of 5-amino-salicylic acid and sulphapyridine joined by an azo bond. It is metabolised into these two forms by colonic bacteria. Sulphasalazine crosses the placenta attaining concentrations similar to those in maternal blood. Sulphasalazine is also reported to displace bilirubin from its protein-bound form but no cases of neonatal jaundice have been reported. Some experts also recommend stopping this drug in the third trimester. There is no effect on the foetus. Sulphasalazine is considered safe during pregnancy. Since it is a folate antagonist, daily supplementation of folic acid (5 mg/day) is recommended. Negligible amounts of sulphasalazine are found in breast milk, so lactation is considered safe. Only one case of an infant developing bloody diarrhoea has been reported.

Men taking sulphasalazine can develop oligospermia, reduced sperm motility and abnormal morphology of the sperms [11]. This is reversible and cessation of the drug 3 months before planning pregnancy is recommended. There is no effect on fertility in women.

20.2.7 Azathioprine

Azathioprine (AZA) is the precursor of 6-mercaptopurine. It is a purine analogue. FDA considers it a Category D drug. It does cross the placenta but lower concentrations suggest that there is placental metabolism. The foetal liver also lacks the enzyme inosinato-pyrophosphorylase, which converts AZA to its active form. Results from the French pregnancy database TERAPPEL [12] and the Danish cohort [13] reported no increase in the risk of major birth defects or preterm births in patients on AZA, and that the preterm births were more likely caused by the underlying disease itself. Some cases of intrauterine growth retardation, neonatal leucopenia, lymphopenia, hypogammaglobulinaemia and immunosuppression have been reported. However, they were able to attain normal adolescence. AZA and its metabolites are secreted in breast milk (0.1% of maternal dose). The BSR considers AZA safe during lactation. Similarly, AZA is safe for paternal exposure and has no effect on fertility in both men and women.

20.2.8 Cyclosporine-A

CS-A is an immunosuppressive drug that exerts this action by inhibiting calcineurin, which ultimately inhibits the formation of IL-2 and T-cell activation. The FDA classifies it in Category C. A meta-analysis confirmed that CS-A does not increase the risk of malformations in the foetus as compared to normal population [14]. CS-A can be used in pregnancy at the lowest possible dose. Long-term effects on children with in utero exposure to CS-A have not been reported.

CS-A is secreted in breast milk in small quantities and there has been one report of therapeutic concentrations found in the infant. Overall, the drug is safe during breastfeeding. There have been no reports of reduced fertility of men receiving CS-A.

20.2.9 Cyclophosphamide

Cyclophosphamide (CYC) is an alkylating agent with powerful cytotoxic effect. It is used in oncology and rheumatology. This is a teratogenic and gonadotoxic agent. The risk for ovarian failure in women increases greatly with age and is dose dependent. CYC resulted in amenorrhoea in 27% of patients in one study [15]. This risk should be conveyed to the patient explicitly before initiating therapy.

Although there have been reports of normal infants being born to mothers who were exposed to CYC, the risk of congenital malformations is estimated to be around 20% [16]. These include growth retardation, developmental delays, blepharophimosis, facial deformities, distal limb defects and craniosynostosis. A history of treatment with CYC prior to pregnancy does not affect the outcomes. CYC is secreted in breast milk and is contraindicated during lactation. Paternal exposure to CYC has also been reported to be unsafe.

20.2.10 Mycophenolate Mofetil

MMF interferes with the de novo guanosine synthesis, resulting in inhibition of formation of lymphocytes. It exerts this action by reversibly inhibiting inosine monophosphate dehydrogenase. FDA classified this drug in Category C, but then reclassified it into Category D after 2007. There have been a few case reports of infants born with birth defects to mothers exposed to MMF. Specific abnormalities have been noted, which include microtia, cleft lip and palate, external auditory canal atresia, oesophageal atresia, diaphragmatic hernia, ocular defects, agenesis of corpus callosum and congenital heart defects. MMF undergoes enterohepatic circulation and it is recommended that it should be stopped at least 6 weeks before a planned pregnancy. All women in childbearing age to be initiated on MMF should be counselled regarding contraception.

No data exists regarding the secretion of MMF into breast milk and therefore is not indicated during lactation.

A study from Norway, which included 230 men on immunosuppression including 155 men on MMF, concluded that MMF is compatible with paternal exposure [17].

20.2.11 Tacrolimus

Tacrolimus (TAC) is a macrolide derivative, which is also a potent calcineurin inhibitor. The experience of using TAC comes mostly from studies on transplant recipients. The BSR recommends that TAC may be used during pregnancy in the lowest possible dose. Aktürk et al. in 2015 reported that 68% of patients of renal transplants had successful pregnancies while on TAC [18]. They also reported that higher doses of TAC were needed during pregnancies to maintain the trough levels. Very low levels of TAC (0.02% of maternal dose) are secreted in breast milk. So, breastfeeding should not be discouraged. No effect on male fertility or on pregnancy with paternal exposure to TAC has been reported.

20.3 Intravenous Immunoglobulin

IVIg is considered as a rescue therapy for a variety of rheumatic diseases. IgG does cross the placenta but no adverse effects have been reported in any foetus. No adverse effects on the foetal immune system have been reported. IVIg is considered safe during lactation. No data exists regarding maternal or paternal fertility. It is safe for paternal exposure with regard to foetal outcome.

20.4 Biologicals & Small Molecules

20.4.1 TNF Inhibitors

TNF inhibitors (TNFi) inhibit the action of the cytokine tumour necrosis factor. These are indicated in a variety of rheumatic conditions, particularly in rheumatoid arthritis and spondyloarthritides. FDA classifies these drugs in Category B. All TNFi cross the placenta except certolizumab pegol, and this is the drug that is recommended for use throughout pregnancy. Other TNFi are recommended by some to be withheld after the second trimester. A meta-analysis by Komaki et al. published in 2016 reported that there was no increase in adverse pregnancy outcomes in TNFi users vs. non-users [19]. No evidence exists to discourage the use of TNFi during lactation and it is also considered safe for paternal exposure.

20.4.2 Rituximab

This is an anti-B-cell drug that is directed against CD20 antigen. The FDA classifies it in Category C. The rate of live births after RTX exposure is about 66%. No congenital malformations have been reported [20]. RTX does cross the placenta and Das et al. reported in 2018 that 39% of newborns born to mothers exposed to it had low B-cell counts, which later normalised [21]. The BSR guidelines indicate that RTX should be stopped at least 6 months prior to conception. Unintentional first-trimester exposure is deemed safe. No data exists for the secretion of RTX into breast milk. No adverse effects of paternal exposure have been reported.

20.4.3 Tocilizumab

Tocilizumab (TCZ) inhibits the IL-6-mediated signalling pathway. It is a humanised monoclonal antibody. No pregnancy-related adverse events have been reported from animal studies. The BSR maintains that TCZ should be stopped 3 months prior to a planned pregnancy; however no increased adverse events have been reported with unintentional exposures during the first trimester. TCZ was found to cross the placenta during later part of the pregnancy in an animal model. A study from Japan reported no congenital malformations in newborns born to mothers ($n = 36$) exposed to TCZ. They also continued TCZ during lactation and reported no adverse outcomes in the infants [22]. No data exists on the safety of paternal exposure to TCZ.

20.4.4 JAK Inhibitors

Tofacitinib and baricitinib are small molecules, which inhibit the JAK-STAT signalling pathway. They are both approved for the treatment of RA. Animal models have shown teratogenic effects of tofacitinib when exposed to much higher doses than used for humans. These can potentially cross the placenta [23]. Although the manufacturer's database has documented successful pregnancy outcomes while on tofacitinib, one case of pulmonary valve stenosis in a child was documented. No such data exists for baricitinib.

Because only scarce data exists, JAK inhibitors should be stopped at least 2 months before planning pregnancy. Since these are small molecules and can be secreted in breast milk, lactation should be avoided. No data exists for the safety of paternal exposure.

20.4.5 Secukinumab

This is a monoclonal antibody that binds with IL-17A. No adverse outcomes were reported in animal models relating to fertility, maternal outcome, foetal toxicity and postnatal development. Because no data for humans exists, secukinumab should be stopped 5–6 months before a planned pregnancy due to its long half-life, and should be avoided during lactation [24].

20.5 Apremilast

Apremilast is a selective antagonist of phosphodiesterase-4 (PDE-4) which down-regulates several proinflammatory cytokines. It was found in the breast milk of mice in 1.5 times the concentration in plasma [24]. Given no human data for safety in pregnancy and lactation it is best avoided.

20.6 Chronic Pain Management

20.6.1 Paracetamol

Paracetamol is safe to use for pain relief during pregnancy and lactation. The BSR cautions against prolonged use on account of risk of childhood asthma and a small risk of cryptorchidism [5]. Paternal exposure to paracetamol is deemed safe.

20.6.2 Tramadol

Tramadol is safe during pregnancy and for short-term use during lactation.

20.6.3 Amitriptyline

Low-dose amitriptyline can be used during pregnancy and lactation and is also compatible with paternal exposure.

20.6.4 Gabapentin and Pregabalin

Adequate evidence for the safety of these medicines during pregnancy and lactation is not present and therefore they should not be continued.

20.6.5 SSRI

SSRIs (fluoxetine, sertraline) are considered safe in pregnancy and breastfeeding.

20.7 Anticoagulants

Low-molecular-weight heparin is safe throughout pregnancy. No concerns were raised for its use during lactation, too. Warfarin should be used during pregnancy only in exceptional circumstances. It can be used during lactation. No safety data for newer anticoagulants during pregnancy and lactation exist and therefore they should not be used.

20.8 Antihypertensives

ACE inhibitors should not be used in pregnancy due to the higher risk of congenital malformations reported. Heart defects were reported with exposure during the first trimester and impairment in the foetal renal function was noted with their use during the second and third trimesters [25, 26]. Nifedipine, a calcium channel blocker, is compatible with pregnancy and lactation. Bosentan has been found to have teratogenic effects in animals, even though no such data exists for humans. It should be avoided in pregnancy [27].

20.9 PDE-5 Inhibitors

Tadalafil and sildenafil can be used during pregnancy albeit with caution. There have been successful reports of their use in pregnancy [28].

20.10 Bisphosphonates

Bisphosphonates are used in the management of osteoporosis. Bisphosphonates cross the placenta and higher doses in animals have shown adverse effects on the foetus. Given their long half-life the BSR recommends that these be stopped at least 6 months prior to planned pregnancies. They should be used only in exceptional circumstances. Successful pregnancies have also been reported [29]. No data exist for their safety during lactation. Paternal exposure should be avoided.

References

1. Witzel AJ (2014) Lactation and the use of biologic immunosuppressive medications. Breastfeed Med 9:543–546
2. Soh MC, Nelson-Piercy C (2015) High-risk pregnancy and the rheumatologist. Rheumatology 54:572–587
3. Flint J, Panchal S, Hurrell A et al (2016) BSR and BHPR guideline on prescribing drugs in pregnancy and breastfeeding—part I: standard and biologic disease modifying anti-rheumatic drugs and corticosteroids. Rheumatology (Oxford) 55:1693–1697
4. Flint J, Panchal S, Hurrell A et al (2016) BSR and BHPR guideline on prescribing drugs in pregnancy and breastfeeding—part II: analgesics and other drugs used in rheumatology practice. Rheumatology (Oxford) 55:1698–1702
5. Murphy VE, Fittock RJ, Zarzycki PK, Delahunty MM, Smith R, Clifton VL (2007) Metabolism of synthetic steroids by the human placenta. Placenta 28:39–46
6. Østensen M, Khamashta M, Lockshin M et al (2006) Anti-inflammatory and immunosuppressive drugs and reproduction. Arthritis Res Ther 8:209–227
7. Kozer E, Moldovan Costei A, Boskovic R, Nulman I, Nikfar S, Koren G (2003) Effects of aspirin consumption during pregnancy on pregnancy outcomes: meta-analysis. Birth Defects Res B Dev Reprod Toxicol 68:70–84
8. Clowse ME, Magder L, Witter F, Petri M (2006) Hydroxychloroquine in lupus pregnancy. Arthritis Rheum 54:3640–3647
9. Bawle EV, Conard JV, Weiss L (1998) Adult and two children with fetal methotrexate syndrome. Teratology 57:51–55
10. Chambers CD, Johnson DL, Robinson LK et al (2010) Birth outcomes in women who have taken leflunomide during pregnancy. Arthritis Rheumatol 62:1494–1503
11. O'Morain C, Smethurst P, Doré CJ, Levi AJ (1984) Reversible male infertility due to sulphasalazine: studies in man and rat. Gut 25:1078–1084

12. Alami Z, Agier MS, Ahid S, Vial T, Dautriche A, Lagarce L, Toutain A, Cherrah Y, Jonville-Bera AP (2018) Pregnancy outcome following in utero exposure to azathioprine: a French comparative observational study. Therapie 73:199–207
13. Langagergaard V, Pedersen L, Gislum M, Norgard B, Sorensen HT (2007) Birth outcome in women treated with azathioprine or mercaptopurine during pregnancy: a Danish nationwide cohort study. Aliment Pharmacol Ther 25:73–81
14. Bar Oz B, Hackman R, Einarson T, Koren G (2001) Pregnancy outcome after cyclosporine therapy during pregnancy: a meta-analysis. Transplantation 71:1051–1055
15. Wang CL, Wang F, Bosco JJ (1995) Ovarian failure in oral cyclophosphamide treatment for systemic lupus erythematosus. Lupus 4:11–14
16. Temprano KK, Bandlamudi R, Moore TL (2005) Antirheumatic drugs in pregnancy and lactation. Semin Arthritis Rheum 35:112–121
17. Midtvedt K, Bergan S, Reisæter AV, Vikse BE, Åsberg A (2017) Exposure to mycophenolate and fatherhood. Transplantation 101:e214–e217
18. Akturk S, Celebi ZK, Erdogmus S, Kanmaz AG, Yuce T, Sengul S, Keven K (2015) Pregnancy after kidney transplantation: outcomes, tacrolimus doses, and trough levels. Transplant Proc 47:1442–1444
19. Komaki F, Komaki Y, Micic D, Ido A, Sakuraba A (2017) Outcome of pregnancy and neonatal complications with anti-tumor necrosis factor-α use in females with immune mediated diseases; a systematic review and meta-analysis. J Autoimmun 76:38–52
20. De Cock D, Birmingham L, Watson KD, Kearsley-Fleet L, Symmons DP, Hyrich KL (2017) Pregnancy outcomes in women with rheumatoid arthritis ever treated with rituximab. Rheumatology (Oxford) 56:661–663
21. Das G, Damotte V, Gelfand JM et al (2018) Rituximab before and during pregnancy: a systematic review, and a case series in MS and NMOSD. Neurol Neuroimmunol Neuroinflamm 5:e453
22. Nakajima K, Watanabe O, Mochizuki M, Nakasone A, Ishizuka N, Murashima A (2016) Pregnancy outcomes after exposure to tocilizumab: a retrospective analysis of 61 patients in Japan. Mod Rheumatol 26:667–671
23. Wollenhaupt J, Silverfield J, Lee EB et al (2014) Safety and efficacy of tofacitinib, an oral Janus kinase inhibitor, for the treatment of rheumatoid arthritis in open-label, long term extension studies. J Rheumatol 41:837–852
24. Rademaker M, Agnew K, Andrews M et al (2017) Psoriasis in those planning a family, pregnant or breastfeeding. The Australasian Psoriasis Collaboration. Aust J Dermatol 59:86. https://doi.org/10.1111/ajd.12641
25. Cooper WO, Hernandez-Diaz S, Arbogast PG et al (2006) Major congenital malformations after first-trimester exposure to ACE inhibitors. N Engl J Med 354:2443–2451
26. Shotan A, Widerhorn J, Hurst A, Elkayam U (1994) Risks of angiotensin-converting enzyme inhibition during pregnancy: experimental and clinical evidence, potential mechanisms, and recommendations for use. Am J Med 96:451–456
27. Kurihara Y, Kurihara H, Oda H et al (1995) Aortic arch malformations and ventricular septal defect in mice deficient in endothelin-1. J Clin Investig 96:293–300
28. Običan SG, Cleary KL (2014) Pulmonary arterial hypertension in pregnancy. Semin Perinatol 38:289–294
29. Stathopoulos IP, Liakou CG, Katsalira A et al (2011) The use of bisphosphonates in women prior to or during pregnancy and lactation. Hormones (Athens) 10:280–291

Nonsteroidal Anti-inflammatory Drug Use During Pregnancy and Lactation: Effects on Mother and Child

21

Ghan Shyam Pangtey and Niharika Agarwal

Abstract

Nonsteroidal anti-inflammatory drugs (NSAIDs) are the most frequently prescribed analgesics in pregnant and lactating mother for the management of pain in rheumatic disorders. Whenever any medication is to be prescribed to a pregnant or lactating woman, the relative benefits and risks to the mother and fetus should always be kept in mind. The teratogenicity or adverse effects of medication in pregnancy and lactation are predominantly influenced by gestational age of fetus, permeability of placental barrier to drug, protein binding, and lipid solubility of the drug. Autoimmune disorders are more common in young females of childbearing age; thus, the treatment of such disorders in women during pregnancy and lactation is an important aspect of their management. It is also important to note that, if untreated, the autoimmune disease per se may also lead to risk to life of mother and her fetus. There are very limited studies regarding safety and tolerability of different NSAIDs in pregnancy and lactation. The majority of evidence comes from observational studies and animal research only.

Indiscriminate use of NSAIDs in early pregnancy may be associated with increased risk of miscarriages and birth defects, and poor fetal and maternal outcomes. Use of NSAIDs by breastfeeding mothers is generally considered safe at usual doses, as minimal amount of drug is secreted in breast milk due to lower protein content in human milk.

Keywords

NSAIDs · Pregnancy · Lactation · Teratogenicity

G. S. Pangtey (✉) · N. Agarwal
Department of Medicine, Lady Hardinge Medical College, New Delhi, India

21.1 Introduction

Nonsteroidal anti-inflammatory drugs (NSAIDs) are the most commonly prescribed non-opioid analgesics in pregnant and lactating mother for the management of pain in various conditions, including rheumatic disorders. Whenever any medication is to be prescribed to a pregnant or lactating woman, the relative benefits and risks to the mother and fetus should always be kept in mind. The medication use may also be influenced by gestational age of fetus, drug-crossing of placental barrier, protein binding, and lipid solubility of the drug. Inflammatory disorders such as rheumatoid arthritis (RA), systemic lupus erythematosus (SLE), and other connective tissue disorders often occur in women of childbearing age; thus, the treatment of such disorders in women during pregnancy and lactation is an important aspect of their management. It is also noteworthy, as untreated autoimmune disease per se may also carry its own risks to the mother and fetus.

There are very limited studies regarding safety and tolerability of different NSAIDs in pregnancy and lactation due to ethical issues involved in doing drug studies in this group of subjects. The majority of evidence comes from observational studies and animal research. The information regarding safety and teratogenicity of NSAIDs and other antirheumatic drugs in pregnant females should be interpreted in light of background risk of adverse pregnancy outcome in general population. The estimated prevalence of major birth defects (medical, surgical, or cosmetic significance) is 2–4% among live birth (healthy general population), which does not vary in different ethnic groups [1]. The evaluation of drug's risk to neonate after breastfeeding is estimated by evaluating relative infant dose (RID), which is the dose administered to the infant through breast milk in mg/kg/day. The RID of <10% of maternal dose is generally considered to be safe.

21.2 NSAIDs in Pregnancy

The NSAID mechanism of action is by inhibiting the enzyme cyclooxygenase (COX 1 and 2) involved in the synthesis of key biological mediators prostaglandins and thromboxanes which are responsible for pain, inflammation, swelling, and platelet aggregation; thus, NSAID use ablates pain and inflammation associated with rheumatological disorders.

The safety of low-dose aspirin and NSAIDs in pregnancy is debatable. There are some studies which have found association of NSAID use in and around time of conception with increased incidence of miscarriages [2–4]. On the other hand, low-dose aspirin (acetylsalicylic acid), an NSAID, has been used in preeclampsia, antiphospholipid (APLA) syndrome, as well as assisted reproductive technology (ART)/intracytoplasmic sperm injection (ICSI) in early pregnancy to late pregnancy with improved pregnancy outcome [5]. Kozer et al. published a meta-analysis of 22 studies of aspirin exposure during first trimester of pregnancy and teratogenicity. The study found no evidence of increased risk of congenital malformations with aspirin use, although the analysis found significantly increased risk of gastroschisis [6]. Similarly, another study of 50,282 pregnant females by Slone et al. did not found any increased risk of congenital anomalies with aspirin use in the initial trimester of pregnancy [7].

NSAIDs can cross placenta and enter fetal circulation [8] and its use in first trimester may be associated with increased frequency of birth defects. One case-control study from Swedish Medical Birth Registration reported association of oral clefts with NSAID (naproxen) use in first trimester [9]. A US congenital anomalies registry also showed small-to-moderate association of NSAID (aspirin, ibuprofen, and naproxen) use with cardiac septal defects particularly ventricular septal defects [10]. NSAID use in first trimester has also been found to be associated with other birth defects like neural tube defects, pulmonary valve stenosis, limb reduction defects, amniotic bands, and diaphragmatic hernia [11, 12].

In second trimester, NSAID use is generally considered safe; however their use should be avoided in late pregnancy (third trimester) as they may be associated with premature closure of ductus arteriosus with potential of persistent primary hypertension in newborn [13, 14], decreased fetal renal perfusion resulting in oligohydramnios, necrotizing enterocolitis, and increased chances of intracranial hemorrhage in newborn [15]. In mothers because of its tocolytic effects, NSAIDs can prolong labor and can also cause postpartum hemorrhage (PPH). There is paucity of studies regarding safety of selective COX 2 inhibitors (celecoxib, etoricoxib, etc.) in pregnancy and therefore their use should be done with caution in pregnancy [16].

Given the general lack of qualitative and quantitative data regarding the safety of NSAIDs during pregnancy, avoidance of frequent NSAID use should be a prudent choice, except use of low-dose aspirin in specific indications (preeclampsia, APLA syndrome, ART/ICSI, etc.).

21.3 NSAIDs in Lactation

Present literature suggests that after ingestion of NSAIDs by mother very minimal amount of drug is excreted in milk as human milk is low in protein and most of the NSAIDs are highly protein bound. Therefore, commonly used NSAIDs (ibuprofen, naproxen, and indomethacin) are usually safe for lactating mother and her baby at approved doses [17, 18]. The maximum literature is available for the safety of ibuprofen and it has been seen that the ibuprofen levels were undetectable (0.0008% of maternal adjusted dosage) in breast milk even after taking four tablets of 400 mg of ibuprofen in a day by breastfeeding mother [19]. Therefore, ibuprofen should be the NSAID of choice in breastfeeding women. A recent study of celecoxib 200 mg (selective COX 2 NSAID) use in lactating female volunteers found very low levels of celecoxib in breast milk (relative infant dose: 0.23%) suggesting it to be safe in lactating mother and her infant [20]. Data on the safety of other NSAIDs during lactation are limited, but it has been found that ketorolac, piroxicam, and diclofenac also appear in insignificant amounts in the human breast milk [21].

In breastfeeding mothers who require high doses of aspirin like in rheumatic fever, they should avoid breastfeeding as neonatal salicylate levels may reach toxic levels [22]. There is very scarce literature available regarding safety of higher dose aspirin in breastfeeding neonates, compared with the available information regarding other NSAIDs and low-dose aspirin regimens. As an example, there has been a case report of metabolic acidosis in an infant whose mother was taking 2.4 g of aspirin a day [23].

21.4 Conclusion

Indiscriminate use of NSAIDs in early pregnancy may be associated with increased risk of miscarriages and birth defects, and poor fetal and maternal outcomes. Selective use of low-dose aspirin, ibuprofen, and naproxen is considered to be of low risk (relatively safe) in first and second trimesters of pregnancy. Use of moderate-to-high dose of aspirin and selective COX 2 inhibitors in any trimester should be avoided, unless benefits outweigh the risks to mother and fetus. NSAIDs should be avoided in the third trimester of pregnancy because of the risk of premature closure of the ductus arteriosus and are considered unsafe. NSAIDs are classified as pregnancy category C drugs under US FDA classification.

Use of NSAIDs by breastfeeding mothers is generally considered safe at usual doses, as minimal amount of drug is secreted in breast milk due to lower protein content in human milk. Low-dose aspirin (up to 81 mg/day) is also considered to be safe in breastfeeding mothers. American Academy of Pediatrics has considered ibuprofen, indomethacin, and naproxen to be safe in lactation [24].

References

1. Bermaas BL. Safety of rheumatic disease medication use during pregnancy and lactation. https://www.uptodate.com/.../safety-of-antiinflammatory-and-immunosuppressive-drug
2. Nielsen G, Sorensen H, Larsen H (2001) Risk of adverse birth outcome and miscarriage in pregnant users of non-steroidal anti-inflammatory drugs: population based observational study and case-control study. BMJ 322(7281):266–270
3. Li D, Liu L, Odouli R (2003) Exposure to non-steroidal anti-inflammatory drugs during pregnancy and risk of miscarriage: population based cohort study. BMJ 327(7411):368–360
4. Li D, Ferber J, Odouli R et al (2018) Use of nonsteroidal antiinflammatory drugs during pregnancy and the risk of miscarriage. Am J Obstet Gynecol 219(3):275.e1–275.e8
5. Wang L, Huang X, Li X et al (2017) Efficacy evaluation of low-dose aspirin in IVF/ICSI patients evidence from 13 RCTs: a systematic review and meta-analysis. Medicine (Baltimore) 96:e7720
6. Kozer E, Nikfar S, Costei A et al (2002) Aspirin consumption during the first trimester of pregnancy and congenital anomalies: a meta-analysis. Am J Obstet Gynecol 187(6):1623
7. Slone D, Siskind V, Heinonen OP et al (1976) Aspirin and congenital malformations. Lancet 1(7974):1373–1375
8. Moise K, Ou C, Kirshon B et al (1990) Placental transfer of indomethacin in the human pregnancy. Am J Obstet Gynecol 162(2):549–554
9. Ericson A, Källén B (2001) Nonsteroidal anti-inflammatory drugs in early pregnancy. Reprod Toxicol 15(4):371–375
10. Källén B, Otterblad-Olausson P (2003) Maternal drug use in early pregnancy and infant cardiovascular defect. Reprod Toxicol 17(3):255–261

11. Chambers C (2012) Pregnancy and NSAIDs. Mdedge.com [cited 11 Jun 2019]. Available from https://www.mdedge.com/obgyn/article/52546/obstetrics/pregnancy-and-nsaids
12. Antonucci R, Zaffanello M, Puxeddu E et al (2012) Use of non-steroidal anti-inflammatory drugs in pregnancy: impact on the fetus and newborn. Curr Drug Metab 13(4):474–490
13. Vermillion S, Scardo J, Lashus A et al (1997) The effect of indomethacin tocolysis on fetal ductus arteriosus constriction with advancing gestational age. Am J Obstet Gynecol 177(2):256–261
14. Stuart M, Gross S, Elrad H et al (1982) Effects of acetylsalicylic acid ingestion on maternal and neonatal hemostasis. N Engl J Med 307(15):909–912
15. Bloor M, Paech M (2013) Nonsteroidal anti-inflammatory drugs during pregnancy and the initiation of lactation. Anesth Analg 116(5):1063–1075
16. Pangtey GS, Anandh K, Sharma SK (2014) Antirheumatic drugs in pregnancy. In: Sharma SK, Sawhney S (eds) Rheumatic diseases in women & children current perspectives. Jaypee, New Delhi, pp 50–61
17. Beaulac-Baillargeon L, Allard G (1993) Distribution of indomethacin in human milk and estimation of its milk to plasma ratio in vitro. Br J Clin Pharmacol 36(5):413–416
18. Walter K, Dilger C (1997) Ibuprofen in human milk. Br J Clin Pharmacol 44(2):211–212
19. Townsend RJ, Benedetti TJ, Erickson SH et al (1984) Excretion of ibuprofen into breast milk. Am J Obstet Gynecol 149:184
20. Gardiner SJ, Doogue MP, Zhang M et al (2006) Quantification of infant exposure to celecoxib through breast milk. Br J Clin Pharmacol 61(1):101–104
21. Thabah MM, Vinod KV (2014) Use of Antirheumatic drugs in lactation. In: Sharma SK, Sawhney S (eds) Rheumatic diseases in women & children current perspectives. Jaypee, New Delhi, pp 62–72
22. Unsworth J, d'Assis-Fonseca A, Beswick D et al (1987) Serum salicylate levels in a breast fed infant. Ann Rheum Dis 46(8):638–639, 56
23. Clark JH, Wilson WG (1981) A 16-day-old breast-fed infant with metabolic acidosis caused by salicylate. Clin Pediatr (Phila) 20:53
24. American Academy of Pediatrics (2001) Committee on drugs. The transfer of drugs and other chemicals into human milk. Pediatrics 108(3):776–789

Management of Neonate with Heart Block

22

Parag Barwad and Lipi Uppal

Abstract

Complete heart block is a rare disease encountered in 1 in 15,000 births. It is mostly seen in babies with structurally normal heart, and its strong association with maternal anti-Ro/SSA and anti-La/SSB antibodies has been established. Once diagnosed, management include insertion of a permanent pacemaker in neonatal period which has shown to have excellent outcomes. Other therapies include in utero corticosteroids administration which may be considered for incomplete varieties in early gestational period.

Keywords

Congenital complete atrioventricular block (CCAVB) · Neonatal pacemaker · Anti-Ro/SSA · Anti-La/SSB

22.1 Introduction

Heart block is an abnormal cardiac rhythm manifesting as interruption or delay of electrical conduction from atria to the ventricles. Complete atrioventricular block (CAVB) or third-degree AV block is the complete failure of the conduction of the sinus impulse to the ventricles. Atrial impulses are not conducted to the ventricles leading to complete dissociation of the atria and the ventricles. Complete AV block is regarded as congenital when it is diagnosed in utero, at birth or within the neonatal period.

P. Barwad (✉) · L. Uppal
Department of Cardiology, Post Graduate Institute of Medical Education and Research, Chandigarh, India

© Springer Nature Singapore Pte Ltd. 2020
S. K. Sharma (ed.), *Women's Health in Autoimmune Diseases*,
https://doi.org/10.1007/978-981-15-0114-2_22

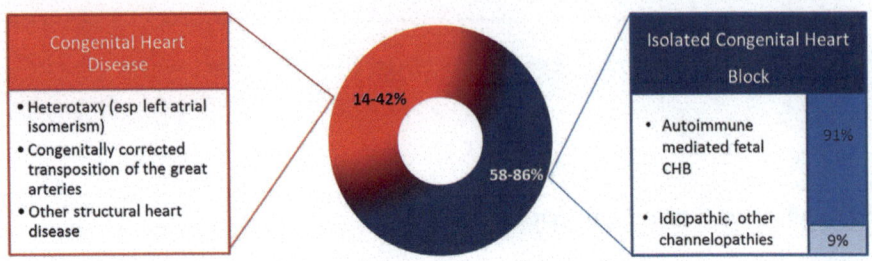

Fig. 22.1 Various causative mechanism of congenital complete heart block

Congenital complete atrioventricular block (CCAVB) is a rare disease with estimated incidence reported between 1 in 15,000 and 1 in 20,000 births [1, 2]. 58–86% of CCAVB is seen in structurally normal heart, also known as isolated congenital complete heart block. It has been found to be strongly associated with the presence of anti-Ro/SSA and anti-La/SSB antibodies, detected in mothers of 91% of the affected children [3, 4]. 14–42% of CCAVB is seen in children having complex structural heart diseases (like left atrial isomerism, L-transposition of great arteries or AV canal defects). Other rare causes being idiopathic and different channelopathies [5] (Fig. 22.1).

22.2 Immune-Mediated CCAVB

Immune-mediated CCAVB is the most common cause of isolated congenital complete heart block. It occurs as a result of passive transplacental passage of maternal IgG anti-Ro/SSA and anti-La/SSB antibodies and can occur as early as 11 weeks of gestation. The mother may have clinical manifestations of autoimmune disorders like systemic lupus erythematosus or Sjogren's syndrome, or may be asymptomatic as seen in about one-third of the cases [4]. These antibodies are believed to trigger cascade of inflammation leading to tissue injury, fibrosis and scarring of the conduction system with foetuses developing congenital heart block in 2–5% of these pregnancies [5]. Another hypothesis suggests that antibodies directly damage the conduction system via disturbing the calcium homeostasis. However, development of CHB in only a small percentage of these patients suggests that multiple factors are involved in the disease development and progression. The familial recurrence rate of autoimmune CCAVB is estimated to be 12–25% [4].

Other cardiac manifestation of neonatal lupus includes diffuse myocardial involvement with LV systolic dysfunction, endocardial fibroelastosis, valvular involvement which may lead to severe valvular regurgitations and pericardial effusion which may occur independent of conduction abnormalities [6]. Non-cardiac manifestations of neonatal lupus includes transient rash, hepatobiliary dysfunction, neurological and pulmonary abnormalities. While most of these abnormalities are corrected by 6 months of age with clearance of the antibodies, the cardiac manifestations are permanent and persist indefinitely.

22.3 Natural History of CCAVB

Most cases are diagnosed in utero with screening obstetric ultrasound, between 18 and 24 weeks of gestation. In other children, CCAVB can have variable presentation ranging from foetal hydrops in utero, congestive heart failure in infants, to poor exercise tolerance, recurrent syncope and sudden cardiac death in older children. Perinatal and neonatal period have the greatest risk of mortality which is estimated to be between 15 and 20% [4, 7]. Poor prognosis is seen in hydrops fetalis, low heart rate (<50–55/min), premature newborn and those who have associated LV dysfunction or endocardial fibroelastosis [4]. Around 10% of the children would be born with hydrops or congestive heart failure secondary to intrauterine myocarditis or severe bradycardia [4]. The choice of therapy remains pacemaker implantation, and almost two-third of the patients will require pacemaker during their lifetime. Majority of patients will undergo pacemaker implantation during the neonatal period and can be expected to have near normal life expectancy [8].

22.4 Cardiac Evaluation of Complete Heart Block in Prenatal Period

Foetal echocardiography is the imaging modality of choice for perinatal cardiac evaluation in foetus. Foetal echocardiography and colour doppler can identify any structural abnormalities. It also recognises other associated functional abnormalities like pericardial effusion, atrioventricular valve regurgitation and is useful for assessment of left ventricular function.

The various techniques on foetal echocardiography include M-Mode, Tissue Doppler and Pulsed wave Doppler. These techniques can accurately assess the time intervals and dissociation of atrial inflow with ventricular outflow.

Simultaneous Doppler flow measurement across mitral valve and aortic valve demonstrates the dissociation between atrial and ventricular rhythms in complete heart block. Atrioventricular contraction Time Interval (AVCTI) is the mechanical representation of electrical PR interval. It is measured between the onset of the A wave (atrial systole) and the onset of the ejection outflow Doppler (ventricular systole). Measurement of AVCTI facilitates the recognition of lower grades of heart block, thus assisting in subsequent follow up and risk assessment.

Mechanical assessment of wall motion by M mode demonstrates sequential contraction of atrial and ventricular myocardium and demonstrates electrical activity.

Tissue Doppler imaging can directly record the mechanical activity of the atria and ventricle during cardiac cycle leading to accurate measurement of cardiac intervals [9]. Other modalities like foetal electrocardiography and foetal magnetography are limited in their utility.

Foetal ECG: Foetal electrocardiogram (fECG) can detect QRS signals in foetuses from as early as 17 weeks gestation. However, this technique is limited by foetal movements and in differentiating foetal from maternal ECG signals. Moreover, fECG is not feasible after 28 weeks of gestation. A fECG with scalp electrodes can be helpful in peripartum management of CHB; however, it cannot be used in screening for foetal arrhythmias.

Foetal magnetography: Foetal magnetography uses the magnetic field created by the electrical signals of the foetal heart. It requires magnetically isolated room and is currently used in research settings.

Since the first degree AVB can rapidly progress to CAVB, early diagnosis, prenatal evaluation and proper management are critical to prevent progression and avoid irreversible damage. The first sign of foetal heart block is seen between 18th and 24th gestational week and is rapidly progressive thereafter.

Initial diagnosis of foetal bradycardia by either auscultation or abnormal obstetric ultrasound is generally the first sign for foetal cardiac evaluation. Since many of these mothers may be asymptomatic, it also prompts screening of mothers for presence of IgG antibodies and other manifestations of autoimmune diseases. For pregnant patients with presence of antibodies or previous child with congenital heart block, evaluation is routinely started at 18 weeks. Because of high risk and rapid progression, foetal echocardiography is carried out weekly till 24th week and monthly thereafter till delivery. In babies diagnosed to have first degree heart block, weekly foetal echocardiography is carried out till elective termination of pregnancy. Echocardiography also helps to rule out presence of cardiac structural abnormalities and myocardial involvement.

22.5 Pharmacotherapy

Corticosteroids may reduce immune-mediated damage to the conduction tissue and decrease inflammation in foetuses with progressive heart block. Fluorinated steroids like dexamethasone and betamethasone have the ability to cross placenta and reach foetus in the active stage. The timely administration of these drugs prevents the progression to higher degrees of AV block and progression of cardiomyopathy and also minimises the clinical morbidity [10, 11]. However, a recent meta-analysis comparing data from eight studies demonstrated no benefit of steroids in patients with AV block with no difference in progression to third-degree heart block or mortality in steroid-treated patients when compared to non-treated patients [12]. Moreover, corticosteroid administration can have negative side effects on both mother and the foetus including hypertension, maternal diabetes, intrauterine growth retardation and foetal neurological abnormalities. Thus, in view of lack of definite evidence, corticosteroids can be considered in first- or second-degree heart block in attempts to reduce progression to complete heart block since development of complete heart block is often irreversible.

22.6 Beta Agonists

Two small retrospective cohort studies evaluated the treatment of patients with dexamethasone along with beta agonist where strict monitoring and concomitant use of dexamethasone with beta agonist had resulted in better outcomes [11, 13]. In both the studies beta agonists were used in patient with foetal heart rate <55/min.

Other experimental therapies including plasmapheresis, digoxin and foetal pacing have no definite data and are only reserved for cases where the foetus is in life threatening situation with hydrops and cardiac dysfunction.

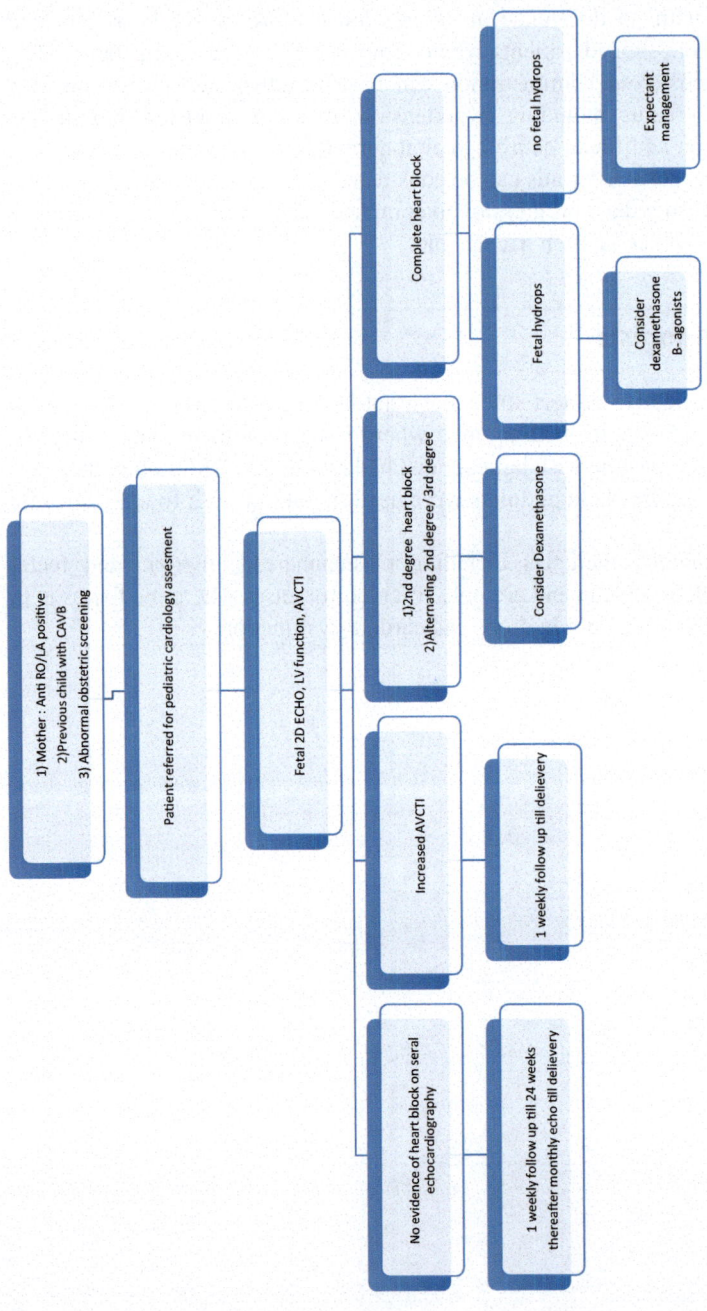

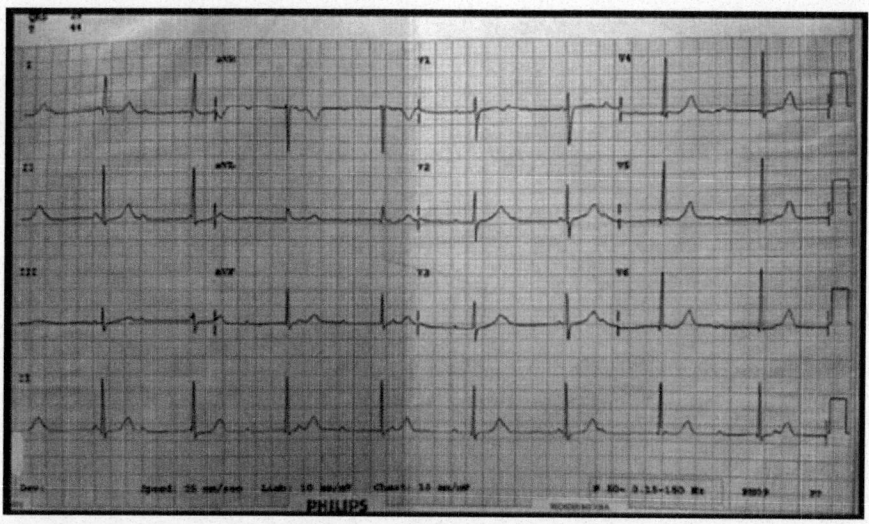

Fig. 22.2 ECG of a child with complete heart block shows atrial rate of 120/min with ventricular rate of 50 beats/min. ECG shows complete atrioventricular dissociation. Narrow QRS complexes suggest origin of ventricular escape rhythm above the bundle of HIS

22.7 Post-natal Management

Most of the neonates developing complete heart block would require a pacemaker in their lifetime. The decision regarding implantation of pacemaker in a neonate depends upon the clinical stability of the child. Newborn with AV block should be managed in intensive care units for optimising acid/base status, inotropic drug infusion and mechanical ventilation. Early pacing of high-risk neonates reduces the adverse effects of low cardiac output. Temporary epicardial pacemaker as a bridge to permanent pacemaker is a feasible option to achieve clinical stability and weight gain. The hemodynamic function of a neonate with complete heart block depends upon one critical factor, i.e. ventricular rate. In addition to heart rate, other factors like absence of structural heart disease and presence of inherently normal myocardium determine the clinical stability of the infant.

Clinical examination generally reveals a low heart rate, ranging from 40 to 90 beats/min. Definitive diagnosis of complete heart block is made on ECG which shows p wave of atrial depolarisation independent of the QRS complexes of ventricular depolarisation. The p–p interval is constant and R–R interval is constant with variable PR interval example shown in Fig. 22.2. Subsidiary pacemakers proximal to HIS bundle produce narrow QRS escape rhythm, whereas those at or below HIS bundle produce a wide QRS complex.

Decision regarding the timing of pacemaker must consider the indications and technical feasibility of putting pacemaker in a neonate. The indications for pacing in congenital complete heart block in a neonate relatively similar to those of adult patient are as follows [14].

22.7.1 Class I

1. Permanent pacemaker implantation is indicated for advanced second- or third-degree AV block associated with symptomatic bradycardia, ventricular dysfunction or low cardiac output (*LOE: C*).
2. Permanent pacemaker implantation is indicated for congenital third-degree AV block with a wide QRS escape rhythm, complex ventricular ectopy or ventricular dysfunction (*LOE: B*).
3. Permanent pacemaker implantation is indicated for congenital third-degree AV block in the infant with a ventricular rate less than 55 bpm or with congenital heart disease and a ventricular rate less than 70 bpm (*LOE: C*).

22.7.2 Class IIa

Permanent pacemaker implantation is reasonable for congenital third-degree AV block beyond the first year of life with an average heart rate less than 50 bpm, abrupt pauses in ventricular rate that are two or three times the basic cycle length, or associated with symptoms due to chronotropic incompetence (*LOE: C*).

22.7.3 Class IIb

Permanent pacemaker implantation may be considered for congenital third-degree AV block in asymptomatic children or adolescents with an acceptable rate, a narrow QRS complex and normal ventricular function (*LOE: B*).

22.8 Choice of Pacemaker

In contrast to adult patients, pacemaker implantation in children requires individual assessment of access (epicardial vs. endocardial), of implantation site (infraclavicular vs. abdominal) and associated structural abnormalities. Also, the expected growth of the child has to be considered, as the lifelong dependency of the patient and multiple revisions that would be required for battery or lead replacements.

Currently it is recommended to use epicardial pacemaker in infants till 2 years of age. High incidence of venous occlusion of small venous structures and concern over loss of venous access in future leads to preference of epicardial pacemaker in this age group. Endocardial pacing is reserved for children who are at least >10 kg or >2 years of age.

Epicardial pacemakers are inserted via a subxiphoid approach or lateral thoracotomy approach, and most patients with pacemaker will require 100% pacing. This allows direct access to RV apex or RA appendage. Alternative sites for lead placement LV apex or biventricular pacing are thought to have better ventricular synchrony and long-term myocardial performance. Various side effects including higher lead threshold, surgical mortality and increased risk of lead fracture are seen with epicardial deployment of pacemaker. With availability of leads with lower profile and smaller generator size, many centres are now exploring the possibility of endocardial placement [15].

Key Points

1. Isolated CCAVB is a rare congenital heart disease mainly seen in pregnant women positive for IgG antibodies.
2. Perinatal diagnosis and strict monitoring is the key to management.
3. Role of fluorinated steroids remains controversial in incomplete forms of CHB, which is not recommended in complete form.
4. Timely pacemaker implantation is the management of choice.
5. Epicardial pacemaker implantation is the currently practised approach for neonatal age group; however, with availability of low profile leads and generators, trans-venous approach is rapidly gaining momentum.

References

1. Michaelsson M, Riesenfeld T, Jonzon A (1997) Natural history of congenital complete atrioventricular block. Pacing Clin Electrophysiol 20(8 Pt 2):2098–2101
2. Yater WM (1929) Congenital heart-block: review of the literature; report of a case with incomplete heterotaxy; the electrocardiogram in dextrocardia. Am J Dis Child 38(1):112–136
3. Pregnancy outcomes in patients with autoimmune diseases and anti-Ro/SSA antibodies [cited 15 May 2019]. Available from https://www.ncbi.nlm.nih.gov/pubmed/20012231
4. Buyon JP, Hiebert R, Copel J, Craft J, Friedman D, Katholi M et al (1998) Autoimmune-associated congenital heart block: demographics, mortality, morbidity and recurrence rates obtained from a National Neonatal Lupus Registry. J Am Coll Cardiol 31(7):1658–1666
5. Brucato A, Frassi M, Franceschini F, Cimaz R, Faden D, Pisoni MP et al (2001) Risk of congenital complete heart block in newborns of mothers with anti-Ro/SSA antibodies detected by counter immunoelectrophoresis: a prospective study of 100 women. Arthritis Rheum 44(8):1832–1835
6. Cardiac manifestations of neonatal lupus: a review of autoantibody associated congenital heart block and its impact in an adult population [cited 13 May 2019]. Available from https://www.ncbi.nlm.nih.gov/pmc/articles/PMC3275696/
7. McCune AB. Maternal and fetal outcome in neonatal lupus erythematosus [cited 13 May 2019]. Available from https://scholar.google.com/scholar_lookup?title=Maternal%20and%20fetal%20outcome%20in%20neonatal%20lupus%20erythematosus&publication_year=1987&author=A.B.%20McCune&author=W.L.%20Weston&author=L.A.%20Lee
8. Brito-Zerón P, Izmirly P, Ramos-Casals M, Buyon J, Khamashta M (2016) Autoimmune congenital heart block: complex and unusual situations. Lupus 25(2):116–128

9. Rein AJJT, O'Donnell C, Geva T, Nir A, Perles Z, Hashimoto I et al (2002) Use of tissue velocity imaging in the diagnosis of fetal cardiac arrhythmias. Circulation 106(14):1827–1833
10. Saleeb S, Copel J, Friedman D, Buyon JP (1999) Comparison of treatment with fluorinated glucocorticoids to the natural history of autoantibody-associated congenital heart block: retrospective review of the research registry for neonatal lupus. Arthritis Rheum 42(11):2335–2345
11. Jaeggi ET, Fouron J-C, Silverman ED, Ryan G, Smallhorn J, Hornberger LK (2004) Transplacental fetal treatment improves the outcome of prenatally diagnosed complete atrioventricular block without structural heart disease. Circulation 110(12):1542–1548
12. Ciardulli A, D'Antonio F, Magro-Malosso ER, Saccone G, Manzoli L, Radolec M et al (2019) Maternal steroid therapy for fetuses with immune-mediated complete atrioventricular block: a systematic review and meta-analysis. J Matern Fetal Neonatal Med 32(11):1884–1892
13. Cuneo BF, Lee M, Roberson D, Niksch A, Ovadia M, Parilla BV et al (2010) A management strategy for fetal immune-mediated atrioventricular block. J Matern Fetal Neonatal Med 23(12):1400–1405
14. Epstein AE, DiMarco JP, Ellenbogen KA, Estes NA, Freedman RA et al (2008) ACC/AHA/HRS 2008 guidelines for device-based therapy of cardiac rhythm abnormalities. Circulation 117(21):e350–e408
15. Robledo-Nolasco R, Ortiz-Avalos M, Rodriguez-Diez G, Jimenez-Carrillo C, Ramírez-Machuca J, De Haro S et al (2009) Transvenous pacing in children weighing less than 10 kilograms. Pacing Clin Electrophysiol 32(Suppl 1):S177–S181

Women Issues in Autoimmune Diseases: Compilation of Indian Data

23

Kaushik S. Bhojani

Abstract

Autoimmune diseases occur more commonly in females of child-bearing age. The diseases with their systemic nature play a role in menstrual irregularities, fertility and may cause complications in pregnancy and delivery. Moreover some medications are contraindicated during conception, pregnancy and breast feeding. Epidemiological data available from India on autoimmune diseases is sparse. The Multicentric COPCORD study reports prevalence of various rheumatological diseases in India. A study by Prem Kumar et al. attempts to give male to female ratio. Kudial et al. have thrown light on the burden of rheumatological disorders in postmenopausal women.

After an extensive search, on these issues in individual rheumatological diseases, we present herewith a compilation of Indian data in this chapter.

Keywords

Autoimmune disease · India · SLE · Rheumatoid arthritis · Vasculitis · Pregnancy

23.1 Introduction

Autoimmune diseases occur significantly more commonly in women than in men (frequency about 78%). They occur predominantly in the childbearing age, i.e. 20–40 [1]. Whilst the disease itself with its systemic features may play a role in causing menstrual irregularities, infertility, pregnancy and delivery, some medications may be contraindicated in conception, pregnancy and breast feeding.

K. S. Bhojani (✉)
Kennisha Rheumatology Care and Diagnostics, Mumbai, India
e-mail: dr.ksbhojani@kennisha.com

High disease activity has an inversely proportional relationship with sexual function secondary to chronic pain, stiffness, fatigue, impaired quality of life, depression or reduced libido. Additionally fecundity (time to achieve pregnancy) may also be affected [2].

23.2 Epidemiology of Rheumatic Diseases in Women in India

Epidemiological data available in India on autoimmune diseases is sparse. The maximum data available is from Dr. Arvind Chopra's article based on the multicentric copcord study which attempted to assess the burden of various rheumatological disorders in India. Data from 55,000 people over 12 sites in various surveys from Bone and Joint decade (2004–2010) reported prevalence of RA in 0.34, undifferentiated arthritis in 0.23, spondyloarthritis in 0.2 (of which incidence of ankylosing spondylitis found to be 0.02), SLE in 0.1 and OA knee in 3.34. Though we know that most autoimmune diseases are prevalent in females, the exact female to male ratio is not available from this study [3].

Mahajan et al. studied 529 males and 485 females and found 245 patients with rheumatic diseases (132 females/113 males) [4]. Kudial et al. reported the prevalence of rheumatic disorders in Indian menopausal women significant enough to draw attention of health care providers to this subsegment of patients. The most common afflictions noted were low backache followed by osteoarthritis, fibromyalgia and rheumatoid arthritis affecting women above the age of 40 years. Hypertension, anaemia and diabetes mellitus were found to be commonly associated comorbidities [5].

Prem Kumar studied 1481 patients attending orthopaedic and rheumatic unit, and the epidemiology of autoimmune diseases found by them is as given in Table 23.1 [6].

Successful pregnancy is largely dependent on a TH2 cytokine profile, whereas spontaneous abortion shows a TH1 cytokine pattern. Evidence for this shift of the TH response is strongest at the maternal–foetal interface. However, a modulation

Table 23.1 Epidemiology of autoimmune diseases

Disease	Percentage	Female to male ratio
Rheumatoid arthritis	39	3.35:1
Spondyloarthropathy	9	0.92:1
Psoriatic arthritis	6	2.42:1
Systemic lupus erythematosus	6	1.9:1
Sjogren's syndrome	5	
Reactive arthritis	5	
Scleroderma	2	10:1
Takayasu's arteritis	1	
Dermatomyositis	1	
Gout	3	1:7.2
Osteoarthritis	3	0.28:1
Fibromyalgia	13	4.79:1

Indian data from Prem Kumar et al.

takes place in synchrony with the stage of pregnancy and a persistent domination of a TH2 cytokine pattern is not seen throughout pregnancy. Studies have shown an increase of anti-inflammatory cytokines in pregnancy such as IL 10, IL 4 and transforming growth factor B and the production of inflammatory cytokines such as interferon gamma and IL 12 is suppressed and immune tolerance is induced. The increase of regulatory T-cells suppresses the proliferation of interferon gamma and interleukin-12 (IL-12) producing effector T-cells and promotes the secretion of IL-10, IL-4 and transforming growth factor-beta [7].

The interaction of paternal HLA antigens with maternal peripheral blood mononuclear cells stimulates the production of IL-4, thereby promoting a TH2 response. Serum levels of cortisol, catecholamines and other factors decrease postpartum leading to an increase of pro-inflammatory cytokines and more vigorous B-cell responses causing an immunological rebound [7].

As mentioned earlier, there is paucity of Indian data on pregnancy and rheumatic diseases and is mainly restricted to SLE (systemic lupus erythematosus). Most of these studies are small in number and hence the interpretation of these or the impact of their conclusions, so as to aid derivation of some form of guidelines for the clinician, is open to debate. Nevertheless the available data has been reviewed and presented disease wise in this chapter.

23.3 Systemic Lupus Erythematosus (SLE)

It is well known that menstrual irregularities occur both due to disease activity and use of cyclophosphamide. Amenorrhoea due to cyclophosphamide may be reversible or irreversible. The chances of irreversibility increase proportionate to increasing age and are significant beyond 30 years of age.

Kothari et al. in 2016 reported 52 patients with SLE of which menstrual irregularities were recorded in 19/52 (36.51%), 10 patients (19.2%) with amenorrhoea at the onset which was attributed to disease activity. Twenty-seven patients received cyclophosphamide pulse doses of which 13 were reported to have developed amenorrhoea post cyclophosphamide therapy (these 13 included the 10 patients who had amenorrhoea at the onset), of these 3 developed irreversible amenorrhoea all being above the age of 30 years. The conclusion therefore is that higher pulse cyclophosphamide dose and age above 30 are the known risk factors [8].

Singh et al. reported 29.4% incidence of amenorrhoea and premature menopause in 17.2% following cyclophosphamide therapy in SLE vs 4% and 2%, respectively, in no cyclo group [9]. In both these studies FSH, LH levels and AMH levels were not checked. Whilst fertility in SLE is not usually compromised, pregnancy losses, preterm deliveries, intrauterine growth retardation (IUGR), low gestational age and low birthweight are not uncommon complications either in SLE [10]. Table 23.2 gives comparative data of various Indian studies. SLE being rare disease, most of the studies even from large centres have small numbers. The higher number of patients are over long periods of time. Since treatment strategies have evolved over

Table 23.2 Showing pregnancy outcomes in SLE patients in India

Study	Disease activity status			Preg/ women	Abortions					Live	Premature	IUGR	LBW	Intervention and comments
	Active	Inactive	Flare		1st	2nd	3rd	Total	MTP					
Aggarwal et al., 1999 [11]	11	4	2	15/15								40%		2 stillbirth, Gest age wks—35.9 ± 2.5
Mittal et al., 2001 [12]	10		9	42/25				13	4	16(38%)	4			4 stillbirths
Gupta et al., 2005 [13]	19	14	9	33/17				12	6	15(45.45%)		4		Lack of tertiary care access
Chandran et al., 2005 [14]	21	31	3	52/31				12(29%)	11	24(58.5%)				
Parkodi et al., 2005 [15]	16(72.8%)	6(27.2%)	4	22	1	6	1	8	0	13(59%)				PIH-1, FND-50%
Gupta et al., 2010 [16]				121/210		34%		64(53%)		30(25%)				
Aggarwal et al., 2011 [17]				71/35				33%		47(66%)	33%			18% CS, perinatal loss 13%
Kothari et al., 2016 [8]	10	6	7	16/16	3		2	5	1	9(56.3%)	1	4		ND-7, Cs-2
Ravindran, 2017 [18]			16(30%)	53				8		44(85%)		10		Cs/Instru-28
Khan et al., 2018 [19]										14%				

time, it is difficult to interpret results from these studies in the current context. Overall studies show the incidence of lupus flare in about 20–40% of patients during pregnancy, whilst the incidence of foetal loss, spontaneous abortions and IUFD is estimated to be around 35–40%, 25–40% and 9.5–18%, respectively. Status of disease activity in the 6 months prior to conception was predictive of lupus flare in pregnancy [8, 12]. Active disease, renal involvement, anti Ro/La, APLA positivity and preclampsia are risk factors for complications during pregnancy.

Leelavati et al. from Mysore presented their experience of 11 pregnant SLE patients wherein the incidence of pre-eclampsia was noted to be 54.54%, HELLP syndrome in 9.09%, PPH in 50%. Seventy-five per cent of patients had LSCS caesarean section and 62.5% had preterm deliveries [20]. Ravindran in 2016 convincingly showed that prenatal counselling, risk stratification, periodic antenatal visits for the monitoring of pregnancy and disease activity along with changes in therapy as required, 2D echocardiogram at weeks 18 and 32 in Ro/LA positive patients and postnatal contraception advice can improve pregnancy outcome suggesting a 'treat to target' protocol [10]. The same conclusion is seen with other tertiary centre multidisciplinary care [20].

23.4 Antiphospholipid Syndrome (APLS)

Antiphospholipid antibodies are reported as one of the important risk factors in adverse outcome. Dadhawal et al. reported 42 pregnant women with a mean age of 30 years who presented between 2007 and 2009 in antenatal clinic that a large proportion of patients developed complications despite treatment. These comprised of missed abortions in 4 (9.5%), intrauterine growth retardation (IUGR) in 9 (21.4%) and pre-eclampsia in 13 (30.9%), abruption placentae in 3 (7.1%) and intrauterine foetal death (IUFD) in 2 (4.7%). Despite these complications, the birth rate improved from 4.6% before treatment to 85.7% after treatment. Early foetal loss reduced from 76.1% to 9.5% and late foetal loss reduced from 19.6% to 4% [21].

Findings of the Euro-Phospholipid study suggest there was early foetal loss (before 10 weeks) in 35.5% as against incidence of late foetal loss in 16.9%. Pre-eclampsia occurred in 9.5% of pregnant women, eclampsia in 4.4% and placental abruption in 2%. The improvement in birth rate is comparable with the international data [22–24].

23.5 Rheumatoid Arthritis

Compared to the national average in India, the average number of living children is observed to be lesser in patients of RA (2.39 ± 1.39), though this fact is applicable more so in patients with SLE (1.44 ± 1.35) which is in concordance with international observations [25]. Reduced fecundity with a duration more than 12 months has been observed in a Dutch study [2]. Factors responsible for the same could be higher maternal age, disease severity and higher steroid dose. In addition to delayed conception, low birth weight and premature delivery are known to occur with active disease [2]. However, no Indian date available on this aspect.

23.6 Vasculitis

23.6.1 ANCA-Associated Vasculitis (AAV)

Singh et al. have reported 137 pregnancies in 110 patients of AAV with mean age of 29.3($\pm$5.3) years. Vasculitis was diagnosed before pregnancy in 69, during pregnancy in 32 and post-partum in 9 patients. There were 91 full-term pregnancies, 28 preterm, 15 abortions and 3 stillbirths; 78 had normal delivery while 26 patients delivered via caesarean section [26].

The study by Veltri et al. included 27 cases of newly diagnosed ANCA-associated vasculitis. The patients ranged from 5 to 39 weeks of gestation, and most were in the second trimester (median 20 weeks). These patients received various modalities of treatment based on severity of the vasculitis and the clinicians' judgement. The vast majority were treated with steroids (89%), whilst some patients also received combination treatment with immunosuppressants such as cyclophosphamide (CYC) (37%), azathioprine (AZA), IVIG, plasma exchange (PLEX) or no therapy (11%) [27].

Not surprisingly, high rates of serious complications such as pre-eclampsia (29%) and maternal death (7%) were noted. Given the gravity of the disease and the complications associated with treatment, the rate of successful pregnancies resulting in live births was satisfactory (73%). Rate of premature delivery was significant with 73% deliveries at less than 37 weeks and 40% less than 34 weeks of pregnancy state. However the majority of infants were born in the third trimester (median 34.5 weeks). Not surprisingly the rates of pregnancy termination were high (23%) with one intrauterine death shortly after initiation of therapy (4%). Encouragingly the incidence of congenital abnormalities was not significant, barring one infant having a solitary, pelvic kidney (6%) after maternal treatment with steroids, CYC and PLEX. Remission of vasculitis was observed in 60% of patients postpartum. Interestingly the use of PLEX, IVIG and AZA has increased after 2005, with corresponding reduction in CYC use [27].

In a British cohort, 51 pregnancies in 29 women with systemic vasculitis were compared to 156 pregnancies in 62 age-, body mass index- and ethnicity-matched healthy pregnant controls. Babies of mothers with vasculitis were born at a median gestational age of 36 weeks versus 40 weeks for controls ($P < 0.03$). The median birth weight for the babies with affected mothers was 3.0 kg versus 3.5 kg for the control babies ($P = 0.004$). Affected mothers suffered 13 miscarriages, 3 had pre-eclampsia and 2 had an intrauterine death [28].

23.6.2 Takayasu's Arteritis

A 13-fold higher rate of obstetric complications was noted in women with aortoarteritis compared to pregnancies in normal young women. Good outcomes have been reported with type I and type II aortoarteritis with a low incidence of secondary hypertension and IUGR; however, perinatal outcomes in types III, IV and V were noted to be poor [29].

Sharma et al. noted the incidence of renovascular hypertension in 3.8% of young hypertensives. Of these 59.4% of them were found to have aortoarteritis [30]. Suri et al. reported 37 pregnancies in 15 patients of aortoarteritis over 9 years from North India. Twenty-seven per cent of women had hypertension at initial presentation. Sixty-two per cent of pregnancies were complicated by pre-eclampsia and IUGR was reported in 16% patients. There was one maternal death due to accelerated hypertension and six preterm deliveries [31]. Garikapati et al. have reported pregnancy outcomes in four patients with Takayasu's arteritis. All these patients had chronic hypertension with renal artery stenosis treated with labetalol. One patient developed pre-eclampsia, one developed peripartum cardiomyopathy and pulmonary oedema. All patients underwent caesarean section for obstetric complications (foetal distress = 1, oligohydramnios = 2 and breech = 2). Of these four, one had IUGR [29].

23.6.3 Scleroderma

Pregnancy and fertility issues in systemic sclerosis have been discussed in depth by Rao et al. [7]. Data from Pradhan from western part of India has presented clinical profile of 110 scleroderma patients in 2014. In this study the mean age of evaluation was 34.7, duration was 43.7 ± 35.4 year, but there is no discussion on pregnancy-related outcomes which could be due to higher age of presentation, ±10.7, and mean disease [32].

There is no Indian data available in systemic sclerosis.

Other autoimmune diseases causing primary ovarian failure (POF): POF is associated with autoimmune diseases and endocrinopathies in 20–30% of cases. POF is reported in patients with Addison's disease (20%), thyroid diseases (9%), polyglandular syndromes (2%), rheumatoid disease (1%) and in less than 1% cases of systemic lupus erythematosus, vitiligo, myasthenia gravis, insulin-dependent diabetes mellitus and Crohn's disease. Ayesha et al. in their study found 35% (7/20) patients with secondary amenorrhoea due to thyroid disorder. Sixty-five per cent of patients in this study had low DHEAS levels suggestive of adrenal dysfunction and adrenal autoimmunity [33].

To summarise Indian data on pregnancy and rheumatic diseases is scanty at best. As treatment modalities progressively improve resulting in longer lifespans and reduced morbidity, we as clinicians will be increasingly faced with questions regarding a better quality of life and fertility issues. Currently we have mainly questions but hardly any answers and we rely on International studies and our individual clinical judgement to try and provide pregnancy-related issues and peripartum care. Needless to say pregnancy counselling does not figure on our landscape except for advice to avoid pregnancy in these diseases and while on most medications.

Systematic data collection from observational studies could be a stepping stone to a better understanding of the exact incidence and approaches to better outcomes. Alternatively multicentric registries could also be the way forward for us to be able to provide better care to our patients with rheumatic diseases.

Disclosures None.

References

1. Fairweather D, Rose N (2004) Women and autoimmune diseases. Emerg Infect Dis 10(11):2005–2011
2. Østensen M, Wallenius M (2016) Fertility and pregnancy in rheumatoid arthritis. Ind J Rheumatol 11(6):122–127
3. Chopra A (2015) Disease burden of rheumatic diseases in India. COPCORD perspective. Ind J Rheumatol 10(2):70–77
4. Mahajan A, Jasrotia D, Manhas A, Jamwal S (2003) Prevalence of major rheumatic diseases in Jammu. JK Sci 5(2):63–66
5. Kudial S, Tandon V, Mahajan A (2015) Rheumatological disorder (RD) in Indian women above 40 years of age: a cross-sectional WHO-ILAR-COPCORD-based survey. J Midlife Health 6(2):76–78
6. Prem Kumar B, Srinivasa Murthy M, Rajagopal K, Nagaprabu VN, Sree Madhuri P (2014) Epidemiology of autoimmune disorders with special reference to rheumatoid arthritis from a tertiary care center. Ind J Pharm Pract 7(3):50–60
7. Rao VKR (2016) Fertility and pregnancy in systemic sclerosis and other autoimmune diseases. Ind J Rheumatol 11:150–155
8. Kothari R, Digole A, Kamat S, Nandanwar Y, Gokhale Y (2016) Reproductive health in systemic lupus erythematosus, an experience from Government Hospital in Western India. J Assoc Phys India 64:16–20
9. Singh G, Misra R, Aggarwal A (2016) Ovarian insufficiency is major short-term toxicity in systemic lupus erythematosus. Patients treated with cyclophosphamide. J Assoc Phys India 64:28–31
10. Mohan MC, Ravindran V (2016) Lupus pregnancies. An Indian perspective. Indian J Rheumatol 11:135–138
11. Aggarwal N, Sawney H, Chopra S, Bambery P (1999) Pregnancy in patients with systemic lupus erythematosus. Aust N Z J Obstet Gynaecol 39:28–30
12. Mittal G, Sule A, Pathan E, Gaitonde S, Samant R, Joshi VR (2001) Pregnancy in lupus—analysis of 25 cases. JIRA 9(4):69–71
13. Gupta A, Agarwal A, Handa R (2005) Pregnancy in Indian patients with systemic lupus erythematosus. Lupus 14:926–927
14. Chandran V, Aggarwal A, Misra R (2005) Active disease during pregnancy is associated with poor foetal outcome in Indian patients with systemic lupus erythematosus. Rheumatol Int 26:152–156
15. Parkodi R, Manimegalai N, Balmeena S, Vasanthy N, Mahavan R, Rajendran CP (2005) Outcome of pregnancy in lupus. J Indian Rheumatol Assoc 13:83–85
16. Gupta R, Deepanjali S, Kumar A, Dadhwal V, Agarwal SK, Pandey RM et al (2010) A comparative study of pregnancy outcomes and menstrual irregularities in northern Indian patients with systemic lupus erythematosus and rheumatoid arthritis. Rheumatol Int 30:1581–1585

17. Aggarwal N, Raveendran A, Suri V, Chopra S, Sikka P, Sharma A (2011) Pregnancy outcome in systemic lupus erythematosus: Asia's largest single centre study. Arch Gynecol Obstet 284:281–285
18. Ravindran V, Bhadran S. Improved outcomes in high-risk lupus pregnancies: usefulness of a protocol-based multidisciplinary approach in Kerala, India. Poster 318. Downloaded from https://academic.oup.com/rheumatology/article-abstract/56/suppl_2/kex062.320/4106822
19. Khan A, Thomas M, Syamala Devi PK (2018) Pregnancy complicated by systemic lupus erythematosus and its outcome over 10 years. J Obstet Gynaecol 38(4):476–481
20. Leelavathi, Nayana DH, Kondareddy T, Kaytri S (2017) SLE during pregnancy, maternal and perinatal outcome in tertiary hospital. Int J Reprod Contracept Obstet Gynecol 6(2):507–551
21. Dadhwal V, Sharma AK, Deka D, Gupta B, Mittal S (2011) The obstetric outcome following treatment in a cohort of patients with antiphospholipid antibody syndrome in a tertiary care center. J Postgrad Med 57(1):16–19
22. Cervera R, Piette JC, Font J, Khamashta MA, Shoenfeld Y, Camps MT et al (2002) Antiphospholipid syndrome: clinical and immunologic manifestations and patterns of disease expression in a cohort of 1,000 patients. Arthritis Rheum 46:1019–1027
23. Cervera R, Khamashta MA, Shoenfeld Y, Camps MT, Jacobsen S, Kiss E et al (2009) Morbidity and mortality in the antiphospholipid syndrome during a 5-year period: a multicentre prospective study of 1000 patients. Ann Rheum Dis 68:1428–1432
24. Rahman A (2016) Antiphospholipid syndrome in pregnancy. Indian J Rheumatol 11:117–121
25. Gupta R, Deepanjali S, Kumar A, Dhaval V et al (2010) A comparative study of pregnancy outcomes and menstrual irregularities in northern Indian patients with systemic lupus erythematosus and rheumatoid arthritis. Rheum Int 30(12):1581–1585
26. Singh P, Dhooria A, Rathi M, Agarwal R et al (2018) Successful treatment outcomes in pregnant patients with ANCA-associated vasculitides: a systematic review of literature. Int J Rheum Dis 21(9):1734–1740
27. Veltri N, Hladunewich M, Bhasin A, Garland J, Thomson B (2018) De novo antineutrophil cytoplasmic antibody associated vasculitis in pregnancy: a systematic review on maternal, pregnancy and fetal outcomes. Clin Kidney J 11(5):659–666
28. Pathak H, Mukhtyar C (2016) Pregnancy and systemic vasculitis. Indian J Rheumatol 11:145–149
29. Garikapati K, Kota LN, Kodey PD (2016) Pregnancy in Takayasu arteritis—maternal and fetal outcome. Int J Reprod Contracept Obstet Gynecol 5(8):2596–2600
30. Sharma BK, Sagar S, Chugh KS, Sakhuja V, Rajachandran A, Malik N (1985) Spectrum of renovascular hypertension in the young in north India: a hospital based study on occurrence and clinical features. Angiology 36(6):370–378
31. Suri V, Aggarwal N, Keepanasseril A, Chopra S, Vijayvergiya R, Jain S (2010) Pregnancy and Takayasu arteritis: a single centre experience from North India. J Obstet Gynaecol Res 36(3):519–524. https://doi.org/10.1111/j.1447-0756.2010.01226
32. Pradhan V, Rajadhyaksha A, Nadkar M, Pandit P et al (2014) Clinical and autoimmune profile of scleroderma patients from western India. Int J Rheumatol 2014:983781. https://doi.org/10.1155/2014/983781
33. Ayesha JV, Goswami D (2016) Premature ovarian failure: an association with autoimmune diseases. J Clin Diagn Res 10(10):QC10–QC12

Osteoporosis in Autoimmune Rheumatic Diseases

C. Godsave, R. Garner, and Ira Pande

Abstract

Bone loss in rheumatic disorders is multifactorial. Contributing factors are the inflammatory process per se including inflammatory cytokines, traditional clinical risk factors and drugs with glucocorticoids being the leading cause. Furthermore, autoimmune rheumatic diseases affect women of childbearing age and young men, who may not have attained peak bone mass at the time of diagnosis. As rheumatologists we need to be mindful of these factors and optimise bone health by addressing modifiable factors and timely implement primary prevention.

Keywords

Osteoporosis · Rheumatic disorders

24.1 Background

The World Health Organisation defines osteoporosis (OP) as a 'progressive systemic skeletal disease characterised by low bone mass and micro architectural deterioration of bone tissue' thereby resulting in an increased risk of fracture due to bone fragility, in response to minimal or low velocity force [1].

C. Godsave · R. Garner · I. Pande (✉)
Rheumatology Department, Queen's Medical Centre, Nottingham University Hospital's NHS Trust, Nottingham, UK
e-mail: ira.pande@nuh.nhs.uk

© Springer Nature Singapore Pte Ltd. 2020
S. K. Sharma (ed.), *Women's Health in Autoimmune Diseases*,
https://doi.org/10.1007/978-981-15-0114-2_24

> *World Health Organisation (WHO) working definition of osteoporosis*:
>
> Bone mineral density (BMD) that falls 2.5 standard deviations (SD) below the mean for a healthy individual (i.e. a T score <-2.5).

> *Fragility fractures*:
>
> - They occur after a fall from standing height or less, or without preceding trauma.
> - The most common sites involved are vertebral, hip and distal radius, but can occur at any site within the skeletal system.

Osteoporosis was originally considered to be an age-related disorder, but it is clear that this is a heterogeneous condition, involving interplay between endocrine, metabolic and mechanical factors. Bone is a target in many autoimmune rheumatic disorders (ARDs). Increased survival and better outcomes due to improved care in patients with ARDs have brought to light the need for both primary and secondary prevention of osteoporosis in this patient group.

The consequences of an osteoporotic fracture can be life changing more so in patients with an existing rheumatic disease. Patients can experience further deterioration in functional independence and quality of life, together with increased morbidity and mortality [2]. Therefore, a thorough understanding of the pathogenesis, diagnostic strategies, therapeutic options and ultimately prevention of complications will result in improved patient care. Although OP has a high prevalence amongst patients with ARDs, most do not receive timely and adequate attention towards their bone health. This chapter provides an overview of osteoporosis with special reference to patients with ARDs.

24.2 Epidemiology

Wright et al. evaluated the prevalence of osteoporosis in adults in the USA using National Bone Health Alliance (NBHA) diagnostic criteria. Their 2017 study showed that 16% of men and 29.9% of women aged 50 years and over have osteoporosis [3].

Osteoporosis can be classified into primary or secondary. Primary or idiopathic osteoporosis has been historically classified as postmenopausal. This accounts for 80% of women and 60% of men with osteoporosis. It results from a combination of factors including nutrition, peak bone mass, genetics, level of physical activity, age of menopause and oestrogen or testosterone levels. In 20% of women and 40% of men, there is a secondary cause [4].

24.3 Pathophysiology

Bone consists of a mixture of mineral crystals (60%), organic matrix (30%) and cells (10%). It is constantly in a balance between osteoclastic and osteoblastic activity, a process known as bone remodelling, resulting in a negligible change in bone mass. Peak bone mass is reached usually at the end of the third decade. At this point, the balance between bone formation and resorption shifts towards that which results in net bone loss.

Osteoclasts remove old and damaged bone, and osteoblasts replace this with new bone. The osteoblasts secrete matrix, primarily containing collagen and induce calcification. Function and differentiation of these cells is regulated by several transcription factors, growth factors, cytokines and matrix proteins.

Osteocytes are the main cells that regulate mineral metabolism during bone remodelling. They are former osteoblasts that become trapped during the process of bone deposition. They are derived from mononuclear cells of the monocyte/macrophage lineage following stimulation by the macrophage colony-stimulating factor (M-CSF) and the receptor activator or nuclear factor-kappa B (RANK) ligand (RANKL) [5, 6].

Bone remodelling begins with stimulation of quiescent osteoblasts and marks the start of the activation-resorption-formation (ARF) sequence [7]. Osteoclast differentiation factors are released, triggering preosteoclast fusion and differentiation to multinucleated osteoclasts. These osteoclasts then adhere to the bone surface and dissolve bone as part of the resorptive phase. These osteoclasts undergo apoptosis to prevent excessive bone resorption. Bone formation is triggered by various growth factors stored in bone matrix. Osteoblasts initially produce osteoid (non-mineralised) bone matrix and then promote its mineralisation. Regulatory activities of osteoclasts and osteoblasts are constantly controlled through direct cell-to-cell contact, via extracellular matrix interactions and via the immune system.

Recent literature has confirmed an association between inflammation and bone loss. Inflammation has an uncoupling effect on bone resorption and formation. Inflammatory cytokines are closely associated with osteoclast physiology. Several pro-inflammatory cytokines, TNF-alpha, IL-1 and IL-6, increase the activity and maturation of osteoclasts by upregulation of RANKL expression which results in proliferation of precursor osteoclastic cells and activation of differentiated osteoclasts. The key osteoclastogenic cytokine, RANKL, plays an important role in the balance of osteoclasts and osteoblasts. The RANK/RANKL is the central pathway involved in bone loss. RANKL expression has been found on some regulatory T cells and on B lineage cells [7].

Rapid bone loss and increased fracture risk have been implicated in autoimmune rheumatic diseases, for example rheumatoid arthritis, systemic lupus erythematosus and ankylosing spondylitis. In the RA population, it has been observed that in comparison to the general population, they have a twofold increased risk of developing osteoporosis; two- to sixfold increase of sustaining a vertebral fracture and two- to threefold increase of hip fracture. Individuals with SLE have an estimated prevalence of osteoporosis 20% greater than their healthy comparators. Early onset osteoporosis amongst patients with autoimmune conditions can be attributed to a range of factors including inflammatory cytokines, use of medications, in particular glucocorticoids, and sequelae from the autoimmune condition itself which may give rise to immobility and a more sedentary lifestyle. As evidenced by research, various molecules have been implicated in bone integrity. Certain cytokines are elevated in condition such as RA. These same cytokines such as IL-6 and TNFA are also involved in bone regulation. During chronic inflammation, the balance between bone formation and bone resorption has been postulated to be skewed towards osteoclast-mediated bone resorption and therefore increasing the risk of fracture.

24.4 Risk Factors

In order to optimise bone health in any patient, particularly those with new or known ARDs, we need to identify individuals at high risk early and implement measures timely. Validated risk factors for fracture prediction that is independent of BMD are well known [8]. Risk factors and associated conditions with osteoporosis are shown in Tables 24.1 and 24.2. The tables are by no means complete, as they list common causes encountered during routine patient care. It is imperative that an accurate history and assessment is carried out in every patient with ARDs particularly if there is an indication for use of glucocorticoids.

24.5 Osteoporosis and Autoimmune Rheumatic Disease(s)

Autoimmune rheumatic diseases affect bone, periarticular soft tissue structures and muscle. Bone loss in rheumatic disorders is multifactorial: inflammation, traditional clinical risk factors and drug-related factors. Glucocorticoid-induced osteoporosis is the leading cause as many patients will need steroids for managing their disease. These effective treatments are used widely but act as a double-edged sword being implicated with multiple side effects including osteoporosis. It is therefore our responsibility to minimise risks using lowest effective dose. Many patients with

Table 24.1 Risk factors for osteoporosis

Modifiable	Non-modifiable
Smoking	Ethnicity
Alcohol	Gender
Dietary calcium	Age
Sedentary lifestyle	Family history—maternal history of hip fracture
Low BMI/eating disorder	Medical co-morbid conditions
Premature menopause	Late menarche
Medications (see below)	Previous fragility fracture(s)
Chronic malnutrition	

Table 24.2 Associations with osteoporosis

Medical conditions	Drugs
Autoimmune rheumatic diseases	Glucocorticoids
Hypogonadism	GnRH analogues
Coeliac disease	SERMs
Inflammatory bowel disease	Antiandrogen therapy
Hyperparathyroidism	Long-term heparin
Type 1 diabetes	Proton pump inhibitors
Hyperthyroidism	Hypoglycaemic agents
Acromegaly	Chemotherapeutic agents
Hyperprolactinaemia	Thyroxine
Hyper-adrenalism	Antipsychotics
Osteogenesis imperfecta	Selective serotonin reuptake inhibitors
Chronic liver disease	Lithium
Chronic kidney disease	
Malignancy	

ARDs are women of childbearing age and young men, who may not have reached their peak bone mass at the time of diagnosis. We need to be mindful that treatments such as glucocorticoids and the disease itself may limit the maximum bone mass potential [9, 10]. As glucocorticoid use is the leading cause of poor bone health in patients with ARDs, a separate section on glucocorticoid-induced osteoporosis follows.

Osteoporosis in RA is of two types—localised to affected/inflamed joints(s) and generalised (systemic). Localised OP reflects disease activity. Generalised OP is multifactorial: inflammatory cytokines (TNF-alpha, IL1, IL6) affecting osteoclast physiology through RANKL-mediated and Wnt-signalling pathways; drugs used to manage RA (glucocorticoids) and traditional clinical risk factors (reduced mobility, female sex, low BMI, vitamin D deficiency). Effective use of disease modifying drugs antirheumatic drugs (DMARDs) and biologic agents can lead to significant decrease in bone resorption, improve bone formation by controlling active inflammation and inflammatory cytokine production. Poor control of disease or delays in initiating treatment leads to bone erosion, deformity, reduced mobility that impacts outdoor exposure to sunlight and vitamin D synthesis. Furthermore, inability to participate in weight-bearing and muscle-strengthening exercises increases risk of falls and fractures.

SLE predominantly affects women of childbearing age. OP in SLE is multifactorial. Risk factors include traditional clinical risk factors (age, low BMI, irregularities in menstrual cycle due to altered female sex hormone status), metabolic factors (vitamin D deficiency, hyperhomocysteinaemia and altered thyroid hormone), use of drugs (steroids, cyclosporine, tacrolimus) and effects of inflammatory cytokines (TNF-alpha, IL-1, IL-6) on RANKL expression that affects the activity and maturation of osteoclasts. Patients with SLE are advised to use adequate UV sun protection with a high sun protection factor. Whilst this may reduce disease flares, it will limit the amount of sun exposure and vitamin D synthesis. If such patients also have Raynaud's, they are more likely to wrap up warm further reducing sun exposure

[11]. Glucocorticoids are widely used in SLE. Whilst they can be life-saving, dose-dependent bone loss, especially at sites rich in trabecular bone, for example vertebrae, is well known. Use of calcineurin inhibitors (cyclosporine and tacrolimus) that impair vitamin D activation pathway and renal calcium transport can lead to further impairment of the normal physiological effects of vitamin D with detrimental effects on calcium homeostasis, bone mineralisation and remodelling as well as neuromuscular function. Other drugs used in SLE that play a role in bone loss are anticonvulsants, oral anticoagulants and heparin.

Osteoporosis in spondyloarthropathies, of which ankylosing spondylosis is a prototype, is the most prevalent comorbidity with prevalence of spinal osteoporosis reported to range between 19 and 50%. Like other ARDs, OP is multifactorial with inflammatory cytokines playing a key role. There is a strong correlation between bone turnover, pro-inflammatory cytokines and acute phase reactants. Reduced mobility, vitamin D deficiency, low sex hormone levels in addition to traditional clinical risk factors contribute to OP in AS. Glucocorticoids are used sparingly hence do not play a major role. The use of long-term glucocorticoids is less in AS compared to other ARDs; TNF inhibitors have been shown to have a protective effect on bone loss [12].

Data on BMD and rates of fracture in other ARDs is scanty. Patients who have calcinosis as part of systemic sclerosis have higher rates of osteoporosis, despite lower rates of glucocorticoid use than those patients without calcinosis. The pathogenesis of osteoporosis in this group remains unclear, but impaired bone metabolism has been recognised [13].

In summary, OP in ARDs is multifactorial. These include traditional clinical risk factors (age, BMI, gender, mobility, Vitamin D deficiency, menopausal status), drugs used in treating the condition with glucocorticoids being the major contributor, and inflammatory cytokines related to disease activity. Most studies support the role of RANK-mediated and Wnt-signalling pathways in bone loss. Tight control of the underlying inflammatory rheumatic disorder is the first step towards primary prevention in addition to addressing modifiable lifestyle factors and early bone protection when using glucocorticoids.

24.5.1 Assessment

Aim is to identify individual at high risk for OP to guide investigations and draw appropriate management plan for both primary and secondary prevention. This section covers the generic workup of any individual where bone health is an issue and is equally applicable to patients with ARDs. The initial assessment involves a thorough history of past and present medical conditions, lifestyle factors, drug history and family history (refer to Tables 24.1–24.3). Examination (Table 24.4), laboratory tests (Table 24.5) and radiological investigations help identify modifiable factors and exclude OP mimics. This can range from a benign correctable disorder, for example vitamin D deficiency, to a more significant condition like myeloma [14].

Table 24.3 History taking in patients with osteoporosis

Current history	Nature of fall leading to fracture
	History of recurrent falls (>3/year)
	Back pain—acute/acute on chronic
	Loss in height (subclinical vertebral fracture)
	Level of mobility
	Systemic symptoms to exclude malignancy
	Planned dental procedures—implants
Past medical history	Previous low trauma fractures
	Medical conditions increasing risk—see Table 24.2
	Women: Menstrual history (age of menarche/menopause, prolonged periods of amenorrhea, use of Depoprovera)
	Previous surgery: oophorectomy
	History of any malignancy and radiotherapy to skeleton
	Reflux, GI ulcer and/or bleed, DVT/PE (impacts choice of bone agent)
Family history	Osteoporosis
	Maternal hip fracture
Drug history	See Table 24.2
	Previous bone agents and total duration of therapy (assist duration of treatment and drug holiday)
	Men: antiandrogen therapy
	Women: HRT, GNRH analogues, aromatase inhibitors, tamoxifen
Social history	Smoking history
	Alcohol intake
	Diet (calcium/vitamin D)

Table 24.4 Examination specific for bone health assessment

Height (monitor any loss in height over time)
BMI
System review particularly breast examination (in women)
Spinal examination—Dowager's hump
Timed Get up and go test

24.5.2 Laboratory Investigations

If the clinical situation permits and it is feasible, ideally one should aim to obtain serum samples at baseline to exclude any underlying treatable condition that may be associated with osteoporosis (for example Vitamin D deficiency), exclude a disorder mimicking osteoporosis (myeloma) and to assist monitoring therapy with bone agents (bone markers). Table 24.5 lists investigations recommended in all patients and specifies additional that may be considered during special situations.

Table 24.5 Laboratory investigations in a patient suspected may have osteoporosis

Blood tests	Urine tests
In all patients: Full blood count Urea and electrolytes Liver function tests Bone profile—Ca, Vit D, Alk Phos Thyroid Bone turnover markers—CTx, PINP (for teriparatide) Erythrocyte sedimentation rate—suspect myeloma, malignancy	*Special situations*: Bence Jones protein Urinary calcium excretion Urinary bone turnover markers
In the very elderly: Parathyroid hormone	
In men: Male sex hormones—testosterone, SHBG, LH	
In patients with vertebral fracture(s): Serum electrophoresis PSA (in men)	
Special situations: Tissue transglutaminase antibodies Serum tryptase Serum prolactin Genetic testing for osteogenesis imperfecta	

24.5.3 Imaging

The gold standard for assessing bone health is dual energy X-ray absorptiometry (DEXA). BMD is measured at two sites in the hip (total hip and femoral neck) and at the lumbar spine (L1–4). Results need to be interpreted with caution, especially in patients with rheumatic disorders such as osteoarthritis (hip OA, degenerative disc disease) and/or metal work (joint replacement surgery, discectomy) it will affect the results. In patients suspected to have primary hyperparathyroidism, the radius is the preferred site for DEXA. In patients with wrist arthritis and/or reduced upper limb function measurements at this site will need to be interpreted with caution. In the elderly (over 65 years of age), vertebral fracture assessment (VFA) is recommended in all patients due to high risk of subclinical vertebral fractures. This is particularly true for patients with rheumatic disorders on steroids. Knowledge of presence and number of vertebral fractures is vital as it affects choice of bone agent and duration of therapy.

Measurements are given as a total BMD level (g/cm^2), Z score (age-matched standard deviation from the mean) and T score (standard deviation from young adult at peak bone mass). VFA results list site and morphometry of vertebral fracture(s). Diagnosis is based on definitions detailed in Table 24.6. DEXA scans are ideally performed at baseline and then at intervals on treatment, no more frequently than 18 months. Most centres now monitor using bone markers (CTx, PINP) and repeat BMD measurements at 5 years. In young patients with ARDs, use of DEXA and its measurements needs to be interpreted with caution as individuals may not have

Table 24.6 National Osteoporosis Foundation—guidance on T score values

Definition	T scores
Normal bone density	Above -1.0
Osteopenia	Between -1.0 and -2.5
Osteoporosis	Less than -2.5

reached peak bone mass making Z scores a better guide for assessing bone health in these patients.

Plain radiographs may be relevant if clinically indicated in the event of a fracture. Radiographic osteopenia should neither form the basis of the diagnosis nor warrant investigations unless accompanied by traditional clinical risk factors for poor bone health. The latter may prompt further investigation. Lateral spine radiographs may be considered when suspicion of vertebral fracture is high and not definite on VFA. Spinal MRI scan may be required in special situations to distinguish osteoporotic fractures from pathological ones. Plain radiographs are occasionally requested in special situations, for example very high BMD or patients with spondyloarthropathies.

24.6 Glucocorticoid-Induced Osteoporosis

It is estimated that approximately 1–2% of the general population at any given time are receiving long-term glucocorticoid treatment. Amongst patients with ARDs this rate is higher. The effect of glucocorticoids on bone is well known. The biggest contributor to the causes of secondary osteoporosis is now glucocorticoid related. The vast majority of patients with autoimmune conditions will require glucocorticoids at some stage in their disease journey. At the start of treatment, often the steroid dose is at its highest and is then tapered with the aim to discontinue. Within the first 3–6 months of initiation of glucocorticoid therapy, there is rapid bone loss and an increased fracture risk. Vertebral fractures are characteristic, although the overall fracture risk is also increased [15–17].

A review by Balasubramanian et al. showed that the risk of vertebral fractures in this group was highest at the start of treatment and decreased over time. It therefore follows that timely intervention with bone protection (lifestyle and drugs) is key to maintaining long-term bone health in patients with ARDs needing steroids. It is unclear whether the fracture risk returns to the baseline risk after discontinuation of steroid therapy, but Balasubramanian showed that the fracture risk after 12 months of discontinuation of therapy was similar to those who were non-glucocorticoid users [18].

Rapid bone loss can be attributed to a combination of increased bone turnover and negative bone remodelling. There is upregulation of the peroxisome proliferator-activated receptor gamma 2 (PPARG2) and effects on the Wnt/B-catenin signalling pathway, resulting in a favoured differentiation of pluripotent cells to adipocytes rather than osteoblasts. There is increased expression of sclerostin. In mice with sclerostin deficiency, it has been shown that the effects of glucocorticoids on the bone can be mediated [17].

Proposed mechanisms for indirect effects on bone include hypogonadism, reduced physical activity, increased renal and intestinal losses of calcium, and reduced production of growth hormone and insulin-like growth factor. The underlying autoimmune condition itself is associated with pro-inflammatory and pro-resorptive cytokines. It has been well established that long-term glucocorticoid use has been linked to reduced muscle mass and myopathy which further leads to increased falls and fracture.

My approach to patients with ARDs likely to need glucocorticoids (any dose) for duration greater than 3 months is to assess their bone health, and if at high risk of osteoporosis or fractures co-prescribe bone protection. Lifestyle advice, adequate calcium either by diet or by supplements and adequate vitamin D need to be implemented in all individuals prescribed steroids. For those patients with ARDs at high risk of fracture, bone agents are prescribed taking into consideration factors like age, gender, renal function and comorbidities. A more in-depth discussion on therapeutic options is discussed later.

24.7 Fracture Risk Assessment Tools

The National Institute of Clinical and Healthcare Excellence (NICE) [19] recommend the use of assessment tools (FRAX or QFracture) to estimate absolute risk of fracture in individuals at high risk of poor bone health. In the UK since 2008, FRAX score [20] in combination with NOGG (National Osteoporosis Guidance Group) guides clinicians on the threshold for treatment. Like any assessment tool, there are caveats. In the very elderly, FRAX may underestimate the short-term fracture risk [21]. Similarly, FRAX does not take into account multiplicity of fragility fractures, dose and duration of oral glucocorticoids, excess alcohol and falls risk thereby underestimating the absolute risk of fracture [22]. FRAX is not validated for use for those under 40 years of age. These caveats need to be borne in mind in patients with ARDs as they are often young and require high doses of steroids. Compston has postulated that an adjustment be made for those on long-term glucocorticoid therapy, for example if a patient is taking more than 7.5 mg/day of prednisolone, the average adjustment for a major osteoporotic fracture probability is increased by 15% [17].

Fracture risk is an ongoing and potentially changing factor of a person's health that needs to be reviewed. NICE suggests recalculating the fracture risk if either the risk factors have changed or a person has undergone 2 years of treatment [19].

24.8 Management

The mainstay of treatment is early identification of patients at risk of poor bone health and timely intervention using combination of lifestyle advice and pharmacological treatment. This aims to prevent any further bone loss and reduce risk of fractures and associated healthcare and social costs.

24.8.1 Lifestyle Measures

The importance of patient education in the management of osteoporosis is paramount to ensure compliance and adherence to change in lifestyle factors and bone agents. Individuals should be advised to drink in moderation and to quit smoking. Weight-bearing and muscle-strengthening exercise should be encouraged, the simplest being brisk walking. Where required, a falls risk assessment should be performed. Of note, although regular weight-bearing exercise is advised, it has not shown to reduce fracture risk, but does have positive effects on BMD [23].

24.8.2 Vitamin D and Calcium

The ideal calcium intake is between 1000 and 1500 mg/day. Where possible this should be by diet, otherwise supplements. Calcium intake alone has not been shown to reduce fracture risk, but when combined with Vitamin D, there is a small reduction in hip and non-vertebral fractures, possibly extending to vertebral fractures.

Exposure to sunlight half an hour three times a week in summer months should be adequate in most patients to achieve adequate vitamin D levels. However, in populations where vitamin D by natural sunlight is difficult to achieve (frail elderly in nursing homes, patients with limited mobility or wheelchair bound, patients with lupus where sun exposure is not recommended, patients with medical disorders such as chronic kidney disease affecting vitamin D metabolism), Vitamin D supplementation is advised aiming for serum Vitamin D levels above 50 nmol/L. Vitamin D and calcium should be co-prescribed to patients with ARDs starting glucocorticoid therapy.

24.8.3 Bisphosphonates

Bisphosphonates are antiresorptive and the mainstay of pharmacological treatment as they are efficacious in reducing vertebral and hip fracture. Alendronic acid (70 mg) and risedronic acid (35 mg) are weekly oral tablets. For patients that are unable to tolerate oral bisphosphonates or in whom oral are contraindicated (patients with previous gastrointestinal bleed, oesophageal stricture, achalasia or ulcers), intravenous Zoledronic acid infusion is an alternative. Zoledronic acid, a 5 mg intravenous infusion, is administered once yearly or every 18 months. A single infusion of the drug is useful to consider in patients with ARDs where exposure to glucocorticoid is likely for a defined duration, for example polymyalgia rheumatic. It is also a useful choice in the very elderly, patients on polypharmacy and where compliance or adherence to treatment is likely to be an issue.

Bisphosphonates are contraindicated in patients of childbearing potential, those with hypocalcaemia and severe renal impairment (defined as GFR ≤35 mL/min for alendronate, ≤30 mL/min for all other bisphosphonates). Reports of osteonecrosis of the jaw (ONJ) and atypical femoral fractures have led to increased awareness of these rare complications and need for monitoring. Glucocorticoid use increases risk of ONJ in patients with ARDs on bisphosphonates. It is therefore recommended that patients

Table 24.7 Indications for use of teriparatide (NICE, UK)

Age	T score	Number of fractures whilst on treatment
55–64 years	−4 or below	2+
>65 years	−4 or below	Any
>65 years	−3.5 or below	2+

undergo any planned major dental procedure or dental implants prior to commencing treating, and maintain good oral hygiene whilst on treatment. Patients should be encouraged to be vigilant to monitor for symptoms of dental mobility and for symptoms suggestive of an atypical femoral fracture such as thigh, hip or groin pain [24, 25].

Based on expert opinion, bone health in patients on treatment is reviewed after 5 years of oral bisphosphonate therapy, or three infusions of intravenous bisphosphonate or earlier if patient sustains a fragility fracture. Total duration of therapy with bone agent is usually 5 years. In patients with vertebral fracture(s) or ongoing risk factors for osteoporosis (for example ongoing use of glucocorticoids), treatment can be extended for 7–10 years before considering drug holiday.

24.8.4 Parathyroid Hormone (Teriparatide)

Teriparatide is a recombinant human parathyroid hormone [PTH] 1–34 and is available as a self-administered daily subcutaneous injection at a dose of 20 ng/day. It is the only bone-forming agent and hence ideal for subpopulation of patients with ARDs who have severe osteoporosis, multiple vertebral and peripheral fractures and requiring steroids. However, because of its high cost, its use is limited to patients at very high risk of fracture and hence in the UK not permitted for use as first-line therapy for osteoporosis—see Table 24.7. Treatment is limited to 24 months and co-prescribed with vitamin D (800–100 IU/day) and calcium (if not adequate by diet). It is contraindicated in patients with hypercalcemia, pregnancy and lactation, severe renal impairment, metabolic bone disease other than osteoporosis, prior radiation or malignancies affecting the skeleton. Monitoring of compliance and efficacy is best done by measuring bone markers (PINP) at 3 months, 6 months, 1 year and on completion of treatment. Side effects include headaches, nausea, transient hypercalcemia, dizziness and postural hypotension [26].

24.8.5 Denosumab

Denosumab is a fully humanised monoclonal antibody against RANKL and is administered as subcutaneous injection 6 monthly. It is licensed both for primary and secondary prevention of fragility fractures. Common side effects are injection site cellulitis and hypocalcaemia. It is a useful bone agent in patients where bisphosphonates are contraindicated due to poor renal function or the frail elderly with low BMI affecting Cockgroft Gault GFR. Due to high risk of hypocalcaemia with this drug in this group of patients, it is imperative that serum calcium is checked prior to initiation of treatment, and 7–14 days after Denosumab is given. ONJ has been reported similar to other bone agents. Unlike bisphosphonates, BMD increases year on year for total duration of denosumab therapy making it the bone agent of choice in a subgroup of patients with ARDs who have very low T scores. In contrast to bisphosphonates, on cessation of denosumab therapy, rapid bone loss and increased risk of vertebral fracture have been reported. One of the measures employed to overcome this is sealing the gain in BMD with a single infusion of Zoledronic acid.

24.8.6 Raloxifene

Raloxifene is a selective oestrogen receptor modulator which inhibits bone resorption and reduces risk of vertebral but not hip fractures. It is a 60 mg daily tablet, but because of the plethora of bone agents that offer fracture risk reductions at all sites, use of raloxifene is limited to a subgroup of women with high risk of vertebral fractures and who may also have a family history of breast cancer. It should be used with caution in those patients with a history of strokes or risk factors for stroke.

24.9 Conclusion

Osteoporosis in autoimmune rheumatic diseases is common and multifactorial with inflammatory cytokines and glucocorticoid use being the major contributory factors. Osteoimmunology has provided some insights into the pathogenic mechanism of osteoporosis in ARDs with RANKL-mediated and Wnt-signalling pathways affecting osteoclast differentiation, function and apoptosis leading to uncoupling of bone with excess bone resorption. Clinicians involved in the care of patients with ARDs should be proactive in early identification of patients at high risk of osteoporosis. In addition to tight control of the underlying rheumatic disorder, early intervention to address bone health in this high-risk group is paramount. It is regrettable that although osteoporosis has a high prevalence in patients with rheumatic disorders and rheumatologists are the biggest users of steroids, most patients still do not receive timely assessment of their bone health. All patients should be encouraged to lead an active healthy lifestyle, ensure adequate dietary calcium (if not supplements), aim vitamin D levels >50 nmol/L and in the subgroup at high risk initiate bone agents (bisphosphonates, denosumab). With increased survival and better outcome of patients with rheumatic diseases if untreated osteoporosis and its sequelae will constitute the major cause of morbidity and mortality in this population.

References

1. Consensus A (1993) Consensus development conference: diagnosis, prophylaxis and treatment of osteoporosis. Am J Med 94:646–650
2. Cosman F, de Beur SJ, LeBoff MS, Lewiecki EM, Tanner B, Randall S, Lindsay R, National Osteoporosis Foundation (2014) Clinician's guide to prevention and treatment of osteoporosis. Osteoporos Int 25(10):2359–2381

3. Wright NC, Saag KG, Dawson-Hughes B, Khosla S, Siris ES (2017) The impact of the new National Bone Health Alliance (NBHA) diagnostic criteria on the prevalence of osteoporosis in the USA. Osteoporos Int 28(4):1225–1232
4. Löfman O, Larsson L, Toss G (2000) Bone mineral density in diagnosis of osteoporosis: reference population, definition of peak bone mass, and measured site determine prevalence. J Clin Densitom 3(2):177–186
5. Jung Y-K, Kang Y-M, Han S (2019) Osteoclasts in the inflammatory arthritis: implications for pathologic osteolysis. Immune Netw 19(1):e2
6. Amarasekera DS, Yu J, Rho J (2015) Bone loss triggered by the cytokine network in inflammatory autoimmune diseases. J Immunol Res 2015:832127
7. Coury F, Peyruchard O, Machuca-Gayet I (2019) Osteoimmunology of bone loss in inflammatory rheumatic disease. Front Immunol 10:679
8. Liu J, Curtis EM, Cooper C, Harvey NC (2019) State of the art in osteoporosis risk assessment and treatment. J Endocrinol Investig 42:1149–1164
9. Iseme RA, Mcevoy M, Kelly B, Agnew L, Walker FR (2017) Is osteoporosis an immune mediated disorder? Bone Rep 7:121–131
10. Briot K, Geusens P, Em Bultink I, Lems WF, Roux C (2017) Inflammatory diseases and bone fragility. Osteoporos Int 28:3301–3314
11. LUPUS UK (2015) Diet and exercise. Available from: https://www.lupusuk.org.uk/diet-and-exercise/. Accessed 3 May 2019
12. Molto A, Nikiphorou E (2018) Comorbidities in spondyloarthritis. Front Med 5:62
13. Valenzuela A, Baron M, Canadian Scleroderma Research Group, Herrick AL, Proudman S, Stevens W, Australian Scleroderma Interest Group, Rodriguez-Reyna TS, Vacca A, Medsger TA Jr, Hinchcliff M, Hsu V, Wu JY, Fiorentino D, Chung L (2016) Calcinosis is associated with digital ulcers and osteoporosis in patients with systemic sclerosis: a Scleroderma Clinical Trials Consortium Study. Semin Arthritis Rheum 46(3):344–349
14. Sheu A, Diamond T (2016) Secondary osteoporosis. Aust Prescr 39(3):85–87
15. Lane NE (2019) Glucocorticoid-induced osteoporosis: new insights into the pathophysiology and treatments. Curr Osteoporos Rep 17(1):1–7
16. Hsu E, Nanes M (2017) Advances in treatment of glucocorticoid-induced osteoporosis. Curr Opin Endocrinol Diab Obes 24(6):411–417
17. Compston J (2018) Glucocorticoid-induced osteoporosis: and update. Endocrine 61:7–16
18. Balasubramanian A, Wade SW, Adler RA, Saag K, Pannacciulli N, Curtis JR (2018) Glucocorticoid exposure and fracture risk in a cohort of US patients with selected conditions. J Bone Miner Res 33(10):1881–1888
19. National Institute for Health and Care Excellence (NICE) (2012) Osteoporosis: assessing the risk of a fragility fracture: clinical guideline [CG146]. Available from: https://www.nice.org.uk/guidance/cg146. Accessed 15 May 2019
20. Centre for Metabolic Bone Diseases, University of Sheffield, UK. FRAX: fracture risk assessment tool. Available from: https://www.sheffield.ac.uk/FRAX/tool.aspx. Accessed 20 May 2019
21. Kanis JA, Harvey NC, Johansson H, Oden A, McCloskey EV, Leslie WD (2017) Overview of fracture prediction tools. J Clin Densitom 20(3):444–450
22. Kanis JA, Glüer CC (2000) An update on the diagnosis and assessment of osteoporosis with densitometry. Committee of Scientific Advisors, International Osteoporosis Foundation. Osteoporos Int 11(3):192–202
23. Crandall CJ, Newberry SJ, Diamant A, Lim YW, Gellad WF, Booth MJ, Motala A, Shekelle PG (2014) Comparative effectiveness of pharmacologic treatments to prevent fractures: an updated systematic review. Ann Intern Med 161(10):711–723
24. Patrick AR, Brookhart MA, Losina E, Schousboe JT, Cadarette SM, Mogun H, Solomon DH (2010) The complex relation between bisphosphonate adherence and fracture reduction. J Clin Endocrinol Metab 95(7):3251–3259
25. Yates J (2013) A meta-analysis characterizing the dose-response relationships for three oral nitrogen-containing bisphosphonates in postmenopausal women. Osteoporos Int 24(1):253–262
26. Lems WF, Raterman H (2017) Critical issues and current challenges in osteoporosis and fracture prevention. An overview of unmet needs. Therap Adv Musculoskel Dis 9:299–316

Menopause in Autoimmune Disease and Hormone Replacement Therapy

25

Ramandeep Bansal and Neelam Aggarwal

Abstract

The relationship between autoimmune diseases and menopause is complex. While deleterious effects of menopause on cardiovascular, genitourinary, skeletal, and central nervous systems due to deficiency of gonadal hormones can contribute to morbidity in autoimmune diseases, autoimmune diseases as well as their treatment per se can accelerate or predate development of menopause. Furthermore, diagnosis of autoimmune disorders may be difficult in the setting of menopause due to overlapping signs and symptoms. In this chapter we discuss the complex relationship between menopause and common autoimmune diseases. We also discuss the effects of menopause on common autoimmune diseases and vice versa and also menopausal hormone therapy.

Keywords

Menopause · Hormone replacement therapy · Autoimmune disease

25.1 Introduction

Menopause is defined as absence of menses for more than 12 months. The median age of occurrence of menopause in Indian women (45.6 years) is lower when compared to Western women [1, 2]. Occurrence of menopause is a significant event in the life of women because of its impact on their clinical, hormonal and psychological well-being. With increase in life expectancy, an average woman is expected to spend one-third to one-fourth her life in menopausal phase. Thus, need of

R. Bansal · N. Aggarwal (✉)
Department of Obstetrics and Gynaecology, Post Graduate Institute of Medical Education and Research, Chandigarh, India

awareness about problems associated with menopause and their management cannot be overemphasized.

Recent years have seen a renewed interest regarding impact of autoimmune diseases on reproductive health of women especially menopause as this is a period of significant endocrinal transition. This may be due to effect on immune system of deranged hormonal milieu and cytokines. Not only have several autoimmune diseases been reported to be associated with premature menopause, the hormonal changes associated with menopause by themselves may further aggravate dysfunction of organs which have already been affected by autoimmune disease. While relationship between premature menopause and autoimmune disorders is well defined for some autoimmune disorders such as systemic lupus erythematosus (SLE), it remains speculative for some others [3]. In this chapter we briefly review association between various autoimmune disease and menopause.

25.2 Clinical, Hormonal and Immunological Changes Associated with Menopause

Menopause is associated with significant changes in hormonal, clinical and immunological status.

25.2.1 Hormonal Changes

The onset of menopause is characterized by severe reduction in serum levels of estradiol with age owing to depletion of oocytes though apoptosis and resultant decrease in production of estrogens by granulosa cells. However small amounts of estrogen continue to be produced by ovarian stroma. The estrone is decreased to a lesser extent. The decrease in serum levels of estrone is less marked as it is derived from peripheral aromatization of androgens whose levels decline more slowly. Correspondingly there is increase in serum levels of follicular-stimulating hormone (FSH) (>40 IU/mL) and to a lesser extent of luteinizing hormone (LH) (<20 IU/L) due to removal of negative feedback inhibition of estrogens. In addition, there may be slight decrease in serum levels of prolactin [3].

25.2.2 Clinical Changes

The reduction in serum levels of estrogens results in significant effects of skeletal, cardiovascular, genitourinary and central nervous systems. These changes include the following.

25.2.2.1 Skeletal Changes
Menopause is associated with decrease in bone mineral density (BMD). While during the premenopausal years BMD decreases on an average by 0.13% per year,

it decreases by a rate of 2.5% per year during the perimenopausal years and by 1% per year during the postmenopausal years [4]. This rapid loss of BMD predisposes postmenopausal women to increased risk of fractures. As autoimmune diseases themselves pose a high risk of fractures owing to chronic inflammation and use of cytotoxic drugs as well as steroids, the risk of fractures is further increased in postmenopausal women with autoimmune diseases. In addition approximately 48% of menopausal women complaints of rheumatic pains and approximately 34% complain of pain and aches in neck and back [5]. All these symptoms are well known in autoimmune diseases and can lead to diagnostic confusion.

25.2.2.2 Genitourinary Changes
Onset of menopause is associated with up to 30% decrease in collagen mass. This decrease in supporting connective tissue can result in vaginal and/or uterine prolapse, urinary incontinence and bladder irritability. Overall 20–40% of women experience some kind of genitourinary problem during menopause. In addition vaginal dryness and atrophy can result in dyspareunia. All these symptoms can be more troublesome in patients with autoimmune disease such as Sjogren's syndrome or SLE [3, 6].

25.2.2.3 Cardiovascular Effects
Estrogens exert several beneficial effects of cardiovascular system. Accordingly risk of cardiovascular disease is lower in premenopausal women compared to men of same age. Both progesterone and estrogens exert a direct effect on blood vessels through their receptors. Decrease in the levels of estrogens during postmenopausal years is associated with increased low-density cholesterol and serum levels, reduced carbohydrate tolerance, decreased prostacyclins synthesis, increased endothelin levels, decreased nitric oxide synthetase activity as well as decrease in the amount of blood flow in all the major vascular beds. All these result in increased cardiovascular risk in postmenopausal and by 70 years of age risk of cardiovascular events in women reaches the same as in men. Needless to say, cardiovascular risk is further increased in postmenopausal women from autoimmune diseases owing to chronic inflammation, treatment-related side effects as well as direct involvement of cardiovascular in autoimmune disease process [7, 8].

25.2.2.4 Central Nervous System (CNS) Effects
The effects of estrogens on CNS are complex. A positive correlation has been well documented with estrogens and cognition as well as mood. Accordingly decrease in estrogens levels during menopause is often associated with changes in mood [3]. In one study from India, the common neurological symptoms associated with menopause included irritability (36.4%), sleep disturbance (36.4%), forgetfulness (34.1%), depression (29.8%), anxiety (28.9%), poor concentration (13.7%), loss of interest in most things (13.1%), and crying spells (10.7%) [8]. The abnormal hypothalamic thermoregulatory response due to decrease in the levels of estrogens results in hot flushes seen in approximately 53% of menopausal women. Furthermore, approximately 53% of menopausal also complain of cold sweats [5]. All these

symptoms increase the likelihood of mistaking autoimmune disease process for menopause and vice versa. Similarly it may be difficult to differentiate cognitive deficits due to normal menopause from those induced by autoimmune diseases.

25.2.3 Immunological Changes

Estrogen decline associated with menopause leads to several changes in immune system. Notably serum concentrations of pro-inflammatory cytokines such as interleukin 1 and 6 and tumor necrotic factor alpha are increased, while there is concomitant decrease in serum concentrations of anti-inflammatory cytokines. These changes in cytokines are similar to those reported in many autoimmune disorders such as multiple sclerosis [9] and are mediated through estrogen receptors (ERα and ERβ) present on immunocompetent cells such as T and B lymphocytes, macrophages and dendritic cells [10]. In addition there is decrease in concentrations of CD4+ helper T cells, decrease in activity of natural killer cells, while the inflammatory response to pro-inflammatory cytokines is enhanced. All these changes in immune system lead to complex effects on overall inflammatory response. The reduction in T helper cell levels is likely to result in mitigation of disease activity in lupus, but aggravation of disease activity in rheumatoid arthritis. Hormone replacement therapy may mitigate some of these immune changes [9, 10].

25.3 Premature Ovarian Insufficiency (POI) and Autoimmunity

Autoimmunity does play a role in causation of POI in some patients. POI is defined as amenorrhea of at least 4 months duration in women less than 40 years of age in the presence of low serum estrogen levels and high serum gonadotropin levels, i.e., serum FSH levels of >40 mIU/mL on at least two separate occasions. Thus POI is characterized by amenorrhea, anovulation and infertility along with deficiency of female sex hormones [11]. Affecting approximately 0.3% of women in general population, this syndrome can result from a variety of etiologies such as chromosomal aberrations, genetic abnormalities, metabolic problems, environmental issues, toxin exposure, and infections and drugs. However cause remains to be determined in a substantial number of cases and these patients are classified as idiopathic. According to an estimate based on the presence of antiovarian antibodies, lymphocytic oophoritis, and coexistence of other autoimmune disorders, autoimmunity accounts for approximately 4–30% of idiopathic cases of POI [12, 13].

25.3.1 Antiovarian Antibodies

Since first discovery of antiovarian antibodies by Vallotton and Forbes in 1996 [14], several authors have documented the presence of different autoantibodies in sera of women with POI. Presence of these autoantibodies is associated with increased risk of POI. Several different autoantibodies which have been described in association with POI are outlined below.

Steroid cell antibodies are polyclonal IgG immunoglobulins directed against cells of various endocrine glands (adrenal cortex, testicular Leydig cells, placental syncytiotrophoblasts and ovarian theca cells) which produce steroids. Their main antigenic targets include 17-alpha-hydroxylase, 21-hydroxylase, and cytochrome p450 side-chain cleavage. Steroid cell antibodies are present in 60% of autoimmune polyglandular syndrome type 1, 25–40% of patients with 60% of autoimmune polyglandular syndrome type 2, 60–87% of women with POI in association with Addison disease, and 3–10% of patients with isolated POI [13]. Thus, while steroid cell antibodies are often positive in women who develop POI in addition with Addison's disease, these are often absent in women with isolated POI or with autoimmune diseases other than Addison disease. Accordingly the presence of steroid cell antibodies can serve as a marker for development of POI in women with autoimmune Addison disease [15] and not in women with isolated POI or with other autoimmune disorders.

Studies evaluating the presence of *anti-gonadotropin antibodies* (e.g., antibodies against beta subunit of FSH) and *anti-gonadotropin receptor antibodies* in women with idiopathic POI have yielded conflicting results. Accordingly their exact clinical and diagnostic significance remain to be determined [13].

Antibodies directed against zona pellucida (ZP) of oocyte have been reported in sera of patients with POI [16, 17]. Molecular structure of ZP consists of several glycoproteins which can serve as strong antigens for induction of antibodies. Anti-ZP antibodies produce their effects through impaired interaction between oocyte and granulose cells. However exact significance of these antibodies remains to be determined, and future study is needed to further clarify their role in women with POI [16, 17].

Antibodies directed against cytoplasmic components of oocyte are also reported in women with POI. The various targets which can act as a putative antigen include MATER (maternal antigen that embryo require), aldehyde dehydrogenase 1A1, selenium binding protein 1, and heat shock protein 90. These antibodies however can also be found in sera of healthy women as well as in women with other inflammatory, autoimmune and neoplastic illnesses [3].

Overall prevalence of anti-ovarian antibodies varies widely ranging from 3% to 66% of women with POI. This coupled with high false-positive results (poor specificity) and poor correlation between serum antiovarian antibody titer and severity of disease puts a question mark on their diagnostic as well as prognostic utility. Accordingly Khole [18] suggested that it will be wrong to make diagnosis of autoimmune POI based solely on presence or absence of antiovarian antibodies. Thus, currently there is no valid serum biomarker to confirm or refute the diagnosis of autoimmune POI.

25.3.2 Histological Evidence of Lymphocytic Oophoritis in Women with POI

Approximately 10% of ovarian biopsies taken from women with POI with normal karyotype show evidence of autoimmune involvement of ovaries in the form of cells (macrophages, natural killer cells, B lymphocytes, T lymphocytes, and plasma cells) infiltrating ovarian follicles [19]. Notably there is lymphocytic infiltration of theca cells of developing follicles while primary and primordial follicles remain speared. Autoimmune oophoritis is usually present in women having POI in association with Addison disease and only rarely in POI. Though advanced stages of autoimmune oophoritis are characterized by follicle depletion, there are many developing follicles in early stages and this may partly explain the beneficial effects of immunosuppressive therapy in some of these patients [20].

The demonstration of autoimmune oophoritis remains a matter of controversy. Some authors believe ovarian biopsy as gold standard for demonstration of autoimmune oophoritis [20]. They believe that serum hormonal profiles and ultrasonographic assessment of ovary are insufficient for diagnosis. Moreover, ovarian biopsy can act as response to immunosuppressive therapy by showing presence of developing follicles as marker of response to treatment compared to follicular depletion in advanced stages of autoimmune oophoritis [20]. Others believe that this procedure is costly and invasive and biopsy may not be representative of follicular density in entire ovary. They suggest the use of noninvasive tests (ultrasonography of ovaries and anti-ovarian antibodies) for the diagnosis of lymphocytic oophoritis. As per them, anti-ovarian antibodies especially steroid cell autoantibodies are usually positive in women with lymphocytic oophoritis [3, 21]. Others have also suggested use of anti-adrenal cortical autoantibodies as a marker for the presence of lymphocytic oophoritis in women with POI [22].

25.3.3 Presence of Other Autoimmune Diseases in Women with POI

POI has been reported in association with many organ-specific and systemic autoimmune diseases, notably hypothyroidism (25–60%), diabetes mellitus (2.5%), and Addison disease (2.5–20%). Overall approximately 10–55% of women with POI have associated autoimmune disease [18, 19]. Approximately 10–20% of women with Addison disease develop POI, probably due to common autoantigen evoking antibodies against steroid-producing cells in adrenal cortex and ovary. 60–70% of women with Addison disease in association with POI have anti-steroid cell antibodies [3, 23]. In fact antibodies against 17 alpha hydroxylase and cytochrome P450 side chain can predict occurrence of POI in women with Addison disease, while antibodies against 21 hydroxylase can predict occurrence of Addison disease in women with POI. Based on above observations it is prudent to screen all women with POI for adrenal cortical dysfunction, thyroid dysfunction, and glucose intolerance [3, 23]. Other autoimmune diseases with high incidence of POI include autoimmune polyglandular syndrome type 1 and 2, with presence of anti-steroid cell antibodies (especially 17 alpha hydroxylase and cytochrome P450 side-chain autoantibodies) being marker for development of POI in these disorders [3].

(a) *Standard treatment of infertility may fail in presence of autoimmune POI*: It has been widely recognized that results of treatment for infertility are far less impressive in presence of ovarian autoimmunity [24]. This conclusion stems from the fact in vitro fertilization (IVF) procedures often fail in the presence of antiovarian antibodies [16, 24, 25]. Thus, Khole recommended screening for antiovarian antibodies in women who respond poorly to standard IVF protocols [18]. Other authors [12, 26] have recommended antiovarian antibody profile as routine workup for all infertility patients to predict risk of gonadal failure in future and a chance to retrieve oocyte at early stage of illness. However there is need for well-conducted studies before IVF protocols can be developed on basis of antiovarian or other autoantibody profile.

25.3.4 Immunosuppression in POI

Though there is enough evidence for role of autoimmunity in POI in at least some women, immunosuppressive treatment even in this select group of women often fails to yield good results [19]. The current recommendations for use of immunosuppressive agents in management of POI are based on case series, and these recommendations are not based on well-conducted randomized controlled trials. Nevertheless, response to treatment is poor in most instances.

To conclude thought here is ample evidence that autoimmunity does play a role in POI in at least some women; there is lack of well-controlled studies in this subject. Further elucidation of mechanisms of anti-ovarian antibody-mediated ovarian damage in autoimmune POI may help in better development of diagnostic and treatment protocols. There is a need to develop noninvasive tests for the diagnosis of autoimmune POF and noninvasive biomarkers which can predict response to immunosuppressive and other treatment modalities in women with autoimmune POI [3, 18, 19].

25.3.4.1 Cyclophosphamide-Induced Ovarian Insufficiency

Cyclophosphamide, a commonly used drug in autoimmune diseases, may lead to POI. Use of cyclophosphamide in women with SLE is associated with 11–59% risk of POI. The major determinants of cyclophosphamide-induced POI include age and cumulative dose. Cyclophosphamide damages granulosa cells resulting of follicular death with decreased production of gonadal steroids which in turn lead or increased production of pituitary gonadotropins. Raised gonadotropin levels in turn recruit immature follicles into mature phase which are susceptible to cyclophosphamide eventually resulting in follicular depletion and POI [27, 28]. Other risk factors for cyclophosphamide-induced POI include longer disease duration and presence of anti-Ro and anti-U1RNP. On the other hand, presence of CYP2C19*2 allele of cytochrome p450 system protects against development of cyclophosphamide-induced POI [29].

25.4 Menopause and Autoimmune Diseases

Menopause can affect autoimmune diseases in several ways such as

(a) The effects of menopause per se on cardiovascular, muscular, skeletal, genitourinary, and other systems can add to damage inflicted to these systems by autoimmune diseases, thereby adding to morbidity and mortality.
(b) Alterations in the levels of gonadal hormones may trigger or aggravate autoimmune diseases. Increase in estrogen generally has immunostimulatory effects, while increase in androgens and progestogens usually causes immunosuppression [30]. Thus menopause may affect delicate balance between host defense, immunological tolerance, and autoimmunity [9].

25.4.1 Systemic Lupus Erythematosus (SLE)

Age-related incidence of SLE shows bimodal distribution with first peak between ages of 35 and 39 years and second peak between ages of 55 and 59 years. In general activity of disease in SLE is lower after menopause due to decrease in estrogens which are immunostimulant. However each exacerbation after leads to greater damage. Compared to SLE patients who have disease onset before menopause, the women with disease onset after menopause tend to have more insidious disease course with lower incidence of nephritis, malar rash, photosensitivity, arthritis, Reynaud's phenomenon, cutaneous vasculitis, purpura as well as lower titer of anti-dsDNA and Ro antibodies. On the other hand incidence of serositis and pulmonary involvement is higher in women with onset of SLE after menopause [31, 32].

Even in women with onset of SLE before menopause, disease activity may be decreased after menopause in the form of decreased number of flares and decrease in maximum disease activity. Even women with SLE who have undergone hysterectomy before disease onset tend to have milder disease and less nephritis, lower anti-dsDNA antibodies, and late age of onset. SLE women with cyclophosphamide-induced ovarian failure tend to have fewer and less severe flares compared to women who continue menstruating [29]. However some studies [33] have suggested that decrease in disease activity of SLE in postmenopausal women compared to premenopausal women may be related to age and duration of disease and not to menopause per se.

HRT in SLE: Studies of HRT in SLE suggest a modest increase in mild to moderate flares in stable SLE women, this effect being modulated through increase in toll like receptors 3, 7, and 9 on mononuclear cells [34]. Also premenopausal use of HRT is associated with two fold increase in risk of developing SLE in Nurse's health study [35]. However, this study was conducted when use of HRT was much more prevalent than today.

While disease activity of SLE is decreased in postmenopausal women, the overall disease-related damage is higher in them as reflected by higher damage accrual. Lumina investigators also reported higher damage accrual and more arterial vascular events in postmenopausal women with SLE compared to premenopausal women with SLE. Multivariate analysis revealed age and use of cyclophospha[?] better predictor of damage accrual and not menopause [35–37].

To conclude disease activity is lower and overall damage accrual is [?] postmenopausal women with SLE compared to premenopausal women with SLE. However whether this difference is due to menopause per se or due to higher age or longer duration of disease or effects of treatment remains to be determined. HRT in women with SLE is associated with increased risk of mild to moderate flares but not severe flares. While prescribing HRT to women with SLE, this risk should be carefully weighed against possible benefits of HRT on menopausal symptoms and associated improvement in quality of life. There is lack of well-controlled studies to determine exact risk of HRT in SLE women with anticardiolipin antibodies or previous thrombosis, though many physicians avoid prescribing HRT in these women.

25.4.2 Rheumatoid Arthritis (RA)

Similar to SLE, it is difficult to determine if changes in disease course of RA observed in postmenopausal women is related to menopause per se or due to older age or longer duration of disease or due to drug treatment of RA itself. Whatsoever the reason, older onset RA is characterized by much less female predominance (male:female ratio reaches 1:1 in RA with disease onset above age of 60 years), more common acute onset, more frequent involvement of large proximal joints, lower ESR (erythrocyte sedimentation rate), more frequent systemic manifestations, more frequent negative testing for rheumatoid factor, and poor functional outcome [29].

Reproductive hormones are known to affect disease activity and disease course in RA. High serum levels of estrogens and progestins appear to protect against RA as evidence by frequent remission of RA during pregnancy, lower risk of RA onset pregnancy, decreased risk of RA with breast feeding and increased risk of RA with nulliparity, early menarche, and irregular menses [38–41].

Age at menopause is inversely associated with onset of RA. Thus early menopause is associated with increased risk of new onset RA as are other factors such as use of HRT, polycystic ovarian syndrome, and endometriosis [42, 43]. Regarding influence of postmenopausal state on course of disease, postmenopausal state is associated with a higher joint damage score and higher functional disability compared to premenopausal state, with menopause per se accounting for the difference [44].

With regard to HRT in RA, WHI (women's health initiative) [45] study evaluated HRT (both estrogen alone and estrogen and progestin combined) in RA. HRT did not affect risk of RA and was associated with only a nonsignificant improvement in joint pain scores. However it did protect against loss of bone density in women with RA [46, 47].

25.4.3 Scleroderma

Early menopause does play a role in onset of scleroderma. The main underlying pathology in scleroderma involves vascular damage and estrogens do benefit vascular system. The estrogen deficiency secondary to menopause has been attributed to play a role in increasing vascular damage induced by scleroderma. Postmenopausal state [either alone or in combination with CREST (calcinosis, Reynaud's phenomenon, esophageal dysmotility, sclerodactyly, and telangiectasias) or HLA-B35 haplotype] is considered to be one of the most important risk factors for development of pulmonary arterial hypertension (PAH) in scleroderma with relative risk of 5.2. HRT may protect against development of PAH in postmenopausal women with scleroderma [48]. In one study [49] on postmenopausal women with CREST, none of the women who received HRT developed PAH compared to 19.5% of women who did not receive HRT over 7.5 years of follow-up period.

25.4.4 Multiple Sclerosis (MS)

Menopause does seem to have some effects on MS. However contribution of menopause per se to these effects remains unknown. In women with disease onset after age of 50 years, disease type is usually primary progressive with more rapid progression, fewer relapse, fewer new gadolinium-enhancing lesions on magnetic resonance imaging of brain, more frequent symptoms involving motor function and coordination and rapid progression to EDSS (expanded disability severity scale) of 6. There is no data available on use of HRT in MS.

25.4.5 Sjogren's Syndrome (SS)

Though common in postmenopausal years, effects of menopause of SS are little studied. Similarly there is no data on use of HRT in SS.

25.4.6 Giant Cell Arteritis

One small study showed early menopause to be a risk factor for occurrence of GCA, a vasculitis illness characteristically seen in postmenopausal women [50].

25.5 Conclusion

Menopause can interact with autoimmune disease in several complex ways. While there is a no doubt regarding existence of an association between autoimmune diseases and menopause, the data concerning this association is often incomplete and even contradictory in many cases. Future well-conducted studies evaluating effects of menopause as well as HRT on autoimmune diseases are needed to further clarify the complex association between autoimmune diseases and menopause.

References

1. Ahuja M (2016) Age of menopause and determinants of menopause age: a PAN India survey by IMS. J Midlife Health 7(3):126–131
2. Bansal R, Aggarwal N (2019) Menopausal hot flashes: a concise review. J Midlife Health 10:6–13
3. Sammaritano LR (2012) Menopause in women with autoimmune diseases. Autoimmun Rev 11:A430–A436
4. Bultink IEM, Lems WF, Kostense PJ, Dijkmans BAC, Voskuyl AE (2005) Prevalence of and risk factors for low bone mineral density and vertebral fractures in patients with systemic lupus erythematosus. Arthritis Rheum 527:2044–2050
5. Sharma S, Tandon VR, Mahajan A (2007) Menopausal symptoms in urban women. JK Sci 9(1):13–17
6. Lund KJ (2008) Menopause and the menopausal transition. Med Clin North Am 92:1253–1271
7. Lubo RA (2007) Menopause: endocrinology, consequences of estrogen deficiency, effects of hormone replacement therapy, treatment regimens. In: Katz VL, Lentz GM, Lobo RA, Gershenson DM (eds) Comprehensive gynecology, 5th edn. Mosby Elsevier, Philadelphia, PA, pp 1039–1071
8. Stokes J III, Kannel WB, Wolf PA, Cupples LA, D'Agostino RB (1987) The relative importance of selected risk factors for various manifestations of cardiovascular disease among men and women from 35 to 64 years old: 30 years of follow-up in the Framingham Study. Circulation 75(6):V65–V73
9. Desai MK, Brinton RZ (2019) Autoimmune diseases in women: endocrine transition and risk across the life span. Front Endocrinol 10:265
10. Arteni A, Fabiani G, Marchesoni D (2014) Hormone replacement therapy and autoimmune diseases. Giorn It Ost Gin 36(2):322–327
11. Ebrahimi M, Akbari Asbagh F (2011) Pathogenesis and causes of premature ovarian failure: an update. Int J Fertil Steril 5:54–65
12. Forges T, Monnier-Barbarino P, Faure GC, Bene MC (2004) Autoimmunity and antigenic targets in ovarian pathology. Hum Reprod Update 10:163–175
13. Ebrahimi M, Akbari Asbagh F (2015) The role of autoimmunity in premature ovarian failure. Iran J Reprod Med 13(8):461–472
14. Vallotton MB, Forbes AP (1996) Antibodies to cytoplasm of ova. Lancet 2:264–265
15. Reato G, Morlin L, Chen S, Furmaniak J, Smith BR, Masiero S et al (2011) Premature ovarian failure in patients with autoimmune Addison's disease: clinical, genetic, and immunological evaluation. J Clin Endocrinol Metab 96:1255–1261
16. Takamizawa S, Shibahara H, Shibayama T, Suzuki M (2007) Detection of antizona pellucida antibodies in the sera from premature ovarian failure patients by a highly specific test. Fertil Steril 88:925–932
17. Kinoshita A, Tanaka H, Komori S, Hasegawa A, Koyoma K (2006) Autoimmunity to zona pellucida possibly causes premature ovarian failure (POF). J Reprod Immunol 71:155
18. Khole V (2010) Does ovarian autoimmunity play a role in the pathophysiology of premature ovarian insufficiency? J Midlife Health 1:9–13
19. Lebovic DI, Naz R (2004) Premature ovarian failure: think "autoimmune disorder". Sex Reprod Menopause 2:230–233
20. Massin N, Gougeon A, Meduri G, Thibaud E, Laborde K, Matuchansky C et al (2004) Significance of ovarian histology in the management of patients presenting a premature ovarian failure. Hum Reprod 19:2555–2560

21. Lass A (2001) Assessment of ovarian reserve—is there a role for ovarian biopsy? Hum Reprod 16:1055–1057
22. Bakalov VK, Anasti JN, Calis KA, Vanderhoof VH, Premkumar A, Chen S et al (2005) Autoimmune oophoritis as a mechanism of follicular dysfunction in women with 46, XX spontaneous premature ovarian failure. Fertil Steril 84:958–965
23. Betterle C, Dal Pra C, Mantero F, Zanchetta R (2002) Autoimmune adrenal insufficiency and autoimmune polyendocrine syndromes: autoantibodies, autoantigens and their applicability in diagnosis and disease prediction. Endocr Rev 23:327–364
24. Horejesi J, Martinek J, Novakova D, Madar J, Brandejska M (2000) Autoimmune antiovarian antibodies and their impact on the success of an IVF/ET program. Ann N Y Acad Sci 900:351–356
25. Forges T, Monnier-Barbarino P, Guillet-May F, Faure GC, Bene MC (2006) Corticosteroids in patients with antiovarian antibodies undergoing in vitro fertilization: a prospective pilot study. Eur J Clin Pharmacol 62:699–705
26. Edassery SL, Shatavi SV, Kunkel JP, Ch H, Brucker C, Penumatsa K et al (2010) Autoantigens in ovarian autoimmunity associated with unexplained infertility and premature ovarian failure. Fertil Steril 94:2636–2641
27. Mok CC, Lau CS, Wong RWS (1998) Risk factors for ovarian failure in patients with systemic lupus erythematosus receiving cyclophosphamide therapy. Arthritis Rheum 41(5):831–837
28. Katsifis GE, Tzioufas AG (2004) Ovarian failure in systemic lupus erythematosus patients with pulsed intravenous cyclophosphamide. Lupus 13:673–678
29. Ho CTK, Mok CC, Lau CS, Wong RWS (1998) Late onset systemic lupus erythematosus in southern Chinese. Ann Rheum Dis 57:437–440
30. Cutolo M, Capelino S, Sulli A, Serioli B, Secchi M, Villaggio B et al (2006) Estrogens and autoimmune diseases. Ann N Y Acad Sci 1089:538–547
31. Font J, Pallares L, Cervera R, Lopez-Soto A, Navarro M, Bosch X et al (1991) Systemic lupus onset in the elderly: clinical and immunological characteristics. Ann Rheum Dis 50:702–705
32. Boddaert J, Huong DLT, Amoura Z, Wechsler B, Godeau P, Piette JC (2004) Late onset systemic lupus erythematosus: a personal series of 47 patients and pooled analysis of 714 cases in the literature. Medicine 83(6):348–359
33. Urowitz MB, Ibanez D, Jerome D, Gladman DD (2006) The effect of menopause on disease activity in systemic lupus erythematosus. J Rheumatol 33:2192–2198
34. Talsania M, Scofield RH (2017) Menopause and rheumatic disease. Rheum Dis Clin N Am 43(2):287–302
35. Sanchez-Guerrero J, Liang MH, Karlson EW, Hunter DJ, Colditz GA (1995) Postmenopausal estrogen therapy and the risk for developing systemic lupus erythematosus. Ann Intern Med 122(6):430–433
36. Fernandez M, Calvo-Alen J, Alarcon G, Roseman JM, Bastian HM, Fessler BJ et al (2005) Systemic lupus erythematosus in a multiethnic US cohort (LUMINA) XXI. Disease activity, damage accrual and vascular events in pre- and post-menopausal women. Arthritis Rheum 52(6):1655–1664
37. Gonzalez LA, Pons-Estel GJ, Zhang JS, McGwin G, Roseman J, Reveille JD et al (2009) Effect of age, menopause and cyclophosphamide use on damage accrual in SLE patients from LUMINA, a multiethnic lupus cohort (LUMINA LXIII). Lupus 18:184–186
38. Ostenson M, Aune B, Husby G (1983) Effect of pregnancy and hormonal changes on the activity of rheumatoid arthritis. Scand J Rheumatol 12(2):69–72
39. Silman A, Kay A, Brennan P (1992) Timing of pregnancy in relation to the onset of rheumatoid arthritis. Arthritis Rheum 35(2):152–155
40. Spector TD, Roman E, Silman AJ (1990) The pill, parity and rheumatoid arthritis. Arthritis Rheum 33(6):782–789
41. Karlson EW, Mandl LA, Hankinson SE, Grodstein F (2004) Do breastfeeding and other reproductive factors influence future risk of rheumatoid arthritis: results from the Nurses' Health Study. Arthritis Rheum 50(11):3458–3467

42. Merlino CJR, Criswell LA, Mikuls TR, Saag KG (2003) Estrogen and other female reproductive risk factors are not strongly associated with the development of rheumatoid arthritis in elderly women. Semin Arthritis Rheum 33(2):72–82
43. Pikwer M, Bergstrom U, Nilsson J-A, Jacobsson L, Turesson C (2012) Early menopause is a independent predictor of rheumatoid arthritis. Ann Rheum Dis 71(3):378–381
44. Kuiper SA, van Gestel AM, Swinkels HL, de Boo TM, da Silva JAP, van Riel PLCM (2001) Influence of sex, age, and menopausal status on the course of early rheumatoid arthritis. J Rheumatol 28:1809–1816
45. Walitt B, Pettinger M, Weinstein A, Katz J, Torner J, Wasko MC, Howard BV (2008) Effects of postmenopausal hormone therapy on rheumatoid arthritis: the women's health initiative randomized controlled trials. Arthritis Rheum 59:302–310
46. Bove R (2013) Autoimmune disease and reproductive aging. Clin Immunol 149(2):251–264
47. Marder W, Vinet E, Somers EC (2015) Rheumatic autoimmune diseases in women and midlife health. Women's Midlife Health 1:11
48. Scorza R, Caronni M, Bazzi S, Nador F, Beretta L, Antonioli R et al (2002) Post-menopause is the main risk factor for developing isolated pulmonary hypertension in systemic sclerosis. Ann N Y Acad Sci 966:238–246
49. Beretta L, Caronni M, Origgi L, Ponti A, Santaniello A, Scorza R (2006) Hormone replacement therapy may prevent the development of isolated pulmonary hypertension in patients with systemic sclerosis and limited cutaneous involvement. Scand J Rheumatol 35(6):468–471
50. Larsson K, Mellstrom D, Nordborg E, Oden A, Nordborg E (2006) Early menopause, low body mass index, and smoking are independent risk factors for developing giant cell arteritis. Ann Rheum Dis 65(4):529–532

Fibromyalgia

B. G. Dharmanand

Abstract

Fibromyalgia (FM) is a common musculoskeletal disorder affecting predominantly women. The prevalence increases with increasing age with 7% of women affected in 60–79 age group. FM is characterised by widespread aches and pains, fatigue, sleep disturbances and multiple somatic symptoms. Depression and other mood disorders occur commonly in FM. There is no diagnostic test to diagnose FM. Hypothyroidism is a common disorder which share some clinical features of FM. FM can mimic rheumatic diseases and also coexist with rheumatic diseases like systemic lupus erythematosus, rheumatoid arthritis and Sjogren's syndrome. Presence of FM may make interpretation of disease activity scales like DAS 28 difficult. Genetic factors predispose one for low pain threshold and environmental factors including stress can contribute to the development of FM. Patient education is a mainstay of FM management. Graded increase in exercises and cognitive behaviour therapy (CBT) are also very useful therapeutic tools. NSAIDS and steroids are generally not effective in FM. Low-dose antidepressants like amitriptyline, duloxetine and antiepileptics like gabapentin and pregabalin act on central mechanism of pain and may be effective in multiple domains of FM like pain and sleep. FM is compatible with successful pregnancy outcomes and pregnancy should be contemplated when FM is well controlled and when the patient is on no drugs or minimum medicines (tricyclic antidepressants like amitriptyline). FM is the most common non-autoimmune musculoskeletal disorder affecting women.

Keywords

Fibromyalgia · Chronic widespread pains · Central sensitisation

---

B. G. Dharmanand (✉)
Vikram Hospital, Bangalore, India

Fibromyalgia (FM) is a chronic disorder characterised by widespread pains and multiple somatic symptoms. FM is more common in women with a prevalence of 3.4–4.9% vs 0.5–1.6% in men [1–3]. The prevalence increases with age, reaching more than 7% in women aged 60–79 years [1]. Though FM like illness is less likely to start in elderly, older women continue to experience chronic widespread pain (CWP) which had begun few decades ago. FM is also a common illness diagnosed in rheumatology clinics occurring in as high as 20% of outpatients [4]. FM also can coexist with many rheumatological diseases like Sjogren's syndrome, systemic lupus erythematosus and rheumatoid arthritis [5].

Fibromyalgia (FM) could be suspected in any patient, particularly young female who presents with pain in multiple areas (widespread pain), pain all over, neck pain, back pain, pain radiating in non-dermatomal patterns. One could positively suspect FM when the patient has subjective more than objective swelling in joints and/or periarticular regions, fatigue, sleep disturbances, headaches, irritable bowel and bladder symptoms, paraesthesia, brain fog and affective symptoms like low mood. FM patients are likely to have more symptoms than signs. If the patient has multiple symptoms ('too many symptoms'), one could suspect FM [6].

26.1 Clinical Features

Widespread pain is the most common and defining symptom of FM. Pain in both sides of the body and both half of the body defines widespread pains. Pain is usually described in the joints and also away from the joints. There may be subjective sensation of swelling around the joints. FM is also associated with multiple somatic symptoms. Fatigue is an important symptom. It is important to rule out common causes of fatigue like anaemia, hypothyroidism and depression. Headache, usually chronic tension type or migraine like, is another common symptom. Many patients have symptoms suggestive of irritable bowel syndrome and irritable bladder. Non-restorative sleep is also very common. It is essential to consider primary sleep disorder which might co exist with FM. Depression and other mood disorder also occur commonly with FM. Most of the symptoms of FM are common to many diseases. It is essential to look for red flag symptoms and signs and also rule out many endocrine disorders like hypothyroidism. Many drugs also can cause widespread pains, like statins. An algorithmic approach to evaluation for patients with widespread pains is suggested in Fig. 26.1.

It is essential to consider fibromyalgia in the differential diagnosis of rheumatic diseases and vice versa since both are common in younger women. It is also important to recognise fibromyalgianess in rheumatic diseases to avoid misinterpretation of symptoms and signs. FM provides an alternate explanation for pain and systemic symptoms. Thus helps interpretation of disease activity measures like DAS 28. So, unnecessary treatment escalation is avoided and the choice of pain medicine would differ. Pain modifying drugs like pregabalin would be the choice over NSAID or steroids. One could consider non- pharmacological solutions like CBT. It is better to include FM clinical screen and tender point examination as a part of routine examination upfront on first consult.

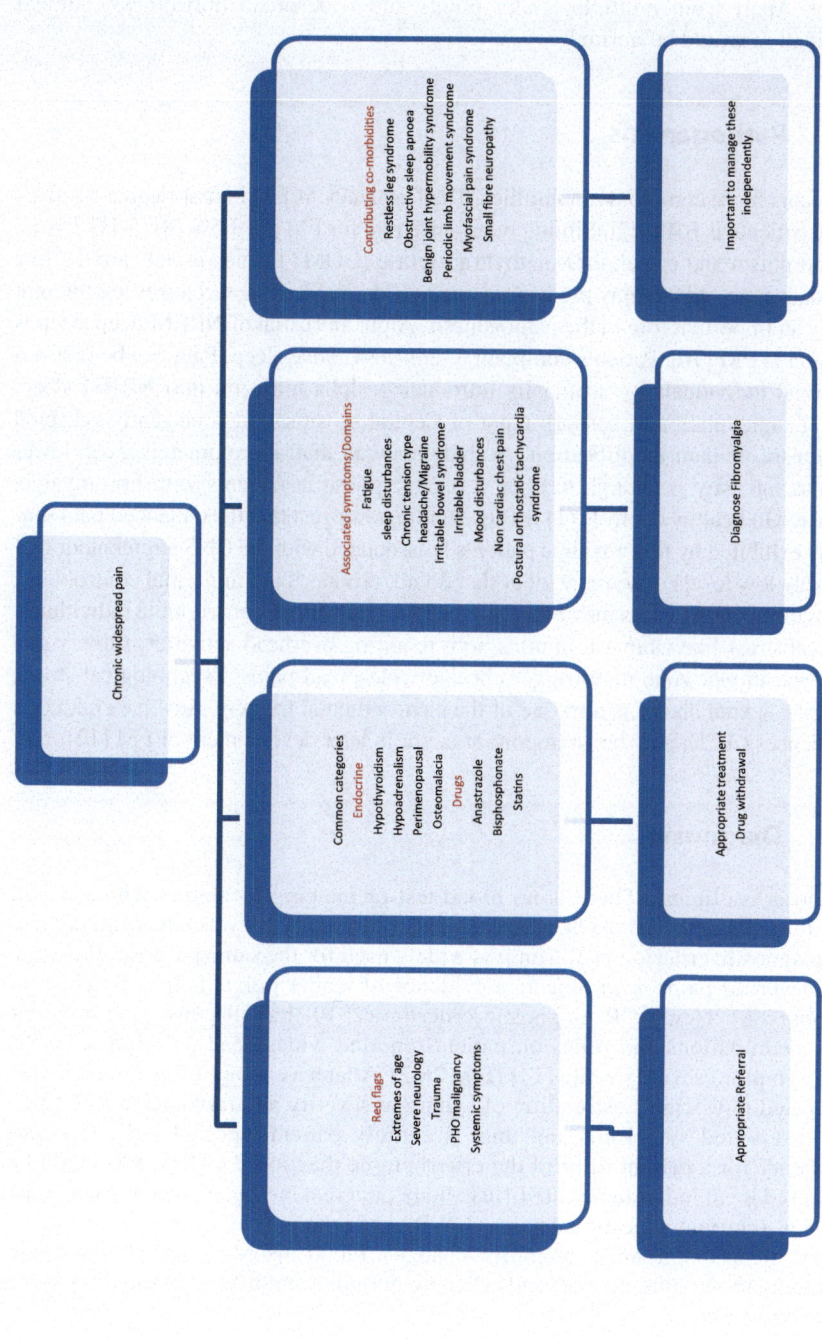

Fig. 26.1 Chronic widespread pain

It is important to perform a thorough physical examination of all the systems. This helps to rule out other illness and also helps to develop a rapport with the patient. Apart from multiple tender points and widespread hurtfulness, clinical examination would be normal.

26.2 Pathogenesis

FM occurs more commonly in families. The frequency of FM in first-degree relatives of FM patients is 6.4% [7]. Sibling recurrence rate for FM is 13.6% [8]. 5-HTT gene polymorphism and catechol-*O*-methyltransferase (COMT) gene variants are the few candidate genes which may predispose one to FM [9]. Sleep disturbances are thought to play an important role in the pathogenesis. Alpha intrusion of NREM deep sleep is common in FM [10]. Patients complain of non-restorative sleep. Pain can be induced in normal individuals by artificially introducing alpha intrusion into NREM sleep. Central augmentation of sensory input or Central sensitisation is currently accepted mechanism of pain amplification. A study showed that approximately 50% lower stimulus intensity is enough to elicit a pain response in patients with fibromyalgia compared to healthy controls [11]. These findings suggest that the enhanced pain sensitivity exhibited by fibromyalgia patients is associated with the CNS augmentation of relatively low levels of sensory input that do not produce pain in normal controls.

Environmental factors may bring out the FM in genetically susceptible individuals. Physical stress like whiplash injuries, jobs requiring overhead activities, surgery and employed in war zone may trigger chronic widespread pains. Psychological stress, including sexual abuse, is also one of the environmental triggers. Adverse childhood experiences (ACE) may be an important factor in later development of FM [12].

26.3 Diagnosis

Diagnosis is clinical. There is no blood test or imaging technique which would help us to diagnose FM. ACR classification criterion (1990) was never intended to be a diagnostic criterion [13]. But it is widely used for the same purpose. Presence of widespread pains with objective evidence of tender points helps clinicians to diagnose FM. New ACR diagnostic criterion (2010) had dispensed with tender point examinations and relies on patient-reported widespread pain index (WPI) and a symptom severity scale [14] (Fig. 26.2). A later version of this criterion had eliminated physician's estimation of symptom severity and replaced it with three patient-reported symptoms and thus is entirely patient-reported [15]. It is not mandatory for a patient to fulfil the criteria to be diagnosed as FM. FM could be diagnosed in an individual with diffuse body pain that has been present for at least 3 months (chronic widespread pain—CWP), and who may also have symptoms of fatigue, sleep disturbance, cognitive changes, mood disorder and other somatic symptoms to variable degree, and when symptoms cannot be explained by some other illness [16].

WPI **Areas looked at for WPI index**	**Symptom Severity scale score:**
Shoulder girdle, left Shoulder girdle, right	Fatigue Waking unrefreshed Cognitive symptoms
Upper arm, left Upper arm, right Lower arm, left Lower arm, right Hip (buttock, trochanter), left Hip (buttock, trochanter), right Upper leg, left Upper leg, right Lower leg, left Lower leg, right	For the each of the 3 symptoms above, indicate the level of severity over the past week using the following scale: 0 = no problem 1 = slight or mild problems, generally mild or intermittent 2 = moderate, considerable problems, often present and/or at a moderate level 3 = severe: pervasive, continuous, life-disturbing problems
Jaw, left Jaw, right Chest Abdomen Upper back Lower back Neck Total score=	Considering somatic symptoms in general, indicate whether the patient has: 0 = no symptoms 1 = few symptoms 2 = a moderate number of symptoms 3 = a great deal of symptoms
	The SS scale score is the sum of the severity of the 3 symptoms (fatigue, waking unrefreshed, cognitive symptoms) plus the extent (severity) of somatic symptoms in general. The final score is between 0 and 12.

Fig. 26.2 2010 ACR preliminary diagnostic criteria. Criteria: A patient satisfies diagnostic criteria for fibromyalgia if the following three conditions are met: (1) Widespread pain index (WPI) 7 and symptom severity (SS) scale score 5 or WPI 3–6 and SS scale score 9. (2) Symptoms have been present at a similar level for at least 3 months. (3) The patient does not have a disorder that would otherwise explain the pain

26.4 Investigations When Evaluating a Patient with CWP

CBC and peripheral smear
ESR & CRP
Thyroid profile
Blood sugars
Liver and renal tests
Bone profile
25 (OH) vitamin D3

Above investigations help in the differential diagnosis and also in identifying treatable elements in patients with FM.

26.5 Management

26.5.1 Education

Patient education forms an important component of management of complex illness like FM. On diagnosis, many would not have heard of fibromyalgia, some might have had some information from friends and the Internet, some would have been told that they do not have any disease and all is in the mind and a few would have researched the subject in a scholarly way. So a useful way to initiate an education session is to ask the patient what they know about fibromyalgia [17].

Points that could be discussed with the patient [18].

- Explain what FM is and what it is not
- Concept of central sensitization and low pain threshold in simple language
- Explain the need to take control of illness (self-management)
- Deleterious effects of deconditioning and need to exercise
- Partial efficacy of current medical therapy
- Concept of cognitive behavioural therapy (CBT)
- Though there is no cure, care is always possible.

26.6 Non-Pharmacological Management

26.6.1 Exercises

The goals of exercise and improved physical fitness for individuals with fibromyalgia are to improve or maintain general fitness, physical function, emotional well-being and gaining control over FM. Pain and deconditioning are potential roadblocks for patients with FM from exercising. FM patients may be more prone to exercise-induced muscle pain due to muscle ischaemia and post-exertional fatigue due to production of inflammatory cytokines after a period of exercise [19]. Following are few important tips for exercises in FM.

- Reasonable pain control has to be achieved before patient could into an exercise program.
- Patients are advised to start slowly and gradually build up (start walking for 5 min and add 1–2 min every week and slowly reach 30–45 min/day).
- Walking, cycling and dancing are the common aerobic exercises tried by patients.
- Gentle weight training is also possible and beneficial in FM.
- Physical activity program should also include a stretching program.
- If hard pressed for time, they could get exercises from activities of daily living (ADL) (climbing stairs, walking to work and walk during work).
- Conserve energy during ADL to be able to exercise.

- Improving physical activity and fitness is one of the important strategies in the management plan of FM.
- 'No pain; no gain' is a useful advice for FM patients who begin exercising. But if it pains for more than 24–48 h, they have to decrease the intensity of exercises.

26.6.2 Cognitive Behavioural Therapy (CBT)

Cognitive behavioural therapy is designed to allow subjects with chronic pain to cope better with their symptoms, which may include formal stress reduction techniques, with a focus on teaching individuals' optimal self-management of chronic illness. There is strong evidence for CBT in the management of fibromyalgia [20]. Improvements were noticed in pain, sleep, fatigue and health-related quality of life (HRQOL). Also there was an improvement in mood, self-efficacy and healthcare-seeking behaviour [20]. Although short-term results are positive, the effect tends to fade after a year. This stresses the importance of continued monitoring and follow-up of patients with FM. CBT is a technique, semi-instructive in nature, where patient plays an active role along with the therapist. This systematically helps the patient to understand the effect of cognition or maladaptive thoughts (perception and beliefs about illness) about the illness and assists in changing the behaviour. It also addresses negativity. CBT requires training in CBT techniques and are generally performed by clinical psychologists. Basic form of CBT could be performed by clinicians. An internet-based CBT-like program has been developed [21]. CBT may not be effective in all. It helps patients with emotional distress and poor coping skills and in those who believe at the onset that treatment would be effective. Though evidence is lacking, CBT is likely to be more useful when combined with drug and exercise therapy.

26.6.3 Diet

There is no standard diet for FM. Recent research suggests that dietary restriction of glutamate, particularly MSG, may be beneficial in decreasing somatic symptoms and increasing well-being in chronic pain conditions [22]. With limited available data, one cannot yet draw definitive conclusions regarding the role of diet in fibromyalgia or make specific dietary recommendations for treatment. More rigorous, controlled trials of dietary intervention in fibromyalgia are warranted. Balanced diet is generally recommended to avoid any micronutrient deficiency.

26.6.4 Drugs

Medications are only partially helpful in relieving FM symptoms. There is no single medication which could address all the domains of FM symptomatology. Pain, sleep disturbances, depression and other somatic symptoms may require different category of medicines. Since most drugs work only in one-third of patients, the best drug for the patient is arrived at by trial and error. The following are the drugs used as per the clinical domains.

Pain
- Analgesics like paracetamol
- NSAIDs
- Tricyclic antidepressants (TCAs) like amitriptyline
- SNRI like duloxetine and milnacipran
- Gabapentinoids like pregabalin and gabapentin
- Alpha blockers like tizanidine
- Muscle relaxants like cyclobenzaprine
- Tramadol

Sleep Disturbance
- Hypnotics like zolpidem, clonazepam
- TCA
- Pregabalin

Depression
- SSRI like fluoxetine, escitalopram
- TCA
- SNRI

Coexisting syndromes like IBS, restless leg syndrome and migraine would respond to specific therapies. Many of the above drugs appear to benefit more than one domain of symptoms. For example, TCA may help pain, sleep and depression. Starting at a small dose and slow escalation of the dose is better tolerated. For example duloxetine may be started at 20 mg bed time and increased every 2 weeks to a maximum of 120 mg or to the dose tolerated.

26.7 FM and Pregnancy

There is scant evidence that fibromyalgia may interfere with a woman's chance to get pregnant (fertility is not affected). Also there is no evidence that FM has any direct effect on the pregnancy outcomes both on the foetus and on the mother. As long as the woman is not completely debilitated with fibromyalgia pain, there is little reason not to consider having children. The main concern is regarding the body's capability to be emotionally, mentally and physically ready to face the stress of pregnancy and also the responsibilities associated with having a baby. Patients are generally advised to consider pregnancy when the symptoms are less severe. Pregnancy is ideal when symptoms of FM could be managed by life style modifications and exercises and other physical measures. Fibromyalgia symptoms tend to worsen with pregnancy, particularly in III trimester and delivery. But this was not associated with hormonal changes [23]. Pregnancy outcome is unaffected by a fibromyalgia diagnosis [24]. Pre-conception discussions should be a routine part of the care of fibromyalgia patients of childbearing potential. Non-drug treatments should be maximised during pregnancy and when nursing, with medications reserved for more disabling and recalcitrant symptoms. FM patients may have difficulties with nursing and caring for the newborn baby because of pain and fatigue [25].

Medications commonly used in FM may not be suitable for someone planning pregnancy. It is ideal to stop all the medications preconception. Patients are generally advised to postpone pregnancy till the symptoms are well controlled and are on minimal medications. Most antidepressants are FDA category C drugs. A prospective study comparing patients taking antidepressants VS non-users did not show difference in the occurrence of major malformations. So drugs like amitriptyline may be used if the benefits outweigh the risks after discussion with the patient and the spouse [26]. There is no data on newer drugs like duloxetine, pregabalin and milnacipran in pregnancy. So they have to be avoided.

References

1. Wolfe F, Ross K, Anderson J, Russell IJ (1995) Aspects of fibromyalgia in the general population: sex, pain threshold, and fibromyalgia symptoms. J Rheumatol 22(1):151–156
2. White KP, Speechley M, Harth M, Ostbye T (1999) The London Fibromyalgia Epidemiology Study: comparing the demographic and clinical characteristics in 100 random community cases of fibromyalgia versus controls. J Rheumatol 26(7):1577–1585
3. Jaime CB, Bernard B et al (2010) Prevalence of fibromyalgia: a survey in five European countries. Semin Arthritis Rheum 39(6):448–453
4. Carol AL, Bruce CG (2010) Fibromyalgia. In: Anthony SF (ed) Harrison's rheumatology, 2nd edn. McGraw-Hill Medical, New York, pp 254–258
5. Bennett RM (2009) Clinical manifestations and diagnosis of fibromyalgia. Rheum Dis Clin N Am 35:215–232
6. Dharmanand BG (2014) In: Chandrashekara S (ed) Managing fibromyalgia. Question & answer. Chanre Healthcare & Research Pvt. Ltd., Bangalore
7. Arnold LM, Hudson JI et al (2004) Family study of fibromyalgia. Arthritis Rheum 50(3):944–952
8. Arnold LM, Fan J et al (2013) The fibromyalgia family study: a genome-wide linkage scan study. Arthritis Rheum 65(4):1122–1128
9. Bradley LA (2009) Pathophysiology of fibromyalgia. Am J Med 122(12 Suppl):S22
10. Roizenblatt S, Moldofsky H et al (2001) Alpha sleep characteristics in fibromyalgia. Arthritis Rheum 44:222–230
11. Gracely RH, Petzke F et al (2002) Functional magnetic resonance imaging evidence of augmented pain processing in fibromyalgia. Arthritis Rheum 46:1333–1343
12. Low AL, Schweinhardt P (2012) Early life adversity as a risk factor for fibromyalgia in later life. Pain Res Treatm 2012:140832, 15 p
13. Wolfe F, Smythe HA et al (1990) The American College of Rheumatology 1990 criteria for the classification of fibromyalgia: report of the Multicenter Criteria Committee. Arthritis Rheum 33:160–172

14. Wolfe F, Clauw D, Fitzcharles MA, Goldenberg DL, Katz RS, Mease P et al (2010) The American College of Rheumatology preliminary diagnostic criteria for fibromyalgia and measurement of symptom severity. Arthritis Care Res 62:600–610
15. Wolfe F, Clauw DJ, Fitzcharles MA et al (2011) Fibromyalgia criteria and severity scales for clinical and epidemiological studies: a modification of the ACR Preliminary Diagnostic Criteria for Fibromyalgia. J Rheumatol 38:1113–1122
16. Fitzcharles MA, Ste-Marie PA et al (2013) 2012 Canadian guidelines for the diagnosis and management of fibromyalgia syndrome. Pain Res Manag 18(3):119–126
17. Bennett RM (2014) Guidelines for the successful management of fibromyalgia patients. Indian J Rheumatol 6(6):13–21
18. Jones KD, Kindler LL et al (2012) Self-management in fibromyalgia. J Clin Rheumatol Musculoskel Med 3(1):59–68
19. Jones KD, Liptan GL (2009) Exercise interventions in fibromyalgia: clinical applications from the evidence. Rheum Dis Clin N Am 35(2):373–391
20. Bernardy K, Fuber N, Kollner V et al (2010) Efficacy of cognitive-behavioral therapies in fibromyalgia syndrome—a systematic review and meta-analysis of randomized controlled trials. J Rheumatol 37:1991–2005
21. https://fibroguide.med.umich.edu/
22. Holton KF, Taren DL et al (2012) The effect of dietary glutamate on fibromyalgia and irritable bowel symptoms. Clin Exp Rheumatol 30(6 Suppl 74):10–17
23. Ostensen M, Rugelsjøen A, Wigers S (1997) The effect of reproductive events and alterations of sex hormone levels on the symptoms of fibromyalgia. Scand J Rheumatol 26:355–360
24. Marcus DA, Deodhar A (2011) Fibromyalgia and pregnancy. In: Marcus DA, Deodhar A (eds) Fibromyalgia. Springer, New York, pp 215–235
25. Schaefer KM (2004) Breastfeeding in chronic illness: the voices of women with fibromyalgia. Am J Matern Child Nurs 29(4):248–253
26. Williams AS (2007) Antidepressants in pregnancy and breastfeeding. Aust Prescr 30:125–127

Printed by Printforce, United Kingdom